Comprehensive Core Clinical Cases Self-Assessment for Medical Students

A Problem-based Learning Approach

Comprehensive Core Clinical Cases Self-Assessment for Medical Students

Andrew Sewart MBChB PhD MRCP MRCGP
GP Partner
Bellingham, Northumberland

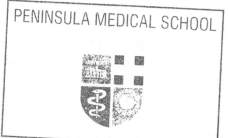

Henriette van Ruiten MBChB MRCPCH
Paediatric Registrar
Northern Deanery

A Problem-based Learning Approach

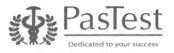

© 2012 PASTEST LTD
Egerton Court
Parkgate Estate
Knutsford
Cheshire
WA16 8DX

Telephone: 01565 752000

A percentage of the questions were previously published in *Core Clinical Cases Problem Based Learning Book 1 2 edition* and *Core Clinical Cases Problem Based Learning Book 2*

First Published 2012

ISBN: 978 1905635 856

A catalogue record for this book is available from the British Library.

The information contained within this book was obtained by the author from reliable sources. However, while every effort has been made to ensure its accuracy, no responsibility for loss, damage or injury occasioned to any person acting or refraining from action as a result of information contained herein can be accepted by the publishers or author.

PasTest Revision Books, Online Revision and Intensive Courses

PasTest has been established in the field of undergraduate and postgraduate medical education since 1972, providing revision books, online revision and intensive study courses for doctors preparing for their professional examinations.

Books, courses and online revision available for:
Medical undergraduates, MRCGP, MRCP Parts 1 and 2, MRCPCH Parts 1 and 2, MRCS, MRCOG, DRCOG, DCH, FRCA, Dentistry.

For further details contact:
PasTest, Freepost, Knutsford, Cheshire WA16 7BR
Tel: 01565 752000   Fax: 01565 650264
www.pastest.co.uk   enquiries@pastest.co.uk

Text prepared by Carnegie Book Production, Lancaster

Contents

Dedication

To Roan and Lotte

Acknowledgements

We would like to thank the following doctors for their invaluable help with reviewing cases:

Francesca Liuzzi, final-year medical student, University of Manchester, Salford Royal Foundation Trust.

Dr Mark Worthington, MBChB MSc MRCPsych, SpR in Old Age Psychiatry, Lancashire, UK.

Dr Ayesha Madan, MRCP MSc, Consultant Rheumatologist, Lancashire Care NHS Foundation Trust

Introduction

We wrote the first edition of *Core Clinical Cases* when we were both fourth-year medical students at Liverpool University. Eight years have now passed of what has been a very steep but thoroughly enjoyable learning curve in our chosen specialties: Henriette is not far off realising her dream of becoming a paediatric consultant while Andy is now a GP partner in a small practice in rural Northumberland.

We remain pleasantly surprised by the continual success of the *Core Clinical Case* series and felt now was the right time to update this book with a new edition, combining the best of Books 1 and 2 to form a comprehensive collection of core clinical cases.

We have intentionally kept to the same format, namely a series of questions to prompt the student through the diagnosis and management of realistic clinical scenarios with the addition of radiographs, CT scans, ECGs and blood results for interpretation. This is quite simply to prepare you for when you start as Foundation Year doctors in a year or so's time because these cases reflect real clinical scenarios, with their management following, where available, national clinical guidelines. As such we hope this book will be used not only as a self-assessment book but also as a core reference guide for your clinical attachments.

Finally, good luck in your future careers and we hope you enjoy medicine as much as we continue to.

Andy and Henriette
October 2012

Abbreviations

ABG	arterial blood gas
ABSPI	ankle–brachial systolic pressure index
ACE	angiotensin-converting enzyme
ACR	albumin:creatinine ratio
ACS	acute coronary syndrome
ACTH	adrenocorticotrophic hormone
ADH	antidiuretic hormone
AF	atrial fibrillation
AFP	α-fetoprotein
AG	anion gap
AIDS	acquired immune deficiency syndrome
ALL	acute lymphoblastic leukaemia
ALP	alkaline phosphatase
ALT	alanine transaminase
AMA	anti-mitochondrial antibody
ANA	anti-nuclear antibody
AP	anteroposterior or action potential
APTT	activated partial thromboplastin time
ARDS	acute respiratory distress syndrome
ARF	acute renal failure
AST	aspartate transaminase
ATN	acute tubular necrosis
AVN	avascular necrosis
bd	twice daily
BMI	body mass index
BNP	brain natriuretic peptide
BP	blood pressure
CHD	coronary heart disease
CMV	cytomegalovirus
CNS	central nervous system
COC	combined oral contraceptive
COPD	chronic obstructive pulmonary disease
CPD	cephalopelvic disproportion
CRF	chronic renal failure
CRP	C-reactive protein
CSF	cerebrospinal fluid
CT	computed tomography

CTG	cardiotocography
CVA	cerebrovascular accident
CVD	cardiovascular disease
CVP	central venous pressure
CVS	chorionic villous sampling
DCT	direct Coombs' test
DDH	developmental dysplasia of the hip
DKA	diabetic ketoacidosis
ECG	electrocardiogram
EEG	electroencephalogram
ERCP	endoscopic retrograde cholangiopancreatography
ESR	erythrocyte sedimentation rate
FBC	full blood count
FTT	failure to thrive
FT3	free triiodothyronine
FT4	free thyroxine
GCS	Glasgow Coma Scale
GGT	γ-glutamyl transferase
GI	gastrointestinal
GnRH	gonadotrophin-releasing hormone
GTN	glyceryl trinitrate
Hb	haemoglobin
hCG	human chorionic gonadotrophin
HIV	human immunodeficiency virus
HLA	human leukocyte antigen
HONK	hyperosmolar non-ketotic
ICP	intracranial pressure
ICU	intensive care unit
INR	international normalised ratio
IUD	intrauterine device
IUGR	intrauterine growth retardation
JVP	jugular venous pressure
LAD	left anterior descending
LBBB	left bundle-branch block
LCPD	leg calf Perthes' disease
LH	luteinising hormone
LP	lumbar puncture
LV	left ventricular
LVH	left ventricular hypertrophy
M3G	morphine-3-glucuronide

M6G	morphine-6-glucuronide
MCP	metacarpophalangeal
MI	myocardial infarction
MMSE	Mini-Mental State Examination
NSTEMI	non-ST-elevation myocardial infarction
NYHA	New York Heart Association
OGTT	oral glucose tolerance test
OHSS	ovarian hyperstimulation syndrome
PCO2	partial pressure of carbon dioxide
PO2	partial pressure of oxygen
PCI	percutaneous coronary intervention
PCOS	polycystic ovarian syndrome
PE	pulmonary embolus
PEA	pulseless electrical activity
PEF	peak expiratory flow
PIP	proximal interphalangeal
RBCs	red blood cells
RF	rheumatoid factor
RSV	respiratory syncytial virus
SaO2	arterial oxygen saturation
SD	standard deviation
SLE	systemic lupus erythematosus
SMA	smooth muscle antibody
STEMI	ST-elevation myocardial infarction
T3	triiodothyronine
T4	thyroxine
TB	tuberculosis
TBG	thyroxine-binding globulin
TC	total cholesterol
TIA	transient ischaemic attack
TSH	thyroid-stimulating hormone
UC	ulcerative colitis
UPSI	unprotected sexual intercourse
VF	ventricular fibrillation
VT	ventricular tachycardia
WBC	white blood cell
WCC	white cell count

CARDIOVASCULAR CASES: QUESTIONS

CARDIOVASCULAR CASE 1

Tim, a 60-year-old solicitor, visits his GP complaining of recent episodes of central chest tightness on exertion, which settles on rest. There is nothing of note in his past medical history. Tim is referred to the rapid-access chest pain clinic, where he is diagnosed with stable angina.

Q 1. **What are the main risk factors for coronary heart disease (CHD)?** 5 marks

Q 2. **List four drugs that may be prescribed to control angina.** 4 marks

Tim is also prescribed a statin and aspirin.

Q 3. **What is the recommended upper limit for fasting total cholesterol (TC) and low-density lipoprotein (LDL) in secondary prevention?** 2 marks

Q 4. **What blood test must you request before prescribing a statin, and what advice must you give to patients on statin therapy?** 2 marks

Despite optimised medical treatment, Tim remains symptomatic, so he undergoes coronary angiography with a view to revascularisation.

Q 5. **What two procedures are used for revascularisation?** 2 marks

Total: 15 marks

CARDIOVASCULAR CASE 2

John, a 72-year-old hypertensive, visits his GP complaining of several months' history of increasing breathlessness. He is now breathless even when doing simple tasks around the home, such as dressing.

Q 1. List four non-cardiac causes of gradually progressive dyspnoea.   4 marks

John's GP suspects heart failure and organises a number of investigations.

Q 2. List four causes of heart failure.   4 marks

Q 3. From the history above classify John's heart failure according to the New York Heart Association (NYHA) criteria.   2 marks

Q 4. **What hormone is significantly raised in heart failure?** 2 marks

Q 5. **Which key investigation would you request to confirm heart failure?** 1 mark

John is diagnosed with left ventricular heart failure.

Q 6. **Which two drugs are the first-line treatment for heart failure?** 2 marks

Total: 15 marks

CARDIOVASCULAR CASE 3

David, a 51-year-old builder, is referred to his GP from the well-man clinic, as his blood pressure was recorded as 164/96 mmHg.

Q 1. Define the systolic/diastolic ranges for mild (phase 1), moderate (phase 2) and severe (phase 3) hypertension. 3 marks

You request an electrocardiogram (ECG), shown in Figure 1.1 below:

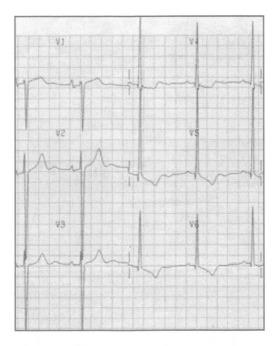

Figure 1.1: David's ECG.

Q 2. What does David's ECG show? 1 mark

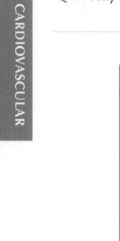

Q 3. Why is this important with regard to hypertension?   1 mark

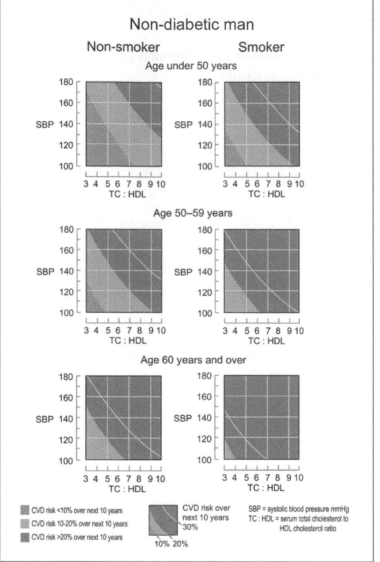

Figure 1.2: CVD risk prediction chart.

Q 4. **List two causes of secondary hypertension.**   2 marks

David smokes ten cigarettes a day, and his fasting bloods are measured: total cholesterol (TC) 6.34 mmol/l, low-density lipoprotein (LDL) 4.22 mmol/l, high-density lipoprotein (HDL) 1.26 mmol/l, triglycerides 2.4 mmol/l, glucose 4.6 mmol/l.

Q 5. **Calculate his 10-year cardiovascular disease (CVD) risk.**   1 mark

You determine that David's blood pressure needs to be treated.

Q 6. **What four lifestyle changes would you recommend?**   2 marks

Q 7. **What antihypertensive treatment would you offer first line?**   1 mark

Q 8. **Name two electrolyte abnormalities caused by thiazide diuretics.** 2 marks

Q 9. Name four complications that might arise if David's hypertension is not treated.

2 marks

Total:

15 marks

CARDIOVASCULAR CASE 4

A GP organises an electrocardiogram (ECG) (shown in Figure 1.3) for one of her patients, 78-year-old Sarah, after checking her pulse during a routine consultation for her hypertension.

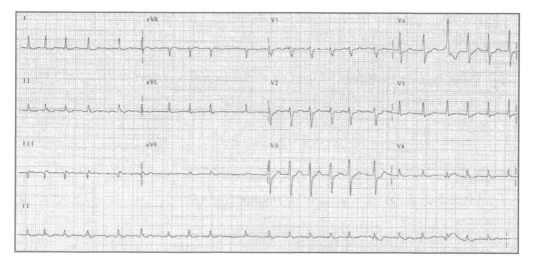

Figure 1.3: Sarah's ECG.

Q 1. What does the ECG show? 1 mark

Q 2. List six causes of this rhythm. 3 marks

Q 3. **What two drugs may be used for rate control?**   2 marks

Q 4. **What two methods may be used to attempt cardioversion?**   2 marks

Q 5. **What two drugs may be used for rhythm control?**   2 marks

Sarah opts for rate control and agrees to be anticoagulated to reduce her risk of stroke.

Q 6. **Name four factors used to stratify stroke risk.**   2 marks

Q 7. **What drug is used for anticoagulation, how is it monitored and what is the target range?**   3 marks

Total: 15 marks

CARDIOVASCULAR CASE 5

James, a 68-year-old lifelong smoker, is brought into the Emergency Department by ambulance. He has a 45-minute history of central, crushing chest pain associated with nausea, dyspnoea and sweating. On cardiovascular examination, his blood pressure is 164/96 mmHg, heart rate 92 bpm and regular; jugular venous pressure is 4 cm above the sternal angle, heart sounds are normal and the chest is clear.

Q 1. **List six differential diagnoses.** 3 marks

James's electrocardiogram (ECG) is shown in Figure 1.6.

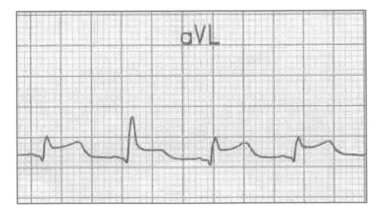

Figure 1.4: James's ECG.

Q 2. What is the abnormality? 1 mark

This abnormality is seen in leads I, aVL, and V5–6.

Q 3. Where is the site of the infarct? 1 mark

Q 4. What other ECG changes may be expected to develop? 1 mark

James undergoes reperfusion therapy and is transferred to coronary care.

Q 5. What are the two options for reperfusion therapy? 2 marks

Q 6. List five complications of myocardial infarction. 5 marks

James makes an uncomplicated recovery and is transferred to the ward before discharge the following week.

Q 7. **What advice, treatment and investigations would you recommend to reduce his risk of a similar episode?** 2 marks

Total: 15 marks

EMERGENCY DEPARTMENT CASES: QUESTIONS

EMERGENCY DEPARTMENT CASE 1

Gary, a 23-year-old man, is brought into the Emergency Department following a high-speed road traffic accident. He has sustained trauma to the left side of his head and has a reduced level of consciousness.

Q 1. List three causes of secondary brain injury. 3 marks

Gary's neck is immobilised, his airway, breathing and circulation is stabilised, and an assessment of his neurological status undertaken. His Glasgow Coma Scale (GCS) score is assessed as follows: his eyes open to pain, he localises pain and his speech is confused.

Q 2. Calculate Gary's GCS.   1 mark

A full examination reveals that Gary has sustained no other major injuries.

Q 3. List four signs on examination of a basal skull fracture.   1 mark

Q 4. List six reasons for admitting a patient following a head injury.   3 marks

Q 5. **List six regular observations Gary should undergo.** 3 marks

Gary undergoes an urgent CT scan of his head (see Figure 2.1).

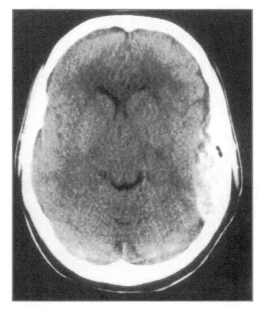

Figure 2.1: Gary's CT brain scan.

Q 6. **Describe two abnormalities seen on his CT scan.** 1 mark

Q 7. What is the diagnosis?

2 marks

Q 8. What further course of action should be undertaken?

1 mark

Total:

15 marks

EMERGENCY DEPARTMENT
CASE 2

Malcolm, a 69-year-old known ischaemic heart disease patient, is brought into the Emergency Department severely dyspnoeic.

Q 1. What is your differential diagnosis?   4 marks

You gain intravenous access, send urgent bloods and request an urgent erect chest X-ray (see Figure 2.2) and electrocardiogram (ECG) (see Figure 2.3).

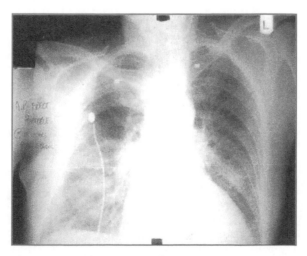

Figure 2.2: Malcom's erect chest X-ray.

Q 2. Identify three abnormalities on his chest X-ray.   3 marks

Q 3. What is your immediate management?   2 marks

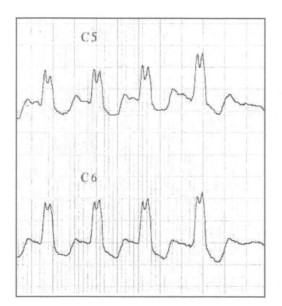

Figure 2.3: Malcolm's ECG.

Q 4. **What does his ECG show?** 1 mark

Q 5. **How could you confirm that this is a new ECG change?** 1 mark

While you are attempting to stabilise Malcolm, he arrests in asystole.

Q 6. **List three other rhythms associated with cardiac arrest.** 3 marks

Q 7. **How would you manage the arrest?** 2 marks

Q 8. **List eight potential reversible causes of cardiac arrest.** 4 marks

Unfortunately cardiopulmonary resuscitation is unsuccessful, and Malcolm is declared dead.

Total: **20 marks**

ENDOCRINE CASES: QUESTIONS

ENDOCRINE CASE 1

Andy, a 47-year-old estate agent, visits his GP complaining of general tiredness. He admits to eating and drinking to excess. On examination, he weighs 95 kg and his height is 1.72 m; blood pressure is 154/92 mmHg.

Q 1. **Calculate Andy's body mass index (BMI).**   1 mark

Urine dipstick is 2+ for glucose.

Q 2. **How would you confirm the diagnosis of diabetes?**   2 marks

Q 3. **List four other presenting symptoms of type 2 diabetes (T2D).**   2 marks

Initially, Andy attempts to manage his diabetes mellitus (DM) by diet and exercise alone, but this fails to control his hyperglycaemia.

Q 4. **What hypoglycaemic agent would you start Andy on?**   1 mark

Andy is reviewed 6-monthly to monitor his glycaemic control and assess the development of any diabetic complications.

Q 5. How do you assess long-term glycaemic control?   1 mark

Q 6. How do you screen for diabetic renal disease?   2 marks

Andy's feet are examined: he has bilateral foot pulses but is unable to perceive the pressure from a 10-g monofilament, so he is at increased risk of developing a 'diabetic foot'.

Q 7. List four pieces of preventive foot-care advice.   4 marks

As part of his diabetes review, Andy also attends the local optometrist.

Q 8. What retinal changes are seen in diabetes?   2 marks

Total: 15 marks

ENDOCRINE

ENDOCRINE CASE 2

Jenny, a 21-year-old type 1 diabetic, is seen by her GP following a 2-day history of nausea and vomiting, and is now complaining of abdominal pain. Urine dipstick showed glycosuria and ketonuria, and she is admitted to the medical assessment unit. On examination her Glasgow Coma Scale (GCS) score is 15/15, heart rate (HR) is 120/min, abdomen is tender throughout, she is hyperventilating and appears dehydrated.

Q 1. **How is diabetic ketoacidosis (DKA) diagnosed biochemically?**   3 marks

ENDOCRINE

Q 2. **List three causes of diabetic ketoacidosis.**   3 marks

Jenny is diagnosed with DKA. Her arterial blood gases (ABG) are shown in Table 3.1.

Q 3. Indicate (↑,↓, or →) where marked '?' for the expected changes.　　4 marks

	Normal range	Jenny's ABG
pH	7.35–7.45	?
pO$_2$	10–12 kPa	11
pCO$_2$	4.7–6 kPa	?
HCO$_3^-$	22–28 mmol/l	?
BE	+/– 2 mmol/l	–9
Anion gap	10–18 mmol/l	?

Table 3.1: Jenny's arterial blood gases.

Q 4. How do you calculate the anion gap?　　1 mark

Q 5. List three causes of metabolic acidosis with an *increased* anion gap.　　3 marks

Jenny is successfully treated with intravenous fluids and sliding scale insulin.

Q 6. List three complications of this treatment.　　3 marks

Once stabilised, Jenny is referred to the diabetic nurse specialist for advice on the management of her diabetes.

Q 7. List four 'illness rules' you would give Jenny. 2 marks

Q 8. List four warning signs of hypoglycaemia. 2 marks

Q 9. What two coexisting conditions should you screen for in Jenny? 2 marks

Q 10. List two challenges facing Jenny. 2 marks

Total: 25 marks

ENDOCRINE CASE 3

Gloria, a 38-year-old woman, is referred by her GP to an endocrinologist with symptoms of hyperthyroidism.

Q 1. Name six symptoms Gloria may be complaining of. 3 marks

On examination she is in sinus tachycardia, has a fine tremor and has bulging eyes (exophthalmos).

Q 2. List two signs specific to Graves' disease. 1 mark

Q 3. What is the underlying cause of Graves' disease? 1 mark

Bloods are taken for thyroid function tests (TFTs), as shown in Table 3.2.

Q 4. In Table 3.2 indicate (with ↑,↓, or →) where marked '?' the expected changes in TFTs.   3 marks

	Normal range	Changes
TSH	0.5–5.7 mU/l	?
Total T$_4$	70–140 nmol/l	?
Total T$_3$	1.2–3.0 nmol/l	?

Table 3.2: Thyroid function tests.

Gloria's symptoms are treated with β-blockers and her hyperthyroidism by a 'block and replace' regimen with carbimazole and thyroxine.

Q 5. Give two complications of untreated hyperthyroidism.   1 mark

Q 6. Give four indications for thyroidectomy in Gloria.   2 marks

Q 7. **Give four complications of surgery.** 2 marks

On cessation of the 'block and replace' regimen, Gloria remains hyperthyroid. She is subsequently treated with radioactive iodine, which initially renders her euthyroid, although eventually it leaves her hypothyroid.

Q 8. **List four other causes of hypothyroidism.** 2 marks

Total: 15 marks

ENDOCRINE

GASTROENTEROLOGY CASES: QUESTIONS

GASTROENTEROLOGY
CASE 1

Henry, a 58-year-old man, presents to the Emergency Department with a 1-hour history of haematemesis, including a severe episode in the ambulance. On examination his blood pressure is 86/44 mmHg, he is cold peripherally and his pulse is 110 bpm.

Q 1. **List six causes of haematemesis.**　　3 marks

Q 2. **What is your immediate management?**　　3 marks

Q 3. **What three brief questions would you ask?**　　3 marks

Q 4. **What four blood tests would you request?**   2 marks

Henry undergoes emergency endoscopy, which diagnoses an actively bleeding gastric ulcer, which is successfully treated by injection of adrenaline.

Q 5. **What factors are used to assess Henry's risk of rebleeding?**   2 marks

Q 6. **List four signs of a rebleed while on the ward.**   2 marks

Total: 15 marks

GASTROENTEROLOGY CASE 2

Rod is admitted to the medical assessment unit complaining of malaise and anorexia. On examination, he is jaundiced with signs of chronic liver disease.

Q 1. List four risk factors for jaundice you would enquire about in the history. 2 marks

Q 2. List three *abdominal* signs of chronic liver disease. 3 marks

Several blood tests are requested to assess the severity of Rod's liver disease.

Q 3. Name two blood tests used to assess liver synthetic function. 2 marks

It is clear that the cause of Rod's liver disease is alcohol excess, and he is given intravenous thiamine and started on a chlordiazepoxide-reducing regimen. He is diagnosed with alcoholic hepatitis and commenced on oral corticosteroids.

Q 4. **What are we trying to prevent by giving thiamine to alcoholics?** 1 mark

Abdominal ultrasound scan reports cirrhotic changes in the liver with gross ascites.

Q 5. **In the absence of obvious risk factors, list three blood tests you would request to identify the cause of Rod's liver disease.** 3 marks

Q 6. **List four complications of liver cirrhosis.** 4 marks

Total: 15 marks

GASTROENTEROLOGY CASE 3

Dennis, a 64-year-old man, is admitted to the surgical assessment unit with several hours' history of severe epigastric pain radiating to his back, associated with nausea and vomiting. His serum amylase is reported as 1170 U/ml (normal range 0–180 U/ml), confirming a diagnosis of acute pancreatitis.

Q 1. List eight criteria used to assess the severity of pancreatitis.   4 marks

Q 2. List six causes of acute pancreatitis.   3 marks

Dennis is given high-flow oxygen therapy and aggressive fluid replacement. A urinary catheter is inserted to monitor his urine output.

Q 3. In fluid replacement, what minimum hourly urinary output do you aim for?   1 mark

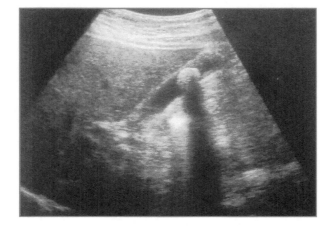

Figure 4.1: Dennis's abdominal ultrasound.

Dennis undergoes an abdominal ultrasound scan, which shows gallbladder stones with their acoustic shadows (see Figure 4.1).

Q 4. Name four additional complications of gallstones.   2 marks

Q 5. **What is the recommended procedure within the first 72 hours?** 1 mark

Dennis undergoes a cholecystectomy before discharge.

Q 6. **List two advantages each of laparoscopic and open cholecystectomy.** 2 marks

Laparoscopic:

Open:

Q 7. **Give four complications of cholecystectomy.** 2 marks

Total: 15 marks

GASTROENTEROLOGY CASE 4

Jennifer, a 25-year-old woman, is referred to gastroenterology with several weeks' history of bloody diarrhoea and general malaise.

Q 1. List four causes of bloody diarrhoea.   4 marks

A flexible sigmoidoscopy is arranged, which reveals a superficial continuous inflammation of the rectum. The mucosa looks reddened and inflamed, consistent with ulcerative colitis (UC), which is confirmed on biopsy.

Q 2. List four pathological differences between UC and Crohn's disease.   4 marks

Q 3. **List four extraintestinal manifestations of inflammatory bowel disease (IBD).**   2 marks

Jennifer is diagnosed with distal UC and responds well to a combination of oral and topical treatment.

Q 4. **What class of drug is prescribed to maintain remission in UC?**   1 mark

Jennifer remains asymptomatic before relapsing, requiring admission to hospital, where she is diagnosed with an attack of her UC.

Q 5. **List six features used to assess the severity of a UC attack.**   3 marks

Q 6. Why would you do a plain abdominal X-ray in an acute attack of UC? 2 marks

Q 7. Give four complications of UC. 4 marks

Total: 20 marks

NEUROLOGY CASES: QUESTIONS

NEUROLOGY CASE 1

George, a 67-year-old smoker, presents to his GP following an episode of slurred speech earlier that day, which resolved in less than 30 minutes. On examination he is in sinus rhythm, blood pressure is 154/83 mmHg and he is neurologically intact. Owing to his high risk of stroke, he is admitted for further assessment.

Q 1. **What should be started immediately?**   1 mark

George undergoes a number of inpatient investigations, including carotid Doppler.

Q 2. **What are the criteria for carotid endarterectomy?**   2 marks

George's blood pressure and cholesterol are optimised, he is commenced on appropriate antiplatelet medication, although he continues to smoke on discharge. Unfortunately, 3 months later he presents with a stroke.

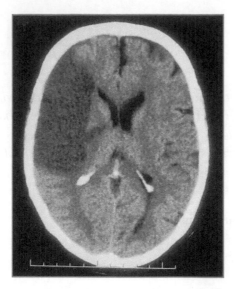

Figure 5.1: George's brain CT scan.

Q 3. **What cerebral artery is affected (please refer to Figure 5.1)?** 1 mark

Q 4. **What features of a stroke may be present?** 2 marks

Q 5. **Is George's stroke due to infarction or haemorrhage?** 1 mark

George is thrombolysed and transferred to the stroke ward for rehabilitation, where over the following weeks he makes good progress.

NEUROLOGY

Q 6. **Name six health professionals involved in George's rehabilitation.**   3 marks

Total: **10 marks**

NEUROLOGY CASE 2

Lisa, a 21-year-old student, is brought into the Emergency Department after having a 'black-out' while watching TV at home with one of her flatmates.

Q 1. **What six questions would you ask Lisa's flatmate?**   3 marks

Lisa's flatmate tells you that she suddenly stopped talking, fell to the floor and then started moving her arms and legs in jerky movements. Lisa has no memory of the attack itself and had no warning of it happening.

Q 2. **List six causes of seizures.**   3 marks

Lisa is discharged the next morning following her suspected seizure, with a neurology outpatient appointment arranged.

Q 3. **What advice should Lisa receive about driving?** 1 mark

Q 4. **What is the most useful investigation to confirm the diagnosis of epilepsy?** 1 mark

Several weeks later Lisa has a second tonic-clonic seizure, and her neurologist decides to start her on anticonvulsive treatment.

Q 5. **What is first-line treatment for Lisa's type of epilepsy?** 1 mark

Q 6. **How would you treat a prolonged seizure?** 3 marks

Q 7. **What advice concerning anti-epileptic drugs do you give women of childbearing age?** 3 marks

Total: 15 marks

NEUROLOGY CASE 3

Harold, a 68-year-old man, is referred to neurology outpatients. As he enters the consultation room, you note that he has a very slow, shuffling gait suggestive of Parkinson's disease.

Q 1. What are the three main features of Parkinson's disease?　　3 marks

Q 2. List three characteristic features of a parkinsonism tremor.　　3 marks

On the basis of the history and examination, you diagnose Parkinson's disease.

Q 3. Other than Parkinson's disease, list two other causes of parkinsonism. 2 marks

Q 4. What is the underlying pathophysiology of Parkinson's disease?　　1 mark

Several months later Harold is started on L-dopa, which greatly improves his motor symptoms.

Q 5. What class of drug is combined with L-dopa to prevent peripheral side-effects?   1 mark

Q 6. Name three limitations of L-dopa therapy.   3 marks

Harold is followed up for his Parkinson's disease by a nurse specialist, who also enquires about common non-motor symptoms.

Q 7. List two non-motor symptoms of Parkinson's disease.   2 marks

Total: 15 marks

NEUROLOGY

OBSTETRICS AND GYNAECOLOGY CASES: QUESTIONS

OBSTETRICS AND GYNAECOLOGY CASE 1

Julie, a 24-year-old teacher, visits her GP on Monday requesting emergency contraception. She recently started a new relationship with a colleague called Paul and had unprotected sexual intercourse on Saturday night. She is on the ninth day of her 28-day cycle.

Q 1. **What would you advise Julie?**   2 marks

Julie chooses the pill for future contraception.

Q 2. **Describe two contraceptive mechanisms of the combined oral contraceptive (COC).**   1 mark

Q 3. **List six contraindications to the COC.**   3 marks

Nothing in Julie's history contraindicates the pill. She is prescribed a 3-month supply of a COC and advised on its side-effects.

Q 4. **Name four *minor* side-effects Julie may experience.**   2 marks

Q 5. **List four pieces of additional advice you would give Julie.**   2 marks

Total: 10 marks

OBSTETRICS AND GYNAECOLOGY CASE 2

Paul and Julie (aged 37 and 33 years, respectively) visit their GP following 2 years of being unable to conceive. A full history is taken from both.

Q 1. What general advice would you give to couples trying to get pregnant? 2 marks

Q 2. List four points that you might elicit in Julie's history that would be suggestive of tubal dysfunction. 2 marks

As an initial assessment the GP organises a semen analysis for Paul and requests a day-21 progesterone level from Julie.

Q 3. List three variables measured in semen analysis. 3 marks

The results come back confirming normal semen analysis. Julie's day-21 progesterone concentration is 8 nmol/l.

Q 4. What is a normal day-21 progesterone concentration?　　1 mark

Q 5. Give two explanations for Julie's low progesterone concentration.　　2 marks

Julie is referred to gynaecology, where she is diagnosed with polycystic ovarian syndrome (PCOS).

Q 6. List three clinical features which Julie might have.　　3 marks

Julie's infertility is treated with clomifene.

Q 7. List two complications associated with this treatment.　　2 marks

Total:　　15 marks

OBS & GYNAE

OBSTETRICS AND GYNAECOLOGY CASE 3

Julie and her husband Paul are both delighted to discover that she is pregnant after many years of trying. Julie is now 10 weeks pregnant (her last menstrual period (LMP) was on 15 July and her cycle is normally a regular 28 days) and she attends the antenatal clinic for her booking visit.

Q 1. **When is Julie's expected date of delivery according to Naegele's rule?** 1 mark

Q 2. **List four blood tests you would offer.** 2 marks

Q 3. **List four examples of dietary advice you would give Julie.** 2 marks

Q 4. List four common minor symptoms of pregnancy Julie may experience.   2 marks

Because of her age, Julie requests screening for Down syndrome.

Q 5. Name two markers measured to screen for trisomy 21.   2 marks

At 34 weeks Julie attends the antenatal clinic for her regular antenatal care. On obstetric examination the midwife finds that the symphysis–fundal height is 30 cm.

Q 6. Give two reasons why Julie may be small for dates.   2 marks

Q 7. List four causes of intrauterine growth restriction (IUGR).   2 marks

Julie's blood pressure (BP) is raised at 154/94 mmHg (her booking BP was 116/78 mmHg) and she has 2+ protein in her urine, so she is admitted to the pregnancy assessment unit with pre-eclampsia.

Q 8. **List four symptoms associated with pre-eclampsia.** 2 marks

Total: 15 marks

OBSTETRICS AND GYNAECOLOGY CASE 4

Julie, who is 34+5 pregnant, is admitted with pre-eclampsia. Fetal monitoring is reassuring, so her hypertension is treated with labetalol, while her blood pressure and bloods are regularly monitored. At 37 weeks it is decided to induce labour, so her cervix is assessed using the Bishop's score.

Q 1. List four features used to assess the Bishop's score.　　　　2 marks

Q 2. What Bishop's score is considered favourable for induction?　　　　1 mark

Q 3. What is used to make the cervix favourable for induction?　　　　1 mark

Induction of labour is successful. Julie's labour is recorded on her partogram, while her baby is monitored by cardiotocography (CTG) to assess fetal distress.

Q 4. List six *maternal* observations recorded on the partogram.   3 marks

Q 5. What four components are used to interpret a CTG?   2 marks

Julie's contractions are inefficient, so she is started with an infusion of oxytocin.

Q 6. List two potential complications of using oxytocin.   1 mark

Julie's contractions become progressively more frequent and painful. Three hours later her cervical dilatation is reassessed (last measurement was 4 cm) and plotted on the partogram, demonstrating that Julie's labour is progressing satisfactorily.

Q 7. By how many centimetres should the cervix be dilated now?   1 mark

Q 8. List four causes of failure to progress in the first stage of labour.   2 marks

Q 9. List four sequential stages in the passage of the fetus through the birth canal, leading up to the delivery of the shoulders.   4 marks

Julie delivers a pink and healthy boy called Alex, who cries immediately.

Q 10. Give two non-pharmacological techniques for reducing postpartum haemorrhage (PPH).   1 mark

Q 11. Name two drugs that are used in the management of postpartum haemorrhage.   2 marks

Total: 20 marks

OBS & GYNAE

PAEDIATRICS
CASES: QUESTIONS

PAEDIATRICS CASE 1

Nathan, an 11-month-old infant, is referred to the paediatric assessment unit with a history of irritability and inconsolable crying for the last 8 hours. His mother has noted that he will settle down for a few minutes, but then wakes up and cries loudly, drawing his legs up to his abdomen. There is no fever, vomiting or diarrhoea. His bowels were last open yesterday and were normal. Past medical history is unremarkable, except that Nathan is recovering from gastroenteritis and remains off his feed.

Q 1. **List four causes of inconsolable crying in an infant.** 2 marks

Nathan is alert, pink and well perfused. His abdomen is not distended and is soft with normal bowel sounds and with a palpable mass in the right upper quadrant.

Q 2. **What is intussusception?** 1 mark

Q 3. **In which part of the bowel does intussusception most commonly occur?** 1 mark

Q 4. **Name four predisposing factors for intussusception.** 2 marks

Q 5. Name four features of intussusception.   2 marks

Suspecting that Nathan has intussusception, you request an abdominal ultrasound scan, shown in Figure 7.1 below.

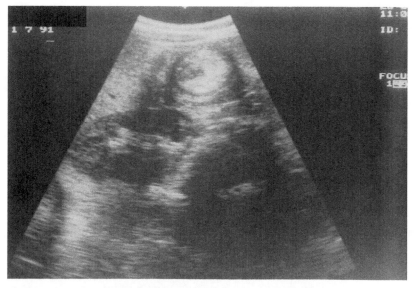

Figure 7.1 Nathan's abdominal ultrasound.

Q 6. **What does the ultrasound show?**   1 mark

Q 7. **How would you treat intussusception in Nathan?**   1 mark

Total: **10 marks**

PAEDIATRICS CASE 2

Rebecca is born at 40 weeks' gestation by normal vaginal delivery weighing 3.2 kg. Her mother (gravida 1, para 1) went into labour spontaneously, and labour was not prolonged. Rebecca's APGAR scores were 9 and 10 at 1 and 5 minutes, respectively, and she was transferred to the postnatal ward together with her mother. At the postnatal check the next day, the midwife notices that Rebecca's skin and sclerae are yellow. Apart from that she appears very well and is breastfeeding satisfactorily.

Q 1. **Are you concerned about Rebecca's jaundice? Briefly explain your reasoning.**   2 marks

Q 2. **Give three reasons why jaundice is common in neonates.**   3 marks

Rebecca's jaundice is investigated. Her blood results are shown below.

Hb	12.2 g/dl (14.5–21.5)	Rebecca's blood group	A, Rh –ve
Platelets	220 x 10⁹/l (150–400)	Maternal blood group	O, Rh –ve
MCV	112 fl (100–135)	Total serum bilirubin	140 μmol/l (3–17) (unconjugated)
WCC	14 x 10⁹/l (10–26)	CRP	< 10 mg/l
Film	Normal RBCs	Direct Coombs' test (DCT)	+ (mildly +ve)

Q 3. **Give three causes of elevated *conjugated* bilirubin in neonates.**   3 marks

Q 4. **What does the direct Coombs' test (DCT) detect and what does it indicate?**   2 marks

Q 5. **From the blood results, what is the cause of her jaundice?**   2 marks

Q 6. **How do you record bilirubin measurements?**   1 mark

Q 7. **How does phototherapy work?**   1 mark

If unconjugated bilirubin reaches high levels, it can become neurotoxic, termed 'kernicterus'.

Q 8. **Give three clinical features of kernicterus.**   3 marks

Q 9. **Give three long-term complications of kernicterus.**   3 marks

---

Fortunately for Rebecca, phototherapy is successful, and she joins her new family at home 4 days later on oral folic acid. She is followed up 2 weeks later in outpatients for a repeat full blood count to ensure late haemolysis is not occurring.

Total: 20 marks

PAEDIATRICS CASE 3

Chelsea, a 3-month old baby girl, is referred to paediatrics with a 2-day history of feeding difficulties and a cough. On examination, she has a runny nose and looks dehydrated. Furthermore she has signs of respiratory distress, with a widespread expiratory wheeze; SaO_2 (on air) 90%.

Q 1. **List six signs of respiratory distress in an infant.**   3 marks

Q 2. **What is the normal heart rate and respiratory rate in infants?**   2 marks

Heart rate:

Respiratory rate:

Chelsea's mum tells you that she is not taking her bottle and her nappies are much drier than normal.

Q 3. **List four signs indicating dehydration in an infant.** 2 marks

Q 4. **How is the maintenance fluid requirement of a child calculated?** 1 mark

You diagnose Chelsea with bronchiolitis and admit her to the ward, where she is barrier-nursed to prevent spread.

Q 5. **List four clinical features of bronchiolitis.** 2 marks

Q 6. **List four types of patients at risk of bronchiolitis.** 2 marks

Q 7. What is the most common cause of bronchiolitis and how is it detected?

2 marks

Q 8. How would you manage Chelsea? 3 marks

Q 9. What is the prophylactic antibody for respiratory syncytial virus (RSV)? 1 mark

Q 10. How would you monitor the effectiveness of treatment? 2 marks

Total: 20 marks

PAEDIATRICS

PAEDIATRICS CASE 4

James, a 3-year-old boy, is referred to the paediatric outpatient clinic because of poor weight gain over the past 6 months. He was born at full term weighing 3.2 kg. However, over the past 6 months his Mum says he has become irritable, his abdomen seems distended, and he has lots of liquid stools that are foul-smelling and difficult to flush. On examination, James is pale and his abdomen is protruded. There is wasting of his muscles (especially buttocks) and his ankles seem swollen.

Q 1. Define failure to thrive.   1 mark

Q 2. List four non-organic causes of failure to thrive.   2 marks

Q 3. What is the likely mechanism of James's diarrhoea?   1 mark

Q 4. Why does James have ankle oedema?   1 mark

As part of his investigations, James is screened for coeliac disease.

Q 5. What is the serological screening test for coeliac disease?　　1 mark

James's serological screening test is positive, and he is referred for a duodenal biopsy, which subsequently confirms coeliac disease.

Q 6. List two histological changes on biopsy seen in coeliac disease.　　2 marks

Q 7. Which rash is associated with coeliac disease?　　1 mark

Q 8. List three food groups James will now have to avoid.　　3 marks

Q 9. Give three complications of coeliac disease.　　3 marks

Total:　　15 marks

PAEDIATRICS CASE 5

Marie, a 17-month-old toddler, is referred by her GP after Mum has noticed that, ever since she started walking, she appears to be limping. Marie appears unaware of this and does not complain of any pain. She was born by elective caesarean section due to breech presentation.

Q 1. **With regards to her motor milestones, at what ages would you expect Marie to do the following?** 7 marks

1. Crawl:

2. Walk:

3. Run:

4. Kick a ball:

5. Ride a tricycle:

6. Hop on one foot:

7. Climbs stairs adult fashion:

Q 2. **Name two pathological gaits in children.** 1 mark

Q 3. **What is your differential diagnosis?** 2 marks

Q 4. **Which non-traumatic cause of a limp needs immediate intervention?** 1 mark

Q 5. **What two manoeuvres can you do to test for congenital hip problems in neonates?** 1 mark

On examination, Marie's left leg is externally rotated and shorter than her right leg. Subsequent X-ray confirms developmental dysplasia of the hip and she is referred to orthopaedics for further management.

Your next patient also presents with a limp, a 12-year-old boy whose weight lies on the 90th centile and who has been complaining for several weeks of an intermittent limp and knee pain, making cycling painful.

Q 6. **What is the most likely diagnosis from this history?** 1 mark

Q 7. **What is the typical finding on examination of the hip?** 1 mark

Q 8. **Which other hip pathology in a child is associated with avascular necrosis?** 1 mark

Total 15 marks

PALLIATIVE CARE CASE: QUESTIONS

PALLIATIVE CARE CASE 1

Margaret, with known inoperable squamous cell bronchial carcinoma, is reviewed by her oncologist with worsening back pain that is no longer eased by paracetamol.

Q 1. **List six 'red flag' back pain features.** 3 marks

Q 2. **Name four primary cancers that metastasise to bone.** 2 marks

A bone scan confirms secondary deposits in the thoracic vertebrae, and she is referred for palliative radiotherapy and commenced on morphine.

Q 3. Describe the three steps of the analgesic ladder.   3 marks

Q 4. List four side-effects of morphine.   2 marks

Q 5. Why should morphine be used with caution in renal failure?   1 mark

Margaret's bone profile is shown below:

Ca²⁺ (mmol/l)	2.7 (2.12–2.65)
Albumin (g/l)	25 (35–50)

Q 6. Calculate Margaret's adjusted calcium.   1 mark

PALLIATIVE CARE

Q 7. **Give four symptoms of hypercalcaemia.** 2 marks

Q 8. **List two further causes of hypercalcaemia.** 1 mark

Q 9. **Name two other palliative care emergencies.** 1 mark

Margaret has had two recent hospital admissions for hypercalcaemia and is now on monthly pamidronate infusions. She takes diclofenac 75 mg bd and morphine sulphate tablets (MST) 120 mg bd for bone pain. Unfortunately, her condition has deteriorated rapidly over the last week, and she is admitted to St John's Hospice. She is nauseous with occasional vomiting, in obvious pain and unable to take oral medications.

Q 10. **Convert her oral morphine to 24-hour diamorphine subcutaneous infusion.** 1 mark

Q 11. Give four potential causes of Margaret's nausea and vomiting.   2 marks

Margaret is prescribed metoclopramide for her nausea and vomiting.

Q 12. Where does metoclopramide exert its anti-emetic effect?   1 mark

Total: 20 marks

PSYCHIATRY
CASE: QUESTIONS

PSYCHIATRY CASE 1

Ethel is 74 and lives alone. She has a fall at home and is admitted to hospital with a fractured neck of femur. Postoperatively she is disoriented and has become increasingly restless and agitated with nursing staff. At times she believes she is being poisoned. She is diagnosed with delirium (acute confusional state).

Q 1. List six possible causes of delirium.   3 marks

Ethel recovers from the episode of delirium and makes a good recovery from her hip fracture before discharge back to her own home. However, her GP is concerned about her increasing forgetfulness and organises a minimental state examination (MMSE) in which she scores 18.

Q 2. What MMSE score supports a diagnosis of dementia?   1 mark

Q 3. What is the commonest cause of dementia?   1 mark

Q 4. **List four blood tests you would request to exclude treatable causes of dementia.**
2 marks

Ethel is referred to the local memory assessment service.

Q 5. **List six potential risks that should be considered in people with dementia.**
3 marks

Total: 10 marks

RENAL CASES: QUESTIONS

RENAL CASE 1

Sheila, a 49-year-old type 1 diabetic, is under the care of the nephrologist. Her current medications include insulin, angiotensin-converting enzyme (ACE) inhibitor (for hypertension) and a non-steroidal anti-inflammatory drug (NSAID) (for chronic back pain). At her annual review her blood pressure is 174/98 mmHg; her blood results are shown in Table 10.1 below.

Hb	8.6 g/dl	Na^+	136 mmol/l
MCV	86 fl	K^+	5.2 mmol/l
WCC	5.2 x 10^9/l	Urea	22.9 mmol/l
Platelets	280 x 10^9/l	Creatinine	246 mmol/l
		eGFR	23 ml/min
HbA_{1c}	11.2%	Adj Ca^{2+}	1.82 mmol/l
		PO_4^{3-}	2.72 mmol/l

Table 10.1: Shelia's blood results.

Q 1. Outline four functions of the kidney.　　　　　**4 marks**

Q 2. List three blood test results suggestive of chronic (as opposed to acute) renal failure.　　　　　**3 marks**

Q 3. Name two factors that might be contributing to her renal failure.   1 mark

Sheila complains of fatigue, which her nephrologist attributes to her anaemia.

Q 4. What is the likely cause of her anaemia?   1 mark

As well as correcting her anaemia, Sheila is commenced on treatment for renal bone disease.

Q 5. List two treatments to prevent renal bone disease.   2 marks

Q 6. How would you monitor the effectiveness of such treatment?   1 mark

RENAL

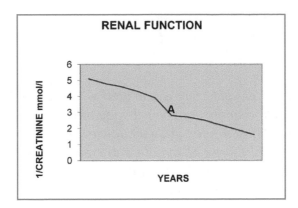

Figure 10.1: A graph of Sheila's reciprocal plasma creatinine against time.

Q 7. **Give three possible generic causes for the sharp decline at time A (please refer to Figure 10.1).** 3 marks

Total: 15 marks

RENAL CASE 2

Christopher, an 84-year-old man, is admitted with a 2-day history of general malaise. On examination, he is hypotensive, pyrexial and clinically dehydrated. His admission urea and electrolytes (U&Es) are: Na^+ 133 mmol/l, K^+ 6.7 mmol/l, urea 41 mmol/l and creatinine 312 micromol/l, and an estimated glomerular filtration rate (eGFR) of 14 ml/min (his eGFR the previous month was 66 ml/min).

Q 1. **List two causes each of prerenal, renal and postrenal causes of renal failure.**
3 marks

Prerenal causes:

Renal causes:

Postrenal causes:

Appropriate investigations are undertaken, including an electrocardiogram (ECG), shown in Figure 10.2 opposite:

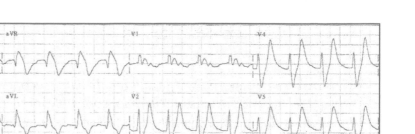

Figure 10.2: Christopher's ECG.

Q 2. **Give two ECG changes associated with hyperkalaemia.**   2 marks

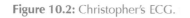

Q 3. **List four causes of hyperkalaemia.**   2 marks

Q 4. **How would you treat life-threatening hyperkalaemia?**   3 marks

Christopher is diagnosed with acute renal failure secondary to urinary sepsis. His hyperkalaemia is treated appropriately, he is resuscitated with intravenous fluids, commenced on broad-spectrum antibiotics and his nephrotoxic drugs stopped.

Q 5. **Outline how ACE inhibitors and NSAIDs cause acute renal failure.** 2 marks

ACE inhibitors:

NSAIDs:

Christopher's blood pressure and urine output respond to fluid resuscitation, and his U&Es subsequently indicate recovery of his renal function.

Q 5. **List four indications for renal replacement therapy.** 2 marks

Q 6. **Name two early complications following recovery from acute tubular necrosis (ATN).** 1 mark

Total: 15 marks

RESPIRATORY
CASES: QUESTIONS

RESPIRATORY CASE 1

*Lucy, a 21-year-old asthmatic, presents to the Emergency Department
with a 2-day history of increased shortness of breath, wheeze and cough.
On examination her pulse is 125 bpm, respiratory rate is 30/min, there is
widespread bilateral expiratory wheeze and air entry is reduced throughout.*

Q 1. **What three brief questions would you ask?**   3 marks

Q 2. **List three criteria used to indicate a severe asthma attack.**   3 marks

Q 3. **List three criteria used to indicate a life-threatening asthma attack.**   3 marks

Q 4. **List two arterial blood gas (ABG) markers of a *life-threatening* attack.**   1 mark

Lucy is diagnosed with a severe asthma attack and is treated appropriately.

Q 5. What is your immediate management in *severe* asthma?   3 marks

Q 6. What additional treatment may be used in life-threatening asthma?   1 mark

Q 7. When would you request a chest X-ray in an asthma attack?   1 mark

Lucy's breathing improves, and she is transferred to the ward.

Q 8. List two ways in which the effects of treatment can be assessed non-invasively.   1 mark

Lucy continues to improve and discharge is planned for the following day.

Q 9. **What four things should Lucy have before discharge?**   4 marks

Total: 20 marks

RESPIRATORY CASE 2

Tom, a 63-year-old lifelong smoker, attends his GP with increasing breathlessness, a chronic cough and regular sputum production. His notes reveal frequent winter chest infections requiring antibiotics. Suspecting a diagnosis of chronic obstructive pulmonary disease (COPD), his GP requests spirometry: FEV_1 54%, $FEV_1/FVC < 0.7$.

Q 1. **On the basis of Tom's spirometry, what is the severity of COPD?**   1 mark

Q 2. **What advice would you offer?**   1 mark

Tom is started on an ipratropium bromide inhaler by his GP.

Q 3. **When are inhaled corticosteroids indicated in COPD?**   1 mark

Q 4. **List two qualifying criteria for home O_2 therapy.**   1 mark

The following winter Tom is admitted to the Emergency Department with severe dyspnoea and cough productive of green sputum. On examination, his temperature is 37 °C, pulse is 95 bpm, respiratory rate 35/min, he has widespread expiratory wheeze, reduced air entry throughout and is cyanosed.

Q 5. **What four brief questions would you ask regarding his COPD?** 2 marks

Q 6. **What is your immediate medical management (including doses, where appropriate)?** 3 marks

The arterial blood gases (ABG) results (on air) are shown below:

pH	7.37	(7.35–7.45)
pO_2	6.9 kPa	(> 10.6)
pCO_2	4.2 kPa	(4.7–6)
HCO_3^-	25 mmol/l	(22–28)
BE	–1.2	(±2)

Q 7. **What type of respiratory failure do the ABGs show?** 1 mark

Q 8. **How will these ABGs influence your immediate management?** 1 mark

Q 9. List four signs of hypercapnia. 2 marks

The diagnosis is made of infective COPD exacerbation, which is successfully treated with amoxicillin.

Q 10. What two organisms are commonly responsible for COPD exacerbations? 2 marks

Total: 15 marks

RESPIRATORY

RESPIRATORY CASE 3

As the surgical FY1, you are bleeped to review Derek, a 76-year-old man, 4 days postop hemicolectomy, who is complaining of right-sided pleuretic chest pain with associated breathlessness. On examination, you find signs of a deep vein in thrombosis (DVT) in his left leg.

Q 1. List three signs of a DVT on examination.   3 marks

Q 2. List six risk factors for pulmonary embolism (PE).   3 marks

Derek undergoes a number of investigations, including an electrocardiogram (ECG). Suspecting a PE, he is commenced on low-molecular-weight heparin (LMWH) while awaiting a CT pulmonary angiogram.

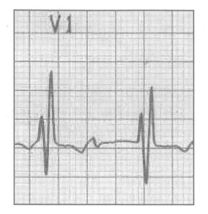

Figure 11.1: Derek's ECG.

Q 3. **What does this ECG show (see Figure 11.1)?**   1 mark

The diagnosis of PE secondary to a DVT is made. Derek is anticoagulated with warfarin, with a target international normalised ratio (INR) of 2–3.

Q 4. **What is the mechanism of action of warfarin?**   1 mark

---

Q 5. **How can you reduce the risk of venous thromboembolism (VTE) in hospital patients?**   2 marks

---

Total: 10 marks

RESPIRATORY CASE 4

Margaret, a 64-year-old heavy smoker, visits her GP complaining of a 3-month history of cough associated with haemoptysis.

Q 1. **List three respiratory causes of haemoptysis.**   3 marks

Q 2. **List two other common presenting lung cancer symptoms.**   2 marks

On examination the only abnormal finding is that she is clubbed.

Q 3. **List two cardiac, two respiratory and two gastrointestinal causes of clubbing.**   3 marks

Cardiac:

Gastrointestinal:

Respiratory:

The GP arranges an urgent chest X-ray (see Figure 11.2). The radiological report notes opacification of the right apex with destruction of the second rib, consistent with bronchial carcinoma.

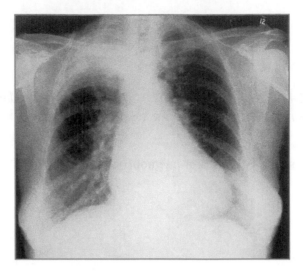

Figure 11.2: Margaret's chest X-ray.

Q 4. **What is this type of lung tumour called?**   1 mark

Q 5. **List four causes of round lesions on the lung on chest X-ray.**   2 marks

Q 6. **Where does lung cancer metastasise to?**   2 marks

Margaret is seen the following week as an outpatient at the respiratory clinic.

Q 7. What two investigations would you arrange to confirm lung cancer?   2 marks

---

Total: **15 marks**

RESPIRATORY CASE 5

John, a 72-year-old insulin-dependent diabetic, visits his GP with a 3-day history of cough, dyspnoea and general malaise. He is prescribed amoxicillin but continues to deteriorate and is admitted to hospital the following day.

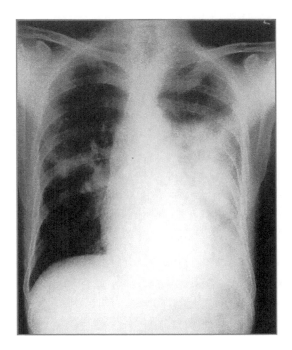

Figure 11.3: John's chest X-ray.

Q 1. **What is your diagnosis (see Figure 11.3).**   2 marks

Q 2. **List two poor prognostic features in the history above.**   2 marks

John is diagnosed with severe pneumonia and treated with intravenous co-amoxiclav and clarithromycin (to cover atypical organisms).

Q 3. **List three causes of 'atypical' pneumonia.** 3 marks

Microbiology call the ward to report Gram-positive cocci in John's blood, while awaiting culture and sensitivity.

Q 4. **What is the most likely cause of John's pneumonia and how can this be prevented?** 2 marks

Q 5. **List six parameters used to assess treatment progress.** 3 marks

John fails to make good progress and clinical examination reveals reduced breath sounds at the right base. His chest X-ray is repeated, which shows a right pleural effusion.

RESPIRATORY

Q 6. What is the most likely complication?   1 mark

Q 7. How should this be treated?   2 marks

Total: 15 marks

RHEUMATOLOGY CASES: QUESTIONS

RHEUMATOLOGY CASE 1

Hayley, a 36-year-old woman, is referred to rheumatology with a 2-month history of stiff, painful, swollen hands associated with general malaise.

Q 1. List four *inflammatory* causes of polyarthropathy.　　　　2 marks

You examine Hayley's hands and wrists.

Q 2. Give four features of rheumatoid arthritis on examination of the hands and wrists.　　　　4 marks

You organise some blood tests and send Hayley for an X-ray of her hands and feet.

Q 3. Give four X-ray changes in the hands in rheumatoid arthritis.   2 marks

You clinically diagnose Hayley with rheumatoid arthritis. You give her an intramuscular glucocorticoid injection, while commencing her on methotrexate.

Q 4. List two side-effects of methotrexate.   2 marks

Q 5. Give four complications of long-term oral steroid treatment.   2 marks

Hayley is followed up by the rheumatology nurse specialist, who monitors her response to treatment.

Q 6. What score is used to monitor disease progression?   1 mark

RHEUMATOLOGY

Q 7. List four features associated with a poor prognosis.   2 marks

Total: 15 marks

RHEUMATOLOGY CASE 2

Julie, a 28-year-old woman, presents with arthralgia and fatigue. On examination, she has a typical butterfly rash. Suspecting a diagnosis of systemic lupus erythematosus (SLE), you request a number of investigations.

Q 1. **List six investigations you would request to help establish the diagnosis.**

3 marks

Julie's urinalysis shows 3+ proteinuria.

Q 2. **What is the likely cause of Julie's proteinuria?**

1 mark

Q 3. **List three treatment options for Julie's joint symptoms.**

3 marks

Two years later Julie speaks to her GP about the possibility of becoming pregnant.

Q 4. What are the potential problems Julie might face during her pregnancy?   3 marks

_____

_____

_____

Total: **10 marks**

SURGICAL
CASES: QUESTIONS

SURGICAL CASE 1

Elizabeth is invited to attend for breast cancer screening at her local unit.

Q 1. From what age are women invited to attend the NHS breast screening programme?   1 mark

Q 2. List six criteria used in deciding whether to screen for a disease.   6 marks

Elizabeth's mammogram (see Figure 13.1) demonstrates an irregular mass in the central part of the left breast, which has spicules radiating from it, and she is urgently referred for triple assessment.

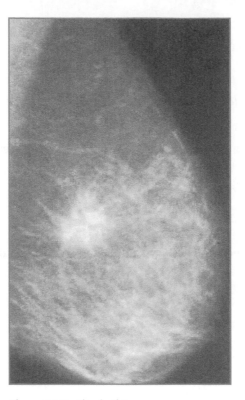

Figure 13.1: Elizabeth's mammogram.

Q 3. What are the three components of the triple assessment?   3 marks

Q 4. List four signs of breast cancer on breast examination.   2 marks

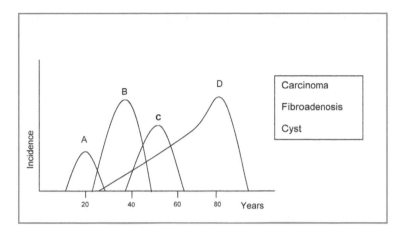

Figure 13.2: Age incidence of common breast lumps.

Q 5. From the graph shown in Figure 13.2 identify which breast lump corresponds to which peak in incidence.   2 marks

A:

B:

C:

D:

Unfortunately, the results of Elizabeth's triple assessment confirm a diagnosis of breast cancer.

Q 6. Name four metastatic sites for breast cancer.   2 marks

Q 7. List four potential treatment options for Elizabeth's breast cancer.   2 marks

Q 8. What is a sentinel node?   1 mark

Q 9. What is the advantage of performing a sentinel node biopsy?   1 mark

Total: **20 marks**

SURGICAL

SURGICAL CASE 2

Ethel, a frail 82-year-old in sheltered accommodation, is brought into the Emergency Department after being found by her carers lying at the side of her bed. On examination, you suspect that she has suffered a fractured hip.

Q 1. What findings would be consistent with a hip fracture? 2 marks

You request anteroposterior (AP) (shown in Figure 13.3) and lateral X-rays to confirm your diagnosis.

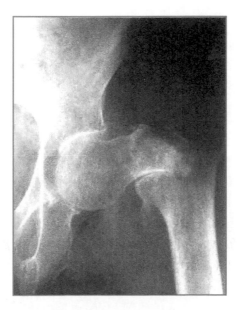

Figure 13.3: Ethel's anteroposterior X-ray.

Q 2. **Is this fracture intra- or extracapsular?** 1 mark

The orthopaedic surgeon elects to fix Ethel's hip fracture with a dynamic hip screw (DHS), and she is scheduled for surgery on the trauma list.

Q 3. **Name two late complications of treating intracapsular fractures by internal fixation, as opposed to hemiarthroplasty.** 2 marks

Q 4. **As the FY1 doctor what eight things should you ensure are done before surgery?** 2 marks

Surgery is successful, and Ethel is encouraged to start partially weight-bearing the following day.

SURGICAL

Q 5. **Give four reasons why Ethel should start weight-bearing as soon as possible.** 2 marks

You note from Ethel's extensive medical history that she has several risk factors for a hip fracture, including osteoporosis and a history of falls.

Q 6. **Give three pieces of *general* advice to help prevent osteoporosis.** 3 marks

Before discharge, you commence Ethel on a bisphosphonate with calcium and vitamin D supplementation.

Q 7. **How do bisphosphonates prevent osteoporosis?** 1 mark

During her inpatient stay Ethel is assessed by the falls intervention team.

SURGICAL

Q 8. List four risk factors for falls in the elderly.　　　　　2 marks

Total:　　　　　15 marks

SURGICAL CASE 3

Doris, a 69-year-old woman, is urgently referred to the lower GI surgeons with suspected colorectal cancer.

Q 1. List four signs, symptoms or investigations that would warrant urgent referral of patients for suspected colorectal cancer.　　　4 marks

Doris undergoes colonoscopy, which identifies a suspicious lesion in the sigmoid colon. This, on biopsy, is diagnosed as cancer. Doris is scheduled for surgery and is counselled about the likelihood of a stoma.

Q 2. Name three complications of a stoma.　　　3 marks

Doris undergoes a sigmoid colectomy. The histopathology findings report that the cancer has extended through the bowel wall, with regional lymph node involvement.

Q 3. What is the Dukes' classification of Doris's colon cancer?　　　1 mark

Eighteen months later Doris is admitted to the surgical assessment unit with a history of colicky lower abdominal pain and increasing constipation for five days.

Q 4. List two causes of *mechanical* large-bowel obstruction.   2 marks

Q 5. What signs would you look for in acute *mechanical* intestinal obstruction?   3 marks

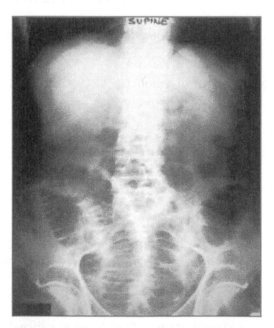

Figure 13.4: Abdominal X-ray from a patient admitted with acute intestinal obstruction.

Q 6. **Is this a small- or large-bowel obstruction (please refer to Figure 13.4)?**
   Explain your answer.   2 marks

Total: 15 marks

SURGICAL CASE 4

Michael, a smoker of 40 cigarettes a day, attends his GP with a history of muscular cramp-like pain, mainly in one calf, on walking a short distance that is rapidly relieved by rest.

Q 1. **What non-invasive test confirms the diagnosis of peripheral vascular disease?**   1 mark

Q 2. **What are the main *modifiable* risk factors for peripheral vascular disease?**

2 marks

Q 3. **What advice would you give Michael?**   2 marks

Twelve months later Michael is urgently referred to the vascular surgeons, describing a history of deteriorating claudication in the same leg, which has recently progressed to nocturnal rest pain. On examination, the affected foot shows signs of critical ischaemia.

Q 4. What are the signs of a critically ischaemic foot?   4 marks

Q 5. Why is pain typically worse at night?   3 marks

Michael undergoes an MR angiogram (shown in Figure 13.5) and his occluded left superficial femoral artery is treated by percutaneous transluminal angioplasty.

SURGICAL

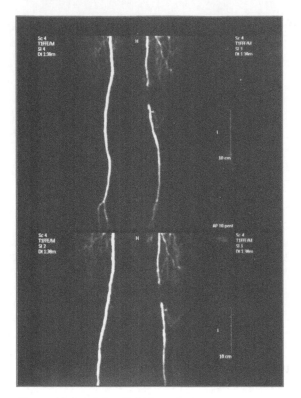

Figure 13.5: Michael's MR angiogram.

Two years later Michael presents to the Emergency Department with features of acute limb ischaemia.

Q 6. List four causes of *embolic* acute lower limb ischaemia. 2 marks

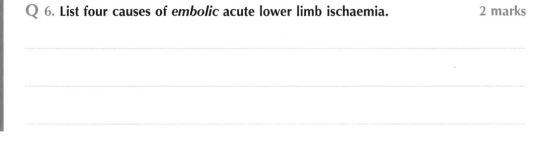

Q 7. Give six features of acute limb ischaemia.   3 marks

Examination is suggestive of complete acute ischaemia. He is given intravenous heparin and taken straight to theatre for revascularisation of his leg.

Q 8. Name three complications of reperfusion.   3 marks

Total: 20 marks

CARDIOVASCULAR CASES: ANSWERS

CARDIOVASCULAR CASE 1

Tim, a 60-year-old solicitor, visits his GP complaining of recent episodes of central chest tightness on exertion, which settles on rest. There is nothing of note in his past medical history. Tim is referred to the rapid-access chest pain clinic, where he is diagnosed with stable angina.

Q 1. **What are the main risk factors for coronary heart disease (CHD)?** 5 marks

A **1 mark each for any of the following:**

- **Age**
- **Diabetes**
- **Smoking**
- **Hyperlipidaemia: total cholesterol > 6.5 mmol/l**
- **Hypertension**
- **Sedentary lifestyle**
- **Diet high in saturated fats (and low in fruit and vegetables)**
- **Family history of CHD**

LEARNING POINTS

❶ Stable anginal pain is: (1) constricting discomfort in the front of the chest, neck, shoulder, jaw and/or arm; (2) precipitated by physical exertion; and (3) relieved by rest or glyceryl trinitrate (GTN). Continuous or very prolonged pain that is not related to activity is unlikely to be stable angina.

❶ The likelihood of suspected stable angina can be estimated from whether the patient has typical symptoms (1–3) and the presence of risk factors such as smoking and diabetes. Clinical assessment alone may be sufficient to diagnose stable angina, although if the diagnosis is less certain it may require further investigations such as angiography, stress echocardiogram (using either exercise or dobutamine), myocardial perfusion scans or CT calcium scoring (CT of coronary arteries for calcified plaques is indicative of CHD). Exercise ECG is not recommended for diagnosing stable angina.

❶ Resting ECG may be normal or may show ischaemia or previous infarction, for example abnormalities in Q waves, left bundle branch block (LBBB), ST-segment or T-wave abnormalities (eg flattening or inversion).

Q 2. **List four drugs that may be prescribed to control angina.** 4 marks

A **1 mark each for any of the following:**

- **Beta-blocker**
- **Calcium-channel blocker: use a dihydropyridine calcium-channel blocker (eg amlodipine)**
- **Long-acting nitrate**
- **Ivabradine: slows down heart rate by inhibiting the sinus node**
- **Nicorandil: vasodilator**
- **Ranolazine**

LEARNING POINTS

🛈 Optimal drug treatment consists of one or two anti-anginal drugs; first-line are β-blockers and/or calcium-channel blockers. Use other anti-anginal drugs if symptoms are not satisfactorily controlled or if β-blockers/calcium-channel blockers are not tolerated or are contraindicated.

🛈 Also give a short-acting nitrate for preventing and treating episodes of angina. Advise patients on common side-effects (headache, flushing, light-headed); use it during episodes of angina and before exercise or exertion; if treating an episode of angina, repeat dose after five minutes if pain persists, and call ambulance if pain is still present five minutes after second dose.

Tim is also prescribed a statin and aspirin.

Q 3. **What is the recommended upper limit for fasting total cholesterol (TC) and low-density lipoprotein (LDL) in secondary prevention?** 2 marks

A **1 mark each for the following:**

- **TC < 4 mmol/l**
- **LDL < 2 mmol/l**

LEARNING POINT

🛈 Patients with existing CHD should ideally have a fasting TC of < 4 mmol/l (or a 25% reduction from baseline, whichever is the greater) and LDL of < 2 mmol/l (or a 30% reduction, whichever is the greater).

Q **4. What blood test must you request before prescribing a statin, and what advice must you give to patients on statin therapy?** 2 marks

A **1 mark each for the following:**

- **Liver function tests (LFTs)**

LEARNING POINT

ⓘ Statins are potentially hepatotoxic (as evidenced by an increase in aminotransferases) and are contraindicated in active liver disease. LFTs should be checked at baseline, at three months and at one year. Discontinue if ALT/AST rise to three times the upper limit (normal range is 3–35 IU/l).

- **Patients should report any unexplained muscle pains, tenderness or weakness.**

LEARNING POINT

ⓘ Although rare, statins may give rise to myositis (diagnosed by raised creatine kinase (CK)), causing muscle pain, weakness and tenderness. In severe cases this can lead to rhabdomyolysis and acute renal failure. Risk is increased in presence of co-morbidities such as renal impairment or if statins are used in combination with other drugs (eg macrolide antibiotics, fibrates).

Despite optimised medical treatment, Tim remains symptomatic, so he undergoes coronary angiography with a view to revascularisation.

Q **5. What two procedures are used for revascularisation?** 2 marks

A **1 mark each for the following:**

- **Percutaneous coronary intervention (PCI): angioplasty (balloon dilatation) and stenting. It improves symptoms but not prognosis.**
- **Coronary artery bypass graft (CABG) (eg using saphenous veins or internal thoracic arteries). It improves prognosis in a subset of patients with CHD (> 65 years old, multi-vessel disease, diabetic).**

LEARNING POINT

ⓘ Stents are either bare-metal or drug-eluting. The latter have a reduced risk of restenosis, although an increased risk of stent thrombosis, so patients are put on both aspirin and clopidogrel (for one year).

Total: **15 marks**

CARDIOVASCULAR CASE 2

John, a 72-year-old hypertensive, visits his GP complaining of several months' history of increasing breathlessness. He is now breathless even when doing simple tasks around the home, such as dressing.

Q 1. **List four non-cardiac causes of gradually progressive dyspnoea.**   4 marks

A **1 mark each for any of the following:**
- **Chronic obstructive pulmonary disease (COPD)**
- **Fibrotic lung disease**
- **Lung cancer**
- **Pleural effusion**
- **Multiple pulmonary emboli**
- **Anaemia**

LEARNING POINT

ⓘ Initial investigations in progressive dyspnoea may include: electrocardiogram (ECG), chest X-ray, spirometry and blood tests, including full blood count, to exclude anaemia.

John's GP suspects heart failure and organises a number of investigations.

Q 2. **List four causes of heart failure.**   4 marks

A **1 mark each for any of the causes listed below:**
Heart failure is caused by structural or functional abnormalities of the heart:
- **Ischaemic heart disease**
- **Hypertension**
- **Cardiomyopathies, eg dilated cardiomyopathy**
- **Valvular heart disease, eg mitral regurgitation (volume overload), aortic stenosis (obstruction to outflow)**
- **High output, eg anaemia, hyperthyroidism**
- **Arrhythmia, eg atrial fibrillation**

- **Cor pulmonale: right heart failure secondary to pulmonary disease, eg COPD**

LEARNING POINTS

🛈 Heart failure itself can be classified in a number of ways, including:

- **Left versus right heart failure**; when occurring together (most commonly) it is termed congestive heart failure. This is useful for understanding clinical symptoms and signs. Symptoms of left heart failure include dyspnoea, orthopnoea, paroxysmal nocturnal dyspnoea (PND) and cardiac wheeze. Symptoms of right-sided failure include peripheral oedema, anorexia and nausea (caused by bowel oedema), and abdominal distension due to ascites.

- **Systolic dysfunction versus diastolic dysfunction** – or left ventricular systolic dysfunction (LVSD) versus heart failure with preserved ejection fraction (HFPEF) – owing to insufficient contraction or relaxation, respectively, of the ventricle, and both causing a reduced stroke volume. The reduced stroke volume in HFPEF is due to a stiff ventricle (eg secondary to hypertension).

Q 3. **From the history above classify John's heart failure according to the New York Heart Classification (NYHA) criteria.** 2 marks

A **Grade III heart failure, ie breathlessness on minimal exertion.**

LEARNING POINT
NYHA heart failure classification

Grade	Extent of breathlessness
I	No undue breathlessness
II	Breathlessness on moderate exertion
III	Breathlessness on minimal exertion
IV	Breathlessness at rest

Q 4. **What hormone is significantly raised in heart failure?** 2 marks

A **B-type (or brain) natriuretic peptide (BNP).**

LEARNING POINT

ⓘ BNP is secreted by the ventricular myocardium in response to distension and acts to reduce circulating volume by inhibiting renin, antidiuretic hormone (ADH) and aldosterone secretion (similar actions to atrial natriuretic peptide (ANP)). BNP levels are raised in heart failure and are used as a screening test for patients with suspected **untreated** heart failure. BNP levels < 100 pg/ml make heart failure unlikely, while high levels (> 400 pg/ml) carry a poor prognosis.

Q 5. **Which key investigation would you request to confirm heart failure?**   1 mark

A **Echocardiogram: this is the key investigation in heart failure. It will confirm the diagnosis and its severity and may indicate the cause.**

LEARNING POINT

ⓘ Parameters assessed by echocardiography include left ventricular systolic and diastolic function, regional/localised hypokinesis (as a result of underlying coronary heart disease) and valvular function.

John is diagnosed with left ventricular heart failure.

Q 6. **Which two drugs are the first-line treatment for heart failure?**   2 marks

A **1 mark each for any of the following:**

- **Angiotensin-converting-enzyme inhibitors (ACEi); angiotensin II receptor blockers (ARBs) are an alternative first-line treatment, but may also be used in combination with ACEi as second-line treatment**
- **Beta-blockers (eg bisoprolol, carvedilol)**

LEARNING POINTS

ⓘ Drug treatment of heart failure is shown in the figure opposite.* ACE inhibitors, β-blockers and aldosterone antagonists improve prognosis. Diuretics and digoxin improve symptoms but do not reduce mortality.

ⓘ Cardiac resynchronisation therapy (CRT) involves implantation of a bi-ventricular pacemaker. By ensuring the heart contracts in synchrony, cardiac function is maximised, thus improving both symptoms and prognosis. CRT is indicated in patients with NYHA grade III–IV symptoms on optimal medical management, an ejection fraction ≤ 35% and a QRS duration > 150 ms (indicating cardiac dys-synchrony).

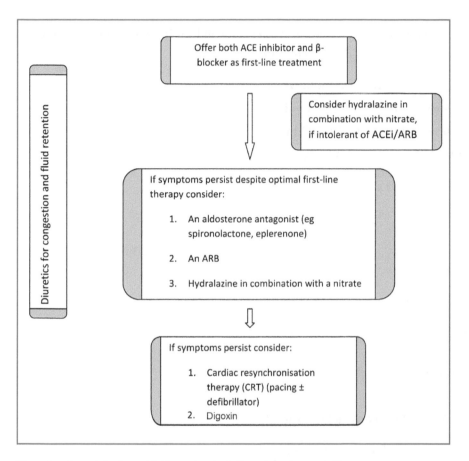

Drug treatment for heart failure due to left ventricular systolic dysfunction

*The treatment flow diagram is for patients with heart failure due to left ventricular systolic dysfunction (LVSD). Management of patients with heart failure with preserved ejection fraction (HFPEF) is primarily aimed at optimising treatment of underlying conditions such as hypertension, diabetes and coronary heart disease.

Total: **15 marks**

CARDIOVASCULAR CASE 3

David, a 51-year-old builder, is referred to his GP from the well-man clinic, as his blood pressure was recorded as 164/96 mmHg.

Q 1. **Define the systolic/diastolic ranges for mild (phase 1), moderate (phase 2) and severe (phase 3) hypertension.**   3 marks

A **1 mark for each of the following:**

- **Phase 1: 140–159/90–99 mmHg**
- **Phase 2: 160–179/100–109 mmHg**
- **Phase 3: ≥ 180/110 mmHg**

LEARNING POINTS

ℹ️ It is recommended to confirm a clinic diagnosis of hypertension with either ambulatory or home blood pressure monitoring, to exclude 'white coat hypertension', defined as a discrepancy of more than 20/10 mmHg between clinic and ambulatory/home readings.

ℹ️ Treat phase 2 and 3 hypertension; treat phase 1 hypertension if there are target organ damage, existing cardiovascular disease, renal disease, diabetes or a ten-year cardiovascular risk ≥ 20%.

You request an ECG, shown opposite.

Q 2. **What does David's ECG show?**   1 mark

A **Left ventricular hypertrophy (LVH).**

LEARNING POINT

ℹ️ LVH causes tall R waves in V5–6 and deep S waves in V1–2 (consider LVH if R wave in V5–6 > 25 mm or combined R wave in V6 and S wave in V1 > 35 mm). May also get T-wave inversion in the lateral leads (ie I, AvL, V5–6) and left axis deviation (ie positive in I, negative in II and III).

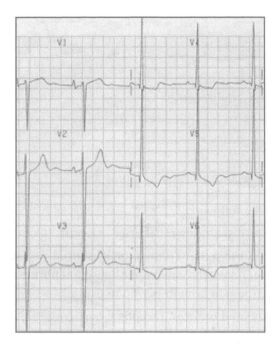

Figure 1.1: David's ECG.

Q 3. **Why is this important with regard to hypertension?**   1 mark

A **LVH indicates hypertensive end-organ damage and is an indication for antihypertensive treatment, even in patients with phase 1 hypertension.**

LEARNING POINTS

🛈 In the presence of LVH, request an echo to assess LV size and function.

🛈 Hypertension may also damage the kidneys, as evidenced by reduced estimated glomerular filtration rate (eGFR) and/or microalbuminuria (ie an albumin to creatinine ratio of ≥30 mg/mmol; in diabetics the ratio is lower at ≥ 2.5 in men and ≥ 3.5 in women).

🛈 Examination should also include fundoscopy, looking for hypertensive retinopathy (see next page).

Grade	Hypertensive retinopathy
I	Tortuous retinal arteries with thick shiny walls (silver wiring)
II	Arteriovenous (AV) nipping (narrowing where arteries cross veins)
III	Flame haemorrhages and cotton-wool spots (small infarcts)
IV	Papilloedema

Q 4. **List two causes of secondary hypertension.**   2 marks

A **1 mark for each of the following:**
- **Renal or renovascular disease (eg renal artery stenosis, glomerulonephritis)**
- **Endocrine disorders: Cushing syndrome (corticosteroid excess), Conn syndrome (hyperaldosteronism), phaeochromocytoma (norepinephrine and epinephrine excess), acromegaly (human growth hormone excess)**
- **Medications (eg combined oral contraceptive, corticosteroids)**
- **Coarctation of the aorta**
- **Pregnancy**

LEARNING POINTS

❶ 95% of patients with hypertension have essential or primary hypertension; 5% of patients have secondary hypertension.

❶ Younger hypertensive patients should have a lower threshold for evaluating secondary causes of hypertension.

David smokes ten cigarettes a day and his fasting bloods are measured: total cholesterol (TC) 6.34 mmol/l, low-densisty lipoprotein (LDL) 4.22 mmol/l, high-density lipoprotein (HDL) 1.26 mmol/l, triglycerides 2.4 mmol/l, glucose 4.6 mmol/l.

Q 5. **Calculate his 10-year cardiovascular disease risk.**   1 mark

A ≥ **30%: male, smoker, aged between 50 and 59 years, systolic BP of 164 mmHg, TC:HDL ratio of 5.**

LEARNING POINT

ℹ️ When investigating hypertension also assess cardiovascular disease (CVD) risk. CVD risk prediction charts (as shown in Figure 1.2) are found at the back of the *British National Formulary* and are used to estimate the risk of CVD (ie fatal and non-fatal myocardial infarction, stroke and angina) in patients with no previous history of CVD or diabetes. High-risk patients are defined as 10-year risk ≥ 20% and should be offered lipid-lowering medication (eg simvastatin 40 mg nocte). Aim to reduce TC to < 4 mmol/l and LDL to < 2 mmol/l, or a 25% reduction in TC and a 30% reduction in LDL from baseline, whichever provides the lowest value.

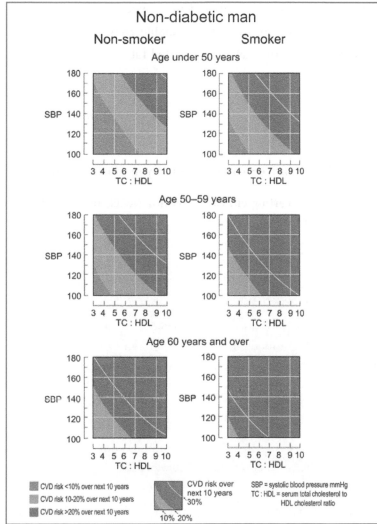

Figure 1.2: CVD risk prediction chart.

You determine that David's blood pressure needs to be treated.

Q 6. **What four lifestyle changes would you recommend?** 2 marks

A **½ mark for each of the following:**

- **Lose weight: aim for body mass index (BMI) 20–25**
- **Stop smoking**
- **Take regular exercise**
- **Reduce salt consumption**
- **Reduce alcohol consumption to ≤ 21 units/week**
- **Consume five portions of fruit and vegetables/day**
- **Reduce consumption of total and saturated fat**

LEARNING POINT

❶ Offer lifestyle advice to patients with hypertension at initial diagnosis and periodically thereafter.

Q 7. **What antihypertensive treatment would you offer first line?** 1 mark

A **An angiotensin-converting enzyme inhibitor (ACEi) or, if not tolerated, an angiotensin II receptor blocker (ARB).**

LEARNING POINTS

❶ For patients aged < 55 years offer ACEi or ARB (though these should not be combined to treat hypertension).

❶ For patients aged > 55 years or black Afro-Caribbean patients, offer a calcium-channel blocker (eg amlodipine). If not tolerated or unsuitable, offer a thiazide-like diuretic (eg chlortalidone or indapamide); bendroflumethiazide is no longer a first-line thiaizide diuretic, although in patients who are already taking it and whose blood pressure is stable and well controlled continue treatment.

❶ If further antihypertensive treatment is required, combine ACEi (or ARB) initially with either a calcium-channel blocker or a thiazide-like diuretic, although some patients may require all three.

❶ If additional treatment is required, consider addition of spironolacatone (25 mg once daily) or higher-dose thiazide-like diuretic; if further diuretic treatment is not tolerated or contraindicated or ineffective, consider an α- (eg doxazosin) or β- (eg atenolol) blocker.

Q 8. Name two electrolyte abnormalities caused by thiazide diuretics.   2 marks

A 1 mark for each of the following:
- Hyponatraemia
- Hypokalaemia: often mild, requiring no correction
- Hyperuricaemia: can precipitate gout
- Hypercalcaemia: thiazide diuretics lower urinary calcium excretion and may be used to prevent formation of calcium-containing kidney stones
- Hyperglycaemia: may impair diabetic control

Q 9. Name four complications if David's hypertension is not treated.   2 marks

A ½ mark for each of the following:
- Stroke: individuals with hypertension have a six-fold increased risk of stroke compared with normotensive individuals
- CVD: individuals with hypertension have a three-fold increased risk of CVD compared with normotensive individuals
- Heart failure
- Peripheral vascular disease (PVD)
- Chronic renal failure: hypertensive nephropathy
- Visual impairment: hypertensive retinopathy

Total: 15 marks

CARDIOVASCULAR CASE 4

A GP organises an electrocardiogram (ECG) (shown in Figure 1.3) for one of her patients, 78-year-old Sarah, after checking her pulse during a routine consultation for her hypertension.

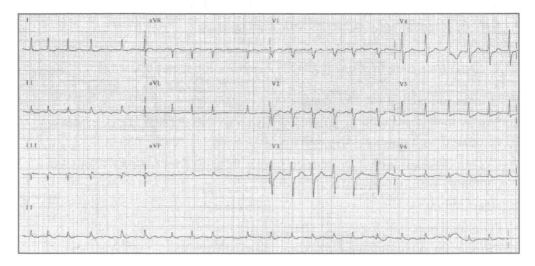

Figure 1.3: Sarah's ECG.

Q 1. What does the ECG show?   1 mark

A Atrial fibrillation.

LEARNING POINTS

- ❶ Atrial fibrillation (AF) is diagnosed by absent P waves and irregular QRS complexes. AF results from a chaotic irregular atrial rhythm (300–600 bpm, of which only a proportion are sufficient to generate an action potential that is conducted to the ventricles, causing an irregular ventricular rate).

- ❶ Atrial fibrillation may present with symptoms of palpitations, breathlessness and chest pain. However, the majority of presentations are clinically silent, with the first presentation as a cerebrovascular accident, heart failure or incidental ECG finding, or following detection of an irregular pulse on examination.

Q 2. **List six causes of this rhythm.** 3 marks

A **½ mark each for any of the following:**
- **Hypertension**
- **Coronary heart disease**
- **Myocardial infarction**
- **Hyperthyroidism**
- **Valvular heart disease (particularly mitral valve disease)**
- **Pneumonia**
- **Pulmonary embolism**
- **Alcohol excess**
- **Heart failure**
- **Lone atrial fibrillation (ie no identifiable cause)**
- **Cardiomyopathy**

LEARNING POINT

❶ Atrial fibrillation can be classified as acute, **paroxysmal** (ie episodes of AF that terminate spontaneously), **persistent** (terminated either pharmacologically or electrically – see below) or **permanent** (fails to respond to attempts to cardiovert or when cardioversion is deemed inappropriate).

Q 3. **What two drugs may be used for rate control?** 2 marks

A **1 mark each for any of the following:**
- **Beta-blockers**
- **(Rate-limiting) calcium-channel blocker: diltiazem or verapamil**
- **Digoxin**

LEARNING POINTS

❶ The treatment of AF involves either **rhythm** or **rate** control. First-line treatment in **paroxysmal** AF is rhythm control; in **permanent** AF it is rate control. The decision whether to rate- or rhythm-control in **persistent** AF depends on age (aim for rhythm control in younger patients), on whether AF is symptomatic, if there is evidence of heart failure (cardioversion improves left ventricular function) and on suitability for cardioversion (eg anticoagulation is contraindicated).

❶ If patients are rate-controlled, first-line treatment is either a standard β-blocker or rate-limiting calcium-channel blocker. If further rate control is needed, consider the addition of digoxin.

Q 4. **What two methods may be used to attempt cardioversion?**   2 marks

A **1 mark for each of the following:**
- **Chemical cardioversion: anti-arrhythmic drugs**
- **DC cardioversion**

LEARNING POINT

❶ If AF is acute (< 48 hours), there is no need to anticoagulate before chemical or DC cardioconversion (haemodynamically compromised patients require urgent DC cardioversion); otherwise, anticoagulate three weeks before and four weeks after cardioconversion (DC cardioversion is first line in persistent AF). If the patient is at high risk of attempted DC cardioversion being unsuccessful (eg previous failure), pre-treatment with anti-arrhythmic drugs before DC cardioversion increases the likelihood of restoring and maintaining sinus rhythm.

Q 5. **What two drugs may be used for rhythm control?**   2 marks

A **1 mark for any 2 of the following:**
- **Standard β-blockers**
- **Class 1 anti-arrhythmic drugs (ie flecainide, propafenone)**
- **Class 3 anti-arrhythmic drugs (ie sotalol, amiodarone)**

LEARNING POINTS

❶ Several anti-arrhythmic drugs can be used to maintain sinus rhythm in patients with paroxysmal or persistent AF who have been successfully cardioverted. First-line treatment is a standard β-blocker; where a standard β-blocker is ineffective, contraindicated or not tolerated, use amiodarone with underlying structural heart disease, or a class 1c agent (eg flecainide) or sotalol without underlying structural heart disease.

❶ Pill-in-the-pocket therapy involves self-administration of an anti-arrhythmic drug in patients with paroxysmal AF to terminate a new episode.

❶ Anti-arrhythmic drugs are classified according to the changes they cause in the action potential or AP (see Figure opposite).

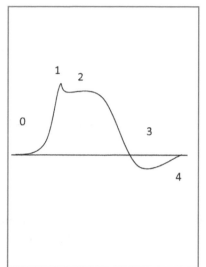

0 – rapid depolarisation due to opening of fast sodium channels

1 – early repolarisation due to closure of sodium channels and opening of potassium channels

2 – plateau phase where potassium outflux equals calcium influx due to opening of slow calcium channels

3 – late repolarisation following closure of calcium channels

4 – return to resting membrane potential by Na/K ATPase

Class 1 (further divided into 1a, b, c): slow phase 0 (eg flecainide (1c))

Class 2: slow phase 4 (ie standard β-blockers)

Class 3: slow phase 3 (eg amiodarone, sotalol)

Class 4: calcium-channel blockers. More effective in supraventricular tachycardia, where the AP in the AV (and SA) node is generated by calcium influx as opposed to calcium influx in the myocardium

Sarah opts for rate control and agrees to be anticoagulated to reduce her risk of stroke.

Q 6. **Name four factors used to stratify stroke risk.** 2 marks

A **½ mark each for any of the following:**
- **Congestive heart failure**
- **Hypertension**
- **Age ≥ 75 years old**
- **Diabetes**
- **Stroke or previous transient ischaemic attack (TIA)**

LEARNING POINTS

❶ The decision whether to anticoagulate a patient in paroxysmal, persistent or permanent AF depends on their risk of stroke, assessed on the basis of the risk factors above. This is termed the **CHADS$_2$** score: each factor scores 1 point (2 points if previous stroke/TIA). Low risk is score 0, intermediate risk is score 1 and high risk is score ≥ 2.

❶ AF carries a risk of embolic stroke of 2–4% per year. Warfarin therapy can reduce this by around 60%, compared to 30% reduction with aspirin alone. Those at high risk should ideally be anticoagulated with warfarin; those at low risk can simply be treated with aspirin (75–300 mg), while intermediate-risk patients can be offered the choice.

Q 7. What drug is used for anticoagulation, how is it monitored and what is the target range? 3 marks

A **1 mark each for the following:**

• **Warfarin**

• **International normalised ratio (INR) (normal range is 0.9–1.2). It is calculated by comparing the prothrombin time (PT) of the patient with a standard value**

• **2–3**

Total: 15 marks

CARDIOVASCULAR CASE 5

James, a 68-year-old lifelong smoker, is brought into the Emergency Department by ambulance. He has a 45-minute history of central, crushing chest pain associated with nausea, dyspnoea and sweating. On cardiovascular examination, his blood pressure is 164/96 mmHg, heart rate 92 bpm and regular; JVP is 4 cm above the sternal angle, heart sounds are normal and the chest is clear.

Q 1. **List six differential diagnoses.**   3 marks

A **½ mark each for any of the following:**
- **Myocardial infarction/acute coronary syndrome (ACS) – see below**
- **Angina pectoris**
- **Pulmonary embolism**
- **Aortic dissection**
- **Gastro-oesophageal reflux disease**
- **Pericarditis**
- **Musculoskeletal chest pain**

LEARNING POINT

ℹ **Acute coronary syndrome** encompasses unstable angina, non-ST-elevation myocardial infarction (NSTEMI) and ST-elevation myocardial infarction (STEMI). While similar in their presentation, their management differs. Therefore the two key investigations are ECG (is there any ST elevation?) and troponin (troponin is elevated 12 hours following myocardial damage); unstable angina is not associated with an elevated troponin, whereas an NSTEMI is.

James's ECG is shown in Figure 1.4.

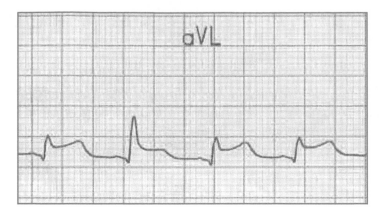

Figure 1.4: James's ECG.

Q 2. What is the abnormality? 1 mark

A **ST-segment elevation.**

LEARNING POINT

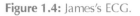 Other causes of ST-segment elevation include acute pericarditis (saddle-shaped ST elevation) and left ventricular aneurysm (ST elevation in leads V1–6).

 Other investigations include chest X-ray (to exclude pulmonary causes of chest pain and signs of left ventricular failure) and bloods (full blood count (FBC), urea and electrolytes (U&Es), glucose, lipids, troponin).

This abnormality is seen in leads I, aVL, and V5-6.

Q 3. Where is the site of the infarct? 1 mark

A **Lateral wall myocardial infarction (MI).**

LEARNING POINT

 The leads affected reflect the site of the infarct: inferior (II, III, aVF), anterior (V1-4), posterior (ST depression in V1-3 with dominant R waves). New-onset left bundle branch block (LBBB) is usually the result of a large anterior infarct.

Q 4. What other ECG changes may be expected to develop? 1 mark

A ½ mark for each of the following:

- **T-wave inversion (within 24 hours)**
- **Pathological Q waves (within days): pathological Q waves do not appear with subendocardial (ie not extending through the ventricular wall) MIs**

LEARNING POINTS

- ST elevation rarely persists, unless a left ventricular aneurysm develops. Patients with persisting ST elevation or LBBB should receive a copy of their ECG in case they should be readmitted with chest pain.

- ECG changes present in other forms of ACS include ST depression, T-wave flattening or inversion, non-specific changes, or normal ECG.

James undergoes reperfusion therapy and is transferred to coronary care.

Q 5. What are the two options for reperfusion therapy? 2 marks

A 1 mark for each of the following:

- **Primary percutaneous coronary intervention (PCI): angioplasty ± stenting – this is the treatment of choice**
- **Thrombolysis**

LEARNING POINTS

- **Initial management of ACS** includes oxygen, analgesia (morphine, nitrates) and aspirin (300 mg chewable aspirin) + clopidogrel (300–600 mg). The MONA acronym refers to **M**orpine, **O**xygen, **N**itrates and **A**spirin.

- Patients with STEMI should undergo reperfusion therapy. While awaiting percutaneous coronary intervention (PCI), give a GPIIb/IIIa receptor inhibitor (eg abciximab), which prevents platelet aggregation. If primary PCI is delayed/ unavailable, consider thrombolysis.

- **Indications for thrombolysis:**
  - ST-segment elevation > 2 mm in two contiguous chest leads
  - ST-segment elevation > 1 mm in two limb leads
  - new-onset LBBB
  - true posterior infarct (ST depression V1–3 with elevation > 1mm in posterior leads V7–9)

❶ Contraindications include previous haemorrhagic stroke, active bleeding, recent surgery. Rescue PCI should be considered if failed thrombolysis (< 50% resolution of ST elevation and ongoing chest pain). Even if successful, thrombolysis should not be considered to be the final treatment, and patients should be considered for angiography ± PCI.

❶ The management of ACS without ST elevation differs from STEMI in that reperfusion is not performed in the acute setting. Instead, patients are anticoagulated (eg unfractionated heparin, fondaparinux) and their risk assessed (eg using GRACE scoring*): low-risk patients can be managed conservatively and only undergo coronary angiography ± PCI if indicated by stress testing (see below) or if there is ongoing ischaemia (evidenced by further chest pain, serial ECG and further rise in troponin). Remaining patients should undergo angiography ± PCI during their inpatient stay.

Q 6. **List five complications of myocardial infarction.**   5 marks

A **1 mark each for any of the following:**

1. **Cardiac arrest**

2. **Arrhythmias/heart block (eg ventricular tachycardias – common during reperfusion), atrial fibrillation, bradyarrhythmias (may require atropine or temporary transcutaneous/intravenous pacemaker if symptomatic). Hence all ACS patients should ideally be managed on coronary care with cardiac monitoring**

3. **Left ventricular failure: usually the result of an anterior MI**

4. **Right ventricular failure: usually the result of an inferior MI; causes hypotension; treatment is fluids**

5. **Cardiogenic shock: extreme form of heart failure. High mortality. May require inotropic support and mechanical assistance to the heart; underlying structural complications (eg severe mitral regurgitation) need surgical correction**

6. **Mitral regurgitation (eg due to papillary muscle rupture)**

7. **Ventricular septal defect (VSD)**

8. **Ventricular rupture and subsequent cardiac tamponade**

9. **Systemic embolism: may arise from a left ventricular mural thrombus**

10. **Left ventricular aneurysm formation**

11. **Pericarditis (Dressler syndrome)**

* Global registry of acute cardiac events (GRACE) risk score estimates six-month mortality and risk of future cardiovascular events on basis of history (age, previous MI), examination (blood pressure, heart rate), ECG and blood tests (creatinine, troponin).

LEARNING POINT

 Complications of MI can be classified as early (1–8), medium (9) and late (10–11).

James makes an uncomplicated recovery and is transferred to the ward before discharge the following week.

Q 7. **What advice, treatment and investigations would you recommend to reduce his risk of a similar episode?** 2 marks

A **½ mark each for any of the following:**

- **Address any modifiable risk factors (eg smoking, diabetes, hypertension)**
- **Advice on lifestyle changes (eg healthy diet, regular physical activity)**
- **Supervised cardiac rehabilitation**
- **Angiotensin-converting enzyme inhibitor (ACEi)**
- **Aspirin (75 mg daily): reduces risk of all vascular events (+ clopidogrel: continue clopidogrel for 28 days following an STEMI and 12 months following an NSTEMI)**
- **Beta-blocker: reduces mortality in patients with MI**
- **Statin therapy: shown to improve prognosis, regardless of baseline cholesterol levels**
- **Echocardiogram: all post-MI patients should have an echocardiogram and, if evidence of left ventricular function, started on an aldosterone antagonist (eg eplerenone)**

LEARNING POINT

 Patients who have not had coronary angiography as part of their ACS management should undergo stress testing (eg exercise ECG, stress echocardiogram, myocardial perfusion scan) to assess whether coronary revascularisation is appropriate.

Total: 15 marks

EMERGENCY DEPARTMENT CASES: ANSWERS

EMERGENCY DEPARTMENT CASE 1

Gary, a 23-year-old man, is brought into the Emergency Department following a high-speed road traffic accident. He has sustained trauma to the left side of his head and has a reduced level of consciousness.

Q 1. List three causes of secondary brain injury. **3 marks**

A 1 mark each for any of the following in list:

Primary brain injury occurs at the time of the head injury (eg axonal injury and haemorrhage, which may be diffuse or localised). The aim of managing head injury is to prevent secondary brain injury caused by raised intracranial pressure (ICP):

- **Blood loss following associated injuries, causing ischaemic cerebral oedema**
- **Hypoxia and hypercapnia (eg due to seizures, chest injury), causing hypoxic and hypercapnic cerebral oedema**
- **Infection (eg via skull fracture), causing inflammatory oedema**
- **Intracranial haemorrhage, causing localised pressure effects and raised ICP**

LEARNING POINT

ℹ️ Secondary brain injury is prevented by managing the patient's airway, breathing and circulation (ABC) – ie maintaining the airway (though immobilising the neck until a potential cervical spine fracture has been cleared; if GCS ≤ 8, the patient will require intubation), high-flow oxygen, and by correcting any hypovolaemia. Patients with compound skull fractures typically receive prophylactic intravenous antibiotics and any seizures are initially treated with intravenous lorazepam. Intracranial haematoma may require drainage.

Gary's neck is immobilised, his airway, breathing and circulation is stabilised, and an assessment of his neurological status undertaken. His Glasgow Coma Scale (GCS) score is assessed as follows: his eyes open to pain, he localises pain and his speech is confused.

EMERGENCY

Component	Response	Score
Eye response	Open spontaneously	4
	Open to verbal command	3
	Open to pain	2
	No response	1
Verbal response	Oriented	5
	Confused conversation	4
	Inappropriate speech	3
	Moaning	2
	None	1
Motor response	Obeys command	6
	Localises pain	5
	Withdraws to pain	4
	Abnormal flexion (ie pressure on nail bed causes upper limbs to flex and adduct (decorticate rigidity)	3
	Abnormal extension (ie pressure on nail bed causes upper limbs to extend, adduct and semipronate (decerebrate rigidity)	2
	No response to pain	1

Table 2.1: Glasgow Coma Score

Q 2. **Calculate Gary's Glasgow Coma Score (please refer to Table 2.1).** 1 mark

A **11/15: E2, V4, M5.**

LEARNING POINT

🟊 The Glasgow Coma Scale (GSC) is a reliable, objective way of recording a patient's conscious state. In a patient with stabilised ABCs, a deteriorating GCS is a medical emergency typically caused by raised ICP. Raised blood pressure and bradycardia (Cushing response) and fixed, dilated pupils are all late signs of raised ICP. Mannitol is an osmotic diuretic that can help reduce ICP while awaiting further management.

A full examination reveals that Gary has sustained no other major injuries.

Q 3. **List four signs on examination of a basal skull fracture.** 1 mark

A **½ mark each for any of the following:**
- **Bilateral orbital bruising (ie panda eyes)**
- **Subconjunctival haemorrhage (with no posterior margin evident)**
- **Haemotympanum (ie blood behind the eardrum)**
- **Otorrhoea (ie cerebrospinal fluid (CSF) discharge from the ears)**
- **Rhinorrhoea (ie CSF discharge from the nose)**
- **Battle's sign (ie bruising over the mastoid process – this is a late sign)**

LEARNING POINTS

❶ Clinical evidence of a skull base fracture is an indication for an urgent (within 1 hour) CT head scan, as is GCS < 13, open or depressed skull fracture, focal neurological deficit, post-traumatic seizure and > 1 episode of vomiting. Amnesia (anterograde ± retrograde amnesia) is an indication for a non-urgent CT brain scan.

❶ Other investigations may include full blood count (FBC), cross-match, urea and electrolytes (U&Es), glucose, arterial blood gases, coagulation screen and radiology (eg chest X-ray, pelvic X-ray, C-spine X-ray), as indicated.

Q 4. **List six reasons for admitting a patient following a head injury.** 3 marks

A **½ mark each for any of the following:**
- **Reduced GCS: NEVER discharge a head injury patient until GCS = 15**
- **History of amnesia (anterograde ± retrograde amnesia)**
- **History of alcohol ingestion or drugs, which impairs ability to assess**
- **Focal neurological deficit (eg hemiparesis, diplopia)**
- **Suspected open or depressed skull fracture, including basal skull fracture**
- **Post-traumatic seizure**
- **Vomiting**
- **Dangerous mechanism of injury (eg thrown from car)**
- **Coagulopathy (eg current treatment with warfarin)**
- **Lack of responsible adult in attendance to observe patient on discharge**
- **Suspicion of non-accidental injury in children**

LEARNING POINT

ⓘ Most patients who present to the Emergency Department with head injury can be safely discharged with head injury advice (most departments have head injury advice cards).

Q 5. **List six regular observations Gary should undergo.** 3 marks

A **½ mark each for any in the list below.**

Patients admitted with head injury require regular neurological observations to detect any complications at an early stage:

- **GCS: see above**
- **Pupil size and response to light: fixed, dilated pupil(s) is a false localising sign indicating raised ICP**
- **Limb power: assessment of any focal neurological deficit**
- **Blood pressure (BP): raised BP may indicate raised ICP (Cushing response); reduced BP may indicate hypovolaemia from other injuries**
- **Pulse: bradycardia may indicate raised ICP (Cushing response); tachycardia may indicate hypovolaemia from other injuries**
- **Respiratory rate: a reduced respiratory rate may reflect CNS depression due to raised ICP**
- **Oxygen saturations**
- **Temperature**

Gary undergoes an urgent CT scan of his head (see Figure 2.1).

Q 6. **Describe two abnormalities seen on his CT scan.** 2 marks

A **1 mark each for any of the following:**

- **A convex area of high attenuation (or hyperdense area consistent with fresh blood) is seen to extend from the inner layer of the skull on the left**
- **This is causing a mass effect with midline shift**
- **A small area of low attenuation (or hypodense area) is seen peripheral to this**

LEARNING POINT

ⓘ No skull fracture is evident, though air within the skull vault (small area of low attenuation) is in keeping with a skull fracture.

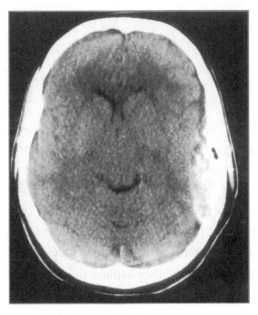

Figure 2.1: Gary's CT brain scan.

Q 7. **What is the diagnosis?**   1 mark

A **Extradural haemorrhage.**

LEARNING POINTS

ⓘ Classically an extradural haemorrhage appears convex, as the dura mater is firmly attached at the suture lines; a subdural haemorrhage appears concave. However, this distinction is not always evident.

ⓘ Extradural haemorrhage is caused by tearing of arteries in close proximity to the skull. For example, tearing of the anterior branch of the middle meningeal artery may be caused by fracture to the temporal bone.

Q 8. **What further course of action should be undertaken?**   1 mark

A **Urgent neurosurgical referral.**

LEARNING POINT

ⓘ Intracranial haemorrhage causes localised pressure effects and generalised raised ICP and may require surgical drainage.

Total: **15 marks**

EMERGENCY DEPARTMENT CASE 2

Malcolm, a 69-year-old known ischaemic heart disease patient, is brought into the Emergency Department severely dyspnoeic.

Q 1. **What is your differential diagnosis?** 4 marks

A **1 mark each for any of the following:**

- **Acute pulmonary oedema (acute left ventricular failure)**
- **Exacerbation of airways disease, either asthma or chronic obstructive pulmonary disease (COPD)**
- **Pneumonia**
- **Pulmonary embolus**
- **Pneumothorax**

LEARNING POINT

❶ Asthma/COPD, pulmonary oedema and pneumonia may be hard to distinguish and can coexist; if in doubt, treat all three simultaneously (eg bronchodilators, antibiotics, diuretics) – although pulmonary oedema/pneumonia should be confirmed on a chest X-ray.

You gain intravenous access, send urgent bloods and request an urgent erect chest X-ray (see Figure 2.2) and electrocardiogram (ECG) (see Figure 2.3).

Q 2. **Identify three abnormalities on his chest X-ray.** 3 marks

A **1 mark each for any in the following list:**

The chest X-ray shows acute pulmonary oedema:

- **Alveolar oedema: diffuse shadowing extending out from both hilar structures into the lung fields (bat's wings), which is more marked on the right**
- **Fluid in the horizontal fissure: seen as horizontal line in right lung field**
- **Upper lobe diversion: prominent pulmonary vessels in the upper lung fields**
- **Chest electrodes**

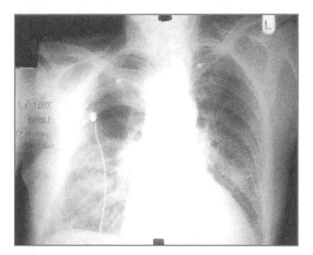

Figure 2.2: Malcom's erect chest X-ray.

LEARNING POINT

ⓘ This is an anteroposterior (AP) film, so cannot comment on the heart size (AP films tend to make the heart look bigger than conventional posteroanterior (PA) films).

Q 3. **What is your immediate management?**   2 marks

A **½ mark for any of the following:**
- **Sit patient upright**
- **High-flow oxygen: by tight-fitting face mask**
- **Intravenous furosemide: 50–100 mg**
- **Glyceryl trinitrate (GTN) spray: two puffs sublingual – reduces preload (though use with caution in hypotension); and commence intravenous GTN infusion (typically start at 10 µg/min and titrate up according to response and blood pressure)**
- **Intravenous diamorphine: 2.5–5 mg if patient is in pain or distressed. This both sedates the patient (so avoid if drowsy or exhausted as it may precipitate respiratory arrest) and causes vasodilatation, reducing both pre- and afterload**

LEARNING POINTS

ⓘ Also give 300 mg aspirin if you suspect myocardial infarction is the precipitating cause.

ⓘ Every Emergency Department will have its own local protocol for managing acute pulmonary oedema.

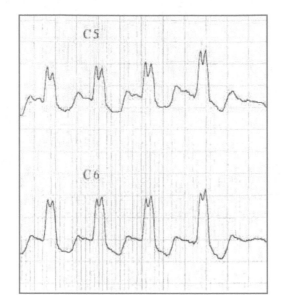

Figure 2.3: Malcolm's ECG.

Q 4. **What does his ECG show?** 1 mark

A **Left bundle branch block (LBBB).**

LEARNING POINT

ⓘ Widened QRS complexes (> 0.12 s), M pattern in V4–6 (the W pattern in V1 is often not developed), inverted T waves in lateral leads (ie I, aVL, V4–6). In the presence of LBBB cannot comment on any other aspects of the ECG, except whether the rhythm is regular or irregular.

Q 5. **How could you confirm that this is a new ECG change?** 1 mark

A **Compare with a previous ECG.**

LEARNING POINTS

ⓘ New-onset LBBB is usually the result of a large anterior infarct.

ⓘ Patients with known LBBB should receive a copy of their ECG in case they should be admitted with chest pain; if not, request Malcolm's old notes.

While you are attempting to stabilise Malcolm, he arrests in asystole.

Q 6. **List three other rhythms associated with cardiac arrest.** 3 marks

A **1 mark each for the following:**
- **Pulseless ventricular tachycardia (VT)**
- **Ventricular fibrillation (VF)**
- **Pulseless electrical activity (PEA): clinical signs of a cardiac arrest with an ECG rhythm compatible with a cardiac output**

LEARNING POINT

ⓘ Whenever a diagnosis of asystole is made, it must be confirmed by ensuring the leads are attached correctly and checking the gain. Fine VF may be misdiagnosed as asystole, but is unlikely to be shocked into a perfusing rhythm; it is best treated by cardiopulmonary resuscitation, so if in doubt follow the non-shockable algorithm (see below).

Q 7. **How would you manage the arrest?** 2 marks

A **1 mark each for any of the following:**
- **Cardiopulmonary resuscitation: 30 compressions to 2 ventilations (though once intubated, is asynchronous – 100 compressions and 12 breaths per minute). Reassess rhythm every 2 minutes**
- **Adrenaline: 1 mg intravenously every 3–5 minutes; administer once intravenous access is secured**
- **Thrombolysis: it is likely that the cause of Malcolm's cardiac arrest is myocardial infarction (see below, reversible causes)**

LEARNING POINTS

ⓘ Heart rhythms associated with cardiac arrest can be divided into two groups: VF/pulseless VT and asystole/PEA. The main difference in their management is the use of defibrillation (patients with VF/VT should receive a single shock of 150 joules biphasic every 2 minutes).

ⓘ **All** patients should receive 1 mg adrenaline every 3–5 minutes (ie during alternate cycles of cardiopulmonary resuscitation): for shockable rhythms adrenaline is given **after** the third shock; in asystole/PEA adrenaline is given once intravenous access is secured.

EMERGENCY

183

EMERGENCY

❶ Also administer 300 mg intravenous amiodarone in shock-refractory VF/VT (ie fails to respond after third shock). Atropine is no longer recommended for asystole or PEA.

Q 8. **List eight potential reversible causes of cardiac arrest.**   4 marks

A **½ mark each for each of the following:**

- **Hypoxia/hypercapnia: ensure adequate oxygenation/ventilation**
- **Hypovolaemia**
- **Hypo/hyperkalaemia and other metabolic disorders – eg acidaemia, hypocalcaemia: either revealed from recent urea and electrolytes or medical history (eg renal failure)**
- **Hypothermia**
- **Tension pneumothorax: diagnose clinically (eg absent breath sounds on ventilation) and insert cannula into second intercostal space, midclavicular line to decompress**
- **Toxic disorders (eg opiates)**
- **Thrombosis – ie pulmonary (ie massive PE) or cardiac (ie myocardial infarction): thrombolysis may be appropriate**
- **Cardiac Tamponade: difficult to diagnose clinically; suspect if penetrating chest wound**

LEARNING POINT

❶ Potential causes must be considered during cardiac arrest. For ease of memory these reversible causes are divided into the four 'H's and four 'T's. Survival following cardiac arrest with asystole or PEA is unlikely, unless a reversible cause can be found and treated effectively.

Unfortunately cardiopulmonary resuscitation is unsuccessful, and Malcolm is declared dead.

Total: 20 marks

ENDOCRINE CASES: ANSWERS

ENDOCRINE CASE 1

Andy, a 47-year-old estate agent, visits his GP complaining of general tiredness. He admits to eating and drinking to excess. On examination, he weighs 95 kg and his height is 1.72 m; blood pressure is 154/92 mmHg.

Q 1. **Calculate his body mass index (BMI).**   1 mark

A **32, ie weight (kg)/height (m)^2 = 95/(1.72)^2 = 32**

LEARNING POINT

 Obesity (ie BMI > 30) is a risk factor for the development of type 2 diabetes (T2D). In obese T2D patients weight loss improves glycaemic control (may achieve normoglycaemic levels) and reduces the risk of diabetic complications. In obese patients who are unable to lose weight by lifestyle changes, consider anti-obesity drugs – eg orlistat (reduces dietary fat absorption) is indicated in T2D patients with BMI ≥ 28.

Urine dipstick is 2+ for glucose.

Q 2. **How would you confirm the diagnosis of diabetes?**   2 marks

A **1 mark each for the following:**
- **Random plasma glucose ≥ 11.1 mmol/l**
- **Fasting plasma glucose ≥ 7.0 mmol/l**

LEARNING POINTS

 If the patient is asymptomatic, repeat the test. If borderline, perform an oral glucose tolerance test (OGTT) with 75 g glucose. A 2-hour plasma glucose ≥ 11.1 mmol/l confirms the diagnosis.

 Impaired fasting glycaemia is where fasting glucose is > 6.1 mmol/l (upper range of normal) but < 7.0 mmol/l. Such patients should have an OGTT to exclude diabetes and given lifestyle advice. Impaired glucose tolerance (IGT) is when the OGTT 2-hour value is > 7.8 mmol/l but < 11.1 mmol/l. Such patients are at higher risk of developing diabetes.

Q 3. **List four other presenting symptoms of type 2 diabetes (T2D).**   2 marks

A **½ mark each for any of the following:**

- **Thirst**
- **Polyuria/nocturia**
- **Blurred vision: due to glucose-induced changes in lens refraction**
- **Infections: candida infection (eg thrush), boils**
- **Weight loss (though conversely may also show weight gain)**
- **Complications of diabetes: cerebrovascular accident (CVA), cardiovascular disease (CVD), neuropathy (eg foot ulcers)**
- **Hyperglycaemic hyperosmolar non-ketotic (HONK) coma**

LEARNING POINTS

❶ HONK affects T2D patients (typically elderly and maybe presenting for the first time), causing dehydration due to severe hyperglycaemia (typically > 30 mmol/l) without acidosis (absence of ketone bodies); plasma osmolality is also high (> 350 mosmol/kg) due to dehydration.

❶ Diabetic ketoacidosis (see Endocrine Case 2) only affects people with type 1 diabetes (T1D), although treatment for both will require fluids and insulin.

Initially, Andy attempts to manage his diabetes mellitus (DM) by diet and exercise alone but this fails to control his hyperglycaemia.

Q 4. **What hypoglycaemic agent would you start Andy on?**   1 mark

A **Metformin (a biguanide).**

LEARNING POINT

❶ Metformin acts by increasing insulin sensitivity and decreasing hepatic gluconeogenesis. It is first-line treatment in T2D, in particular in obese patients, as it does NOT promote weight gain. In non-obese patients or patients contraindicated/unable to tolerate metformin (eg avoid if estimated glomerular filtration rate (eGFR) < 30ml/min or creatinine > 150 mmol/l; gastrointestinal side-effects are common) use sulphonylureas (eg gliclazide), which increase insulin secretion. Initial dose is 500 mg od, although it can be titrated up to 2 g daily in divided doses.

ENDOCRINE

Other hypoglycaemic agents include:

- **Poglitazone: acts by decreasing peripheral insulin resistance. Contraindicated in heart failure**
- **DDP4 (dipeptidylpeptidase-4) inhibitors (eg saxagliptin): increase insulin secretion and inhibit glucagon secretion**
- **GLP-1 (glucagon-like peptide-1) receptor agonists (eg exenatide): increase insulin secretion and inhibit glucagon secretion (administered subcutaneously)**
- **Insulin is indicated if optimal oral hypoglycaemic combination therapy is inadequate: either human neutral protamine Hagedorn (NPH) insulin (eg Insulatard), or long-acting insulin analogues (eg glargine)**

Andy is reviewed 6-monthly to monitor his glycaemic control and assess the development of any diabetic complications.

Q 5. **How do you assess long-term glycaemic control?**   1 mark

A **HbA_{1c}.**

LEARNING POINT

- HbA_{1c} (glycated haemoglobin) indicates average glucose concentrations over the last 8 weeks (ie half-life of RBC). The recommended target is 6.5–7.5% (48–59 mmol/mol) and levels should be measured every 2–6 months, depending on glycaemic control.

Q 6. **How do you screen for diabetic renal disease?**   2 marks

A **1 mark each for the following:**
- **Urinary albumin to creatinine ratio (ACR)**
- **Urinary albumin excretion in 24 hours**

LEARNING POINTS

- The ACR is usually used as it can be done on a 'spot' urine.

- Microalbuminuria is the earliest indicator of diabetic nephropathy and is defined as ACR ≥ 2.5 mg/mmol (men) or ≥ 3.5 mg/mmol (women). Treatment of microalbuminuria (which indicates an increased risk of end-stage renal disease and cardiovascular disease) involves good glycaemic control, treatment of blood pressure (BP) and angiotensin-converting enzyme (ACE) inhibitor or angiotensin II receptor antagonist (even if normotensive as it protects the kidneys).

ⓘ Target BP in diabetic patients depends on whether microalbuminuria is present (≤ 130/80 mmHg) or absent (≤ 140/80 mmHg).

Andy's feet are examined: he has bilateral foot pulses but is unable to perceive the pressure from a 10-g monofilament, so he is at increased risk of developing a 'diabetic foot'.

Q 7. **List four pieces of preventive foot care advice.** 4 marks

A **1 mark each for any of the following:**
- **Wash and inspect feet daily**
- **Use creams/lotions to prevent dry skin/callus formation**
- **Always have feet measured when buying shoes**
- **Avoid walking barefoot**
- **Avoid thermal injury (eg from hot-water bottles)**
- **Seek medical attention for any foot injury (however trivial)**
- **Avoid self-treatment of corns, calluses or other foot problems**

LEARNING POINT

ⓘ Diabetic foot problems (eg ulceration) are caused by neuropathy (causing insensitivity with resulting trauma) and/or peripheral vascular disease. Feet should be inspected annually: signs of neuropathy include dry skin and callus formation at pressure areas; inability to perceive a 10-g monofilament is a sensitive indicator of an 'at-risk' foot. Foot pulses should also be assessed. The best treatment is prevention through good foot care, targeting those at increased risk.

As part of his diabetes review, Andy also attends the local optometrist.

Q 8. **What retinal changes are seen in diabetes?** 2 marks

A ½ **mark for each of the following:**
- **Dots (microaneurysms)**
- **Blots (microhaemorrhages)**
- **Cotton-wool spots (retinal infarcts)**
- **New vessel formation**

ENDOCRINE

LEARNING POINTS

ⓘ Diabetic retinopathy can be classified as:

- Background retinopathy: dots (microaneurysms), blots (microhaemorrhages) and hard exudates. Refer to ophthalmologist if within 1 disc diameter of macula.

- Preproliferative retinopathy: as above but also cotton-wool spots (retinal infarcts). Refer to ophthalmologist.

- Proliferative retinopathy: new vessels form on the retina which may bleed or cause retinal detachment. Urgent referral (eg for laser treatment).

ⓘ All diabetic patients should be screened annually (eg by an optometrist). Good glycaemic control and treatment of hypertension and hyperlipidaemia delay the onset of retinopathy and can slow its progression.

Total: **15 marks**

ENDOCRINE

ENDOCRINE CASE 2

Jenny, a 21-year-old type 1 diabetic, is seen by her GP following a 2-day history of nausea and vomiting, and now complaining of abdominal pain. Urine dipstick showed glycosuria and ketonuria, and she is admitted to the medical assessment unit. On examination her Glasgow Coma Scale (GCS) is 15/15, heart rate (HR) is 120/min, abdomen is tender throughout, she is hyperventilating and appears dehydrated.

ENDOCRINE

Q 1. **How is diabetic ketoacidosis (DKA) diagnosed biochemically?** 3 marks

A **1 mark for each of the following:**
- **Hyperglycaemia: blood glucose typically > 20 mmol/l**
- **Ketonuria**
- **Acidosis: blood pH < 7.35**

LEARNING POINT

ⓘ DKA is due to hyperglycaemia secondary to insulin deficiency, which causes osmotic diuresis, resulting in dehydration; deficiency of intracellular glucose switches energy production to lipolysis, which forms ketone bodies (detected as ketonuria), causing metabolic acidosis (which is associated with abdominal pain, which in turn may be misdiagnosed as an acute abdomen, and vomiting, further exacerbating fluid and electrolyte balance). A diagnosis of DKA requires all three biochemical changes to be present.

Q 2. **List three causes of DKA.** 3 marks

A **1 mark each for any of the following:**
- **Presentation of type 1 diabetes**
- **Interruption of insulin therapy (eg non-compliance)**
- **Infection**
- **Surgery/trauma**
- **Myocardial infarction**

LEARNING POINTS

ⓘ While type 1 diabetes typically presents with the classic symptoms of polyuria, polydipsia, weight loss and lethargy, it may also present with DKA.

ⓘ Examples 3–5 given can cause DKA due to stress increasing insulin demand. The most common cause is for patients to reduce or omit insulin because they are unable to eat, owing to nausea and vomiting; all patients receive illness rules to minimise the risk of DKA (see below). Relevant investigations to identify the underlying cause include septic screen (chest X-ray, urine/blood cultures) and ECG.

ⓘ DKA is not associated with type 2 diabetes (T2D), although this may cause hyperosmolar non-ketotic (HONK) coma: severe hyperglycaemia (> 30 mmol/l) but no acidosis/ketones. Treatment is essentially the same as for DKA, ie less aggressive intravenous fluids and insulin.

Jenny is diagnosed with DKA. Her arterial blood gases (ABG) are shown in Table 3.1.

Q 3. **Indicate (↑,↓, or →) where marked for the expected changes.**　　4 marks

A **1 mark for each of the following:**

	Normal range	Jenny's ABG	Explanation
pH	7.35–7.45	↓	Acidosis due to ketonaemia
pO$_2$	10–12 kPa	11	Depending on whether patient is shocked, hypoxia may or may not be present
pCO$_2$	4.7–6 kPa	↓	Hypocapnia due to respiratory compensation causing hyperventilation (Kussmaul respiration or air hunger)
HCO$_3^-$	22–28 mmol/l	↓	Bicarbonate-depleted, attempting to buffer metabolic acidosis
BE	+/– 2 mmol/l	–9	Base deficit due to HCO$_3^-$ depletion
Anion gap	10–18 mmol/l	↑	Increased due to addition of 'unmeasured' ketones

Table 3.1: Jenny's arterial blood gases.

ENDOCRINE

Q 4. **How do you calculate the anion gap?** 1 mark

A $(Na^+ + K^+) - (HCO_3^- + Cl^-)$.

LEARNING POINTS

❶ The anion gap (AG) is calculated from the difference between plasma cations $(Na^+ + K^+)$ and anions $(HCO_3^- + Cl^-)$; normal range is 10–18 mmol/l. Arterial blood gases (ABG) machines will calculate the AG for you.

❶ This is just an approximation, as there are additional 'unmeasured' cations (eg calcium, magnesium) and anions (eg albumin, lactate); the total (Σ) unmeasured anions > Σunmeasured cations, so there appears to be a positive anion gap (ie Σcations > Σanions), whereas in fact there is a state of electroneutrality (ie Σcations = Σanions).

Q 5. **List three causes of metabolic acidosis with an *increased* anion gap.** 3 marks

A **1 mark each for any of the following:**
- **Lactic acid (eg shock, sepsis)**
- **Renal failure: due to accumulation of sulphate, urate, phosphate**
- **Ketones (eg DKA, alcohol, starvation)**
- **Drugs (eg aspirin, metformin, methanol)**

LEARNING POINTS

❶ The AG is used to help identify the underlying cause of metabolic acidosis. In metabolic acidosis with an increased anion gap there must be more 'unmeasured' anions (ie anions associated with acids).

❶ If the AG is normal, metabolic acidosis is either due to H^+ retention (eg type 1 renal tubular acidosis) or HCO_3^- loss (eg type 2 renal tubular acidosis, diarrhoea). In these conditions plasma bicarbonate is reduced and replaced by chloride to maintain electroneutrality.

❶ Bicarbonate is not routinely used in the treatment of DKA (it worsens intracellular acidosis), but is reserved for severe metabolic acidosis (pH < 7) not responding to treatment.

Jenny is successfully treated with intravenous fluids and sliding scale insulin.

Q 6. **List three complications of this treatment.** 3 marks

A **1 mark for each of the following:**
- **Fluid overload: this may cause pulmonary (and rarely cerebral) oedema**
- **Hypoglycaemia**
- **Hypokalaemia**

LEARNING POINTS

ⓘ Diabetic ketoacidosis (DKA) typically presents with a fluid deficit of 5–12 litres (less in those with an omitted insulin dose). Dehydration is more life-threatening than hyperglycaemia and takes precedence. A typical regimen involves: 1.5 litres in the first hour, 1 litre in next hour, 1 litre in next 2 hours, 2 litres in next 8 hours and then 0.5 litre every 4 hours, although reduced doses may be required in elderly/heart failure patients to avoid fluid overload.

ⓘ Initially rehydration is with normal saline (0.9%) but once blood glucose < 15 mmol/l, switch to dextrose saline or 5% dextrose to prevent hypoglycaemia. The aim of intravenous insulin therapy is to reduce blood glucose by 3–4 mmol/h; initially give 4–6 units per hour and then reduce, aiming to maintain glucose between 5–10 mmol/l. If higher rates of insulin infusion are required, it suggests an underlying cause such as sepsis or myocardial infarction.

ⓘ DKA patients are potassium-depleted, though initial plasma levels maybe high/normal in response to the acidosis (due to cellular exchange of K^+ for H^+). Potassium levels decrease with rehydration (dilutional) and insulin (which drives potassium into the cells) and require replacement (usually with the second or third litre of fluid) and careful monitoring (as it may cause arrhythmias).

ⓘ Once the patient is eating and drinking normally with no ketonuria, restart the normal insulin regimen and take down the insulin infusion after the same meal. It is important to ensure that there is an overlap between restarting subcutaneous insulin and stopping intravenous insulin to prevent rebound hyperglycaemia.

Once stabilised, Jenny is referred to the diabetic nurse specialist for advice on the management of her diabetes.

ENDOCRINE

Q 7. **List four 'illness rules' you would give Jenny.** 2 marks

A **½ mark each for any of the following:**
- **Obtain early treatment for infections**
- **Always take your insulin therapy**
- **Self-monitor more often during illnesses and adjust therapy accordingly (or seek advice if hyperglycaemic): may need to increase insulin by 10–30%**
- **If unable to eat (eg anorexia, nauseous), take sugary fluids (eg Lucozade), in place of meals; if unable to tolerate fluids, will need admission**
- **Take plenty of sugar-free fluids frequently to prevent dehydration**
- **Frequent urinalysis: 1+ ketones is acceptable; ≥ 2+, seek medical advice**

LEARNING POINT

ⓘ Infections, due to the increased stress on the body, increase insulin demand and may lead to a loss of glycaemic control, potentially causing DKA. This may be exacerbated by the common misconception that if the patient is not eating properly, there is no need to take their insulin.

Q 8. **List four warning signs of hypoglycaemia.** 2 marks

A **1 mark for each of any of the following:**
- **Autonomic: sweating, palpitations, shaking, hunger**
- **Neurological: confusion, drowsiness, uncoordination, odd behaviour, slurred speech**

LEARNING POINT

ⓘ The brain depends on a constant supply of glucose to maintain function; concentration < 3.5 mmol/l impairs neurological function. This activates the sympathetic nervous system, which opposes the actions of insulin and warns the patient. Risk is increased by missed meals, unusual exertion. All type 1 diabetics should carry rapidly absorbed carbohydrate and a warning card.

Q 9. **What two coexisting conditions should you screen for in Jenny?** 2 marks

A **1 mark for each of the following:**
- **Hyper- and hypo-thyroidism**
- **Coeliac disease**

LEARNING POINT

🛈 Type 1 diabetes, an autoimmune disease, is associated with thyroid disease and with coeliac disease, the presence of which complicates good glycaemic control. These should be screened for at diagnosis and at regular intervals throughout life.

Q 10. **List two challenges facing Jenny.** 2 marks

A **There are no 'correct' answers to this question. However, it has been included to highlight the fact that diabetes is a self-managed disease, and if the patient is unwilling or unable to self-manage their own diabetes, the outcome is poor. The greatest barriers to good self-management are the challenges posed by diabetes, which may be specific to diabetes or chronic diseases in general. A few examples include the following:**

- **Managing medical treatment – regular blood tests and self-injecting (eg may stigmatise the patient)**
- **Fear regarding the future – both short term (eg regular blood tests) and long term (eg blindness, complications of diabetes)**
- **The need for regular meals takes away spontaneity**

Total: 25 marks

ENDOCRINE CASE 3

Gloria, a 38-year-old woman, is referred by her GP to an endocrinologist with symptoms of hyperthyroidism.

Q 1. **Name six symptoms Gloria may be complaining of.**   3 marks

A **½ mark for any of the following:**
- **Weight loss (despite increased appetite)**
- **Increased appetite**
- **Heat intolerance**
- **Sweating**
- **Fatigue and weakness**
- **Irritability, nervousness, restlessness, insomnia**
- **Diarrhoea**
- **Palpitations, dyspnoea, angina**
- **Oligomenorrhoea, loss of libido, infertility**

LEARNING POINTS

ⓘ The thyroid gland, stimulated by thyroid-stimulating hormone (TSH) from the anterior pituitary, produces and releases thyroxine (T_4) and tri-iodthyronine (T_3), which exert negative feedback on TSH. The thyroid produces more T_4 than T_3, which is more biologically active; most T_4 undergoes peripheral conversion to T_3. Thyroid hormones are over 95% protein-bound, predominantly to thyroxine-binding globulin (TBG), though it is the unbound (ie free) form that is biologically active. Thyroid hormones regulate cell metabolism, enhance the effects of catecholamines and regulate growth and mental development.

ⓘ Thyrotoxicosis is due to excessive levels of circulating free thyroxine (FT_4) and/ or free tri-iodothyronine (FT_3). Hyperthyroidism refers to an overactive thyroid gland, though thyrotoxicosis can occur without hyperthyroidism (eg excessive thyroxine administration).

On examination she is in sinus tachycardia, has a fine tremor and has bulging eyes (exophthalmos).

Q 2. **List two signs specific to Graves' disease.** 1 mark

A **Signs of hyperthyroidism include sinus tachycardia, atrial fibrillation (particularly in older patients), warm moist peripheries, fine tremor, lid lag and goitre (either diffuse – eg Graves, or nodular); note that goitre may be associated with hyper-, hypo- and euthyroid states). Graves' disease is associated with additional signs, including those in the following list (½ mark for each):**

- **Exophthalmos (ie protruding eyes); proptosis refers to eyes protruding beyond the orbit**
- **Opthalmoplegia (ie paralysis of extraocular muscles causing strabismus (squint)): due to muscle swelling and fibrosis. The patient will complain of diplopia (double vision)**
- **Conjunctival oedema**
- **Periorbital oedema**
- **Pretibial myxoedema (ie painless thickening of skin in nodules or plaques over the shins)**
- **Thyroid acropachy (ie clubbing)**

LEARNING POINTS

ⓘ Graves' disease is the most common cause of thyrotoxicosis, causing relapsing and remitting hyperthyroidism that often eventually progresses to hypothyroidism. It is associated with other autoimmune conditions such as pernicious anaemia, vitiligo, type 1 diabetes, coeliac disease and myasthenia gravis.

ⓘ Other causes of thyrotoxicosis include toxic adenoma (a single nodule which is 'hot' on scanning), toxic multinodular goitre (most common cause in the elderly), thyroiditis (transient hyperthyroidism due to acute inflammation of the gland – eg post-viral (de Quervain's), metastatic thyroid cancer and drugs (eg excess thyroxine, amiodarone).

Q 3. **What is the underlying cause of Graves' disease?** 1 mark

A **TSH receptor IgG antibodies binding to the TSH receptor, stimulating production of thyroid hormones.**

LEARNING POINTS

❶ These TSH receptor antibodies are not routinely measured, with the diagnosis of Graves' disease made from the clinical features plus thyroid autoantibody measurement (ie autoantibodies against thyroglobulin and thyroid peroxidise).

❶ These autoantibodies may also occur in healthy individuals and in Hashimoto's thyroiditis (see causes of hypothyroidism below).

Bloods are taken for thyroid function test (TFTs), shown in Table 3.2.

Q 4. **In the table below indicate (↑,↓, or →) where marked '?' the expected changes in TFTs.**   3 marks

A **1 mark for each of the following:**

	Normal range	Hyperthyroidism	Hypothyroidism	Subclinical hypothyroidism
TSH	0.5–5.7 mU/l	↓	↑	↑
Total T$_4$	70–140 nmol/l	↑	↓	→
Total T$_3$	1.2–3.0 nmol/l	↑	↓ →	→

Table 3.2: Thyroid function tests.

LEARNING POINTS

❶ FT$_4$ and FT$_3$ are not routinely measured. However, several factors, including excess oestrogens, pregnancy, nephrotic syndrome and chronic liver disease, alter levels of TBG (and certain drugs also affect TBG binding) and so total T$_4$ levels are inaccurate in these circumstances – you should measure FT$_4$ to assess any thyrotoxicosis.

❶ Raised TSH with normal T$_4$ in an asymptomatic patient indicates subclinical hypothyroidism. The presence of thyroid antibodies increases the risk of developing overt hypothyroidism. T$_3$ levels are often normal in hypothyroidism, reflecting upregulated peripheral conversion of T$_4$.

ⓘ Other investigations in hyperthyroidism may include erythrocyte sedimentation rate (ESR) (increased in thyroiditis), a thyroid ultrasound scan to identify any solitary or multinodular goitre and a radio-labelled iodine scan to assess thyroid uptake (ie hot or cold nodules). Thyroid malignancy usually presents as a cold nodule (ie endocrinologically inactive) and is further investigated by fine-needle aspiration (FNA) or biopsy.

Gloria's symptoms are treated with β blockers and her hyperthyroidism by a 'block and replace' regimen with carbimazole and thyroxine.

Q 5. **Give two complications of untreated hyperthyroidism.**   1 mark

A **½ for any of the following:**
- **Short-term complications:**
  - **atrial fibrillation (AF): the risk of embolic stroke is high in AF associated with hyperthyroidism and anticoagulation is mandatory**
  - **angina**
  - **thyrotoxic storm**
- **Long-term complications:**
  - **osteoporosis**
  - **heart failure: causes thyrotoxic cardiomyopathy**

LEARNING POINTS

ⓘ Thyroid crisis (thyrotoxic storm) is due to a rapid deterioration of hyperthyroidism, causing tachycardia, hyperthermia, confusion and coma. It may be triggered by myocardial infarction, trauma, infection, radioiodine or thyroid surgery (prevented by ensuring the patient is euthyroid before surgery). Urgent treatment involves β blockers, potassium iodide, anti-thyroid drugs and corticosteroids.

ⓘ Treatment options for hyperthyroidism involve the following:
- **Antithyroid drugs** (eg carbimazole): can either be titrated up until adequate control or can be given in large doses to completely block the thyroid, with oral thyroxine to keep patient euthyroid. Propylthiouracil is an alternative. Measure TSH to monitor effectiveness of treatment.

- **Radioactive iodine (¹³¹I) therapy:** single-dose treatment that is concentrated by the thyroid, causing cell death. The patient must stay away from pregnant women or young children for 17 days after the treatment. Patients usually end up hypothyroid, requiring lifelong thyroxine.
- **Surgical resection** (subtotal thyroidectomy) of the thyroid gland (see below).

ⓘ The eye problems of Graves' disease are typically independent of the thyroid status and are therefore not prevented by treating the hyperthyroidism (in fact, radioactive iodine therapy can transiently worsen the eye disease). Treatment may involve taping eyelids closed at night, lubricating eye drops, lateral tarsorrhaphy (to protect the cornea), high-dose corticosteroids, orbital radiotherapy and, occasionally, surgical decompression of the orbit.

Q 6. **Give four indications for thyroidectomy in Gloria.** 2 marks

A **½ mark for any of the following:**
- **Patient choice (eg for cosmetic reasons)**
- **Pressure symptoms from a large goitre (eg dyspnoea, dysphagia)**
- **Intolerable drug side-effects (eg carbimazole may cause agranulocytosis; propylthiouracil may also cause marrow suppression)**
- **Poor compliance with drug therapy**
- **Relapse of hyperthyroidism after withdrawal of medication (patients are usually treated for 12–18 months)**

LEARNING POINT

ⓘ In nodular goitre a further indication for surgery is the risk of thyroid cancer in these patients.

Q 7. **Give four complications of surgery.** 2 marks

A **½ mark each for any of the following:**
- **Early postoperative bleeding, causing dyspnoea due to haematoma pressure effects**
- **Hypothyroidism**
- **Recurrent hyperthyroidism**

- **Hypoparathyroidism, causing hypocalcaemia (due to damage to adjacent parathyroid glands)**
- **Hoarseness due to recurrent laryngeal nerve damage**

On cessation of the 'block and replace' regimen, Gloria remains hyperthyroid. She is subsequently treated with radioactive iodine, which initially renders her euthyroid, although eventually it leaves her hypothyroid.

Q 8. **List four other causes of hypothyroidism.** 2 marks

A **½ mark for any of the following:**
- **Autoimmune hypothyroidism (eg Hashimoto's thyroiditis – causes a goitre: may be hypo-, hyper- or euthyroid at presentation), atrophic hypothyroidism (without the goitre): both associated with thyroid autoantibodies**
- **Iodine deficiency: main cause of goitre and hypothyroidism worldwide**
- **Thyroidectomy or radioiodine treatment**
- **Drugs (eg anti-thyroid drugs, amiodarone)**
- **Congenital hypopthyroidism: screened for by the Guthrie heel-prick test at post-natal day 7 (detects increased TSH in heel-prick sample)**

LEARNING POINT

ⓘ Patients with symptomatic hypothyroidism require T_4. The aim of therapy is to return T_4 and TSH levels to normal (avoid suppressing TSH), although it may take several months before symptoms of hypothyroidism are resolved following biochemical correction. A dose of 100–150 microg/day is effective in most patients, although in older patients or patients with ischaemic heart disease you need to start at 25 microg/day and slowly titrate up to euthyroid levels.

Total : 15 marks

GASTROENTEROLOGY
CASES: ANSWERS

GASTROENTEROLOGY CASE 1

Henry, a 58-year-old man, presents to the Emergency Department with a 1-hour history of haematemesis, including a severe episode in the ambulance. On examination his blood pressure is 86/44 mmHg, he is cold peripherally and his pulse is 110 bpm.

Q 1. **List six causes of haematemesis.**   3 marks

A **1 mark each for any of the following:**
- **Peptic ulcer disease (PUD), the most common cause**
- **Oesophageal varices**
- **Oesophagitis**
- **Gastritis**
- **Mallory–Weiss (oesophageal) tear: due to excessive vomiting (eg due to alcohol, chemotherapy)**
- **Upper gastrointestinal malignancy (eg gastric cancer)**
- **Arteriovenous malformations (AVMs)**

LEARNING POINTS

ⓘ The two main causes of peptic ulcer disease (PUD), which encompasses duodenal and gastric ulcers, are non-steroidal anti-inflammatory drugs (NSAIDs) and *Helicobacter pylori* infection.

ⓘ *H. pylori* infection can be detected on endoscopy (eg rapid urease test, histology, culture) and by non-invasive tests (eg carbon-13 urea breath test, stool antigen test, serology). Serology for *H. pylori* antibodies cannot be used after treatment. It is eradicated by 1-week course of triple therapy (ie proton pump inhibitor and a combination of amoxicillin, clarithromycin or metronidazole).

ⓘ Portal hypertension (eg due to liver cirrhosis) causes dilated collateral veins (varices) at sites of portosystemic anastomosis (eg oesophagus, umbilicus (caput medusae), rectum and stomach). Those at the oesophagus may rupture, causing variceal bleeding; this is prevented by prophylactic β-blockers, which lower portal hypertension.

Q 2. **What is your immediate management?**   3 marks

A **1 mark each for any of the following:**

- **Airway, breathing and circulation (ABC) as the patient is shocked (ie heart rate > systolic blood pressure is a good working definition)**

- **Airways: ascertain that the airway is not compromised and manage in recovery position to protect airway**

- **Breathing: give high-flow O$_2$**

- **Circulation: obtain IV access with two large-bore cannulae and resuscitate with intravenous colloid/crystalloid, while waiting for blood to be cross-matched (in emergencies can give O Rh–ve blood)**

LEARNING POINT

❶ Patients who are shocked and actively bleeding will require transfusion. However, massive transfusions can also cause coagulopathy, requiring additional platelet and fresh frozen plasma (FFP) transfusions.

Q 3. **What three brief questions would you ask?**   3 marks

A **1 mark each for asking about any of the following:**

- **Any previous episodes of haematemesis and/or melaena (both indicate upper GI bleeds), including their cause, severity and treatment**

- **Any known causes of upper GI bleeds (eg peptic ulcer disease, chronic liver disease)**

- **Any dyspeptic symptoms (eg epigastric pain)**

- **Alcohol consumption, intravenous drug use (IVDU): alcohol, hepatitis B and C virus (from IVDU) are the main causes of liver cirrhosis**

- **Medication history (eg NSAIDs, aspirin, warfarin)**

LEARNING POINT

❶ Examination should include rectal examination (for malaena) and for signs (stigmata) of chronic liver disease.

Q 4. **What four blood tests would you request?** 2 marks

A ½ **point each for any of the following:**

- **Full blood count (FBC): anaemia (Hb may not fall until circulating volume is restored), thrombocytopenia (increased risk of bleeding)**

- **Urea and electrolytes (U&Es): may show prerenal failure from hypovolaemia (see above notes on fluid resuscitation); also used to assess risk of re-bleeding (see below)**

- **Clotting screen: any bleeding disorder (eg raised INR)**

- **LFTs: suspect varices if chronic liver disease; liver disease causes increased INR due to reduced clotting factor synthesis, reduced vitamin K absorption (fat-soluble vitamin requiring bile for absorption)**

- **Group and save (G&S)/cross-match: if active bleeding cross-match 4–6 units**

LEARNING POINTS

ℹ In the presence of a bleeding disorder consult a haematologist for advice on intravenous vitamin K, fresh frozen plasma (FFP) and platelet transfusion.

ℹ Endoscopy (OGD) should be performed within 24 hours or urgently in the presence of active bleeding or if variceal haemorrhage is suspected. Endoscopy has three purposes: (1) diagnosis, (2) prognosis (see below), and (3) treatment (eg banding or sclerotherapy of varices, adrenaline injection into bleeding ulcers).

ℹ If variceal haemorrhage is confirmed on endoscopy (or suspected in bleeding associated with stigmata of liver disease), give intravenous terlipressin, which constricts the splanchnic arteries, restricting portal inflow (this is continued 48 hours following endoscopic treatment of bleeding varices). Uncontrolled variceal haemorrhage may require balloon tamponade (with a Sengstaken–Blakemore tube) before transjugular intrahepatic portosystemic stent shunting (TIPSS). Patients should also receive antibiotics (eg IV ceftriaxone), as this has been shown to reduce mortality associated with variceal haemorrhage.

Henry undergoes emergency endoscopy, which diagnoses an actively bleeding gastric ulcer, which in turn is successfully treated by injection of adrenaline.

Q 5. **What factors are used to assess Henry's risk of rebleeding?** 2 marks

A ½ **point for any of the following:**

- **Age**
- **Shock**
- **Co-morbidity: death following an upper GI bleed is usually a result of decompensated co-morbidity rather than exsanguination**
- **Endoscopic findings: presence of blood in upper GI tract, active spurting haemorrhage, non-bleeding visible vessel are all poor prognostic signs**

LEARNING POINT

❶ It is important to identify those patients at risk of continuing bleeding or rebleeding, as they will require more intensive monitoring (see below). The Rockhall score (see Table 4.1) is used to predict those at risk of rebleeding and death; a score ≥ 7 is high risk.

Score	0	1	2	3
Age (years)	< 60	60–79	80	–
Shock systolic BP pulse	None	> 100 mmHg > 100 bpm	< 100 mmHg	–
Co-morbidty	None	–	Cardiac or other major disease	Renal or liver failure; malignancy
Diagnosis on oeophagogastroduodenoscopy (OGD)	None Mallory–Weiss tear No sign of recent bleeding	All other diagnoses	Upper GI malignancy	–
Signs of recent haemorrhage	None Black spots	–	Blood in upper GI tract Clot Spurting haemorrhage Non-bleeding visible vessel	–

Table 4.1: Rockall risk scoring system.

GASTROENTEROLOGY

Q 6. **List four signs of a rebleed while on the ward.** 2 marks

A ½ **mark each for any of the following:**

- **Increasing heart rate**
- **Decreasing blood pressure**
- **Decreasing central venous pressure (although not all patients will have a central line)**
- **Decreasing urine output: hourly urinary output can be monitored in catheterised patients**
- **Haematemesis**
- **Melaena**

LEARNING POINTS

ℹ️ Management following rebleeding usually involves repeat endoscopy. Surgery (eg ulcer excision) or arterial embolisation is indicated when active bleeding cannot be controlled by endoscopic therapy (either at presentation or following re-bleeding) or if there is exsanguinating haemorrhage (ie too fast to replace or requiring > 6 units blood to restore blood pressure), so warn surgeon on call of all serious non-variceal bleeds.

ℹ️ To prevent rebleeding in high-risk cases start intravenous propton pump inhibitor therapy (eg omeprazole infusion, ie 80-mg bolus followed by 8 mg/h for 72 hours (clot formation is impaired in an acid environment).

Total: 15 marks

GASTROENTEROLOGY CASE 2

Rod is admitted to the medical assessment unit complaining of malaise and anorexia. On examination he is jaundiced with signs of chronic liver disease.

Q 1. **List four risk factors for jaundice you would enquire about in the history.** 2 marks

A ½ **mark each for any of the following:**

- **Recent travel abroad: to areas endemic for hepatitis A virus (HAV)**
- **Intravenous drug use (IVDU): increased risk of hepatitis B and C viruses (HBV, HCV)**
- **Excessive alcohol consumption: alcoholic liver disease**
- **Drugs taken: both prescribed and OTC: many drugs cause jaundice (eg paracetamol overdose)**
- **Sexuality: homosexuals/sex workers have an increased risk of HBV**
- **Healthcare worker: increased risk of HBV and HCV**
- **Farm or sewage worker: increased risk of leptospiral infection**
- **Watersports: increased risk of leptospiral infection**

LEARNING POINTS

ⓘ Jaundice can be classified as:

- Prehepatic (unconjugated hyperbilirubinaemia): due to haemolysis
- Hepatocellular: hepatocyte damage ± intrahepatic cholestasis
- Cholestatic (obstructive): intra- and extrahepatic cholestasis. It is important in the history to enquire about obstructive symptoms (ie pale stools and dark urine).

ⓘ Extrahepatic causes of obstructive jaundice include: gallstones; pancreatic cancer; benign stricture of the common bile duct (eg complication of endoscopic retrograde cholangiopancreatography (ERCP)); sclerosing cholangitis (eg associated with inflammatory bowel disease (IBD)); and cholangiocarcinoma.

Q 2. **List three *abdominal* signs of chronic liver disease.** 3 marks

A **1 mark each for any of the following:**
- **Hepatomegaly (or small liver in late disease)**
- **Ascites (see below)**
- **Splenomegaly: due to portal hypertension**
- **Caput medusae (dilated collateral veins around the umbilicus): due to portal hypertension**

LEARNING POINT

❶ Other signs of chronic liver disease include: hands (clubbing, palmar erythema, leuconychia, Dupuytren's contracture), endocrine disturbances (loss of body hair, testicular atrophy, gynaecomastia), peripheral oedema (due to hypoalbuminaemia) and spider naevi (occur on upper body in the drainage of the superior vena cava (SVC); $\geq$ 5 suggests liver disease).

Several blood tests are requested to assess the severity of Rod's liver disease.

Q 3. **Name two blood tests used to assess liver synthetic function.** 2 marks

A **1 mark for each of the following:**
There are only two tests of liver synthetic function:
- **Albumin (normal range 35–50 g/l): albumin is synthesised by the liver, with hypoalbuminaemia seen in chronic liver disease. The resulting reduction in plasma oncotic pressure promotes peripheral oedema and ascites**
- **INR (normal range 0.9–1.2)/prothrombin time (normal range 10–14 s): increased due to impaired synthesis of clotting factors and vitamin K malabsorption (fat-soluble vitamin requiring bile)**

LEARNING POINT

❶ Liver function tests do not actually assess liver function; they are non-specific indicators of liver or biliary disease. For example, raised AST and ALT (aminotransferases) reflect hepatocellular damage, while raised ALP and γGT reflect cholestasis (either intra- or extrahepatic).

It is clear that the cause of Rod's liver disease is alcohol excess, and he is given intravenous thiamine and started on a chlordiazepoxide-reducing regimen. He is diagnosed with alcoholic hepatitis and commenced on oral corticosteroids.

Q 4. **What are we trying to prevent by giving thiamine to alcoholics?** 1 mark

A **Wernicke–Korsakoff syndrome.**

LEARNING POINTS

ⓘ Thiamine (B_1) deficiency in alcoholics, due to dietary deficiency and impaired gut absorption, may cause Wernicke's encephalopathy, characterised by ophthalmoplegia, ataxia and confusion, which if not treated may progress to irreversible Korsakoff syndrome. This causes antegrade amnesia, resulting in confabulation (ie making up stories to fill the gaps in memory).

ⓘ All alcoholics should be given IV thiamine (Pabrinex®) and a chlordiazepoxide (Librium®) reducing regimen (to relieve the symptoms of withdrawal). Thiamine must be given before any intravenous glucose infusion as this may precipitate Wernicke's.

ⓘ Alcoholic hepatitis is due to alcohol binge and may cause jaundice, ascites and hepatic encephalopathy (see below). It is considered an early stage of alcoholic liver disease, but may also occur in patients with established alcoholic liver disease or alcoholic cirrhosis. Its severity can be assessed using modified Maddrey's discriminant function: 4.6 x (PT–control value) + serum bilirubin: a score > 32 indicates severe alcoholic hepatitis, and such patients should be given corticosteroids as their risk of mortality is high.

Abdominal ultrasound scan reports cirrhotic changes in the liver with gross ascites.

Q 5. **In the absence of obvious risk factors, list three blood tests you would request to identify the cause of Rod's liver disease.** 3 marks

A **1 mark each for any of the following:**
- **Full blood count (FBC): raised mean corpuscular volume (MCV) (macrocytosis) is an indicator of alcohol misuse**
- **Hepatitis B and C virus serology**
- **Alpha$_1$-antitrypsin level: to exclude α_1-antitrypsin deficiency**

GASTROENTEROLOGY

- **Copper studies (reduced serum copper and caeruloplasmin, a copper-containing protein synthesised by the liver): to exclude Wilson's disease, resulting in copper deposition in the liver**
- **Iron studies (increased iron and ferritin and reduced total iron-binding capacity (TIBC)): to exclude haemochromatosis, resulting in iron deposition in the liver**
- **Autoantibodies: used to identify autoimmune causes of cirrhosis. AMA (primary biliary cirrhosis (PBC)), ANA and SMA (autoimmune hepatitis)**

LEARNING POINTS

ⓘ Chronic liver disease may progress to cirrhosis owing to irreversible liver damage. This is confirmed on liver biopsy; histologically there is fibrosis and nodular regeneration with loss of normal hepatic architecture.

ⓘ The severity of liver cirrhosis is based on Child–Pugh grading system (see Table 4.2).

Score	1 point	2 points	3 points
Bilirubin (μmol/l)	< 34	34–51	> 51
Albumin (g/l)	> 35	28–35	< 28
Prothrombin time (secs > normal)	1–4	4–6	> 6
Ascites	None	Slight	Moderate
Encephalopathy*	None	Grade 1–2	Grade 3–4

Grade A: < 7; Grade B 7–9; and Grade C > 9

*See over page for grading of encephalopathy.

Table 4.2: Child–Pugh score.

ⓘ **Ascites** (ie accumulation of fluid in peritoneal cavity) indicates a poor prognosis in chronic liver disease and may be demonstrated by shifting dullness or a fluid thrill. It is caused by a combination of splanchnic vasodilatation, resulting in sodium and water retention (exacerbated by secondary hyperaldosteronism) and portal hypertension, forcing transudation of fluid into the peritoneal cavity (exacerbated by hypoalbuminaemia). **Treatment** involves fluid restriction, low-salt diet and spironolactone. Refractory or symptomatic tense ascites can be drained (therapeutic paracentesis) with concomitant albumin infusion (8 g/l fluid removed – use human albumin 20%, not the standard 4.5% bottles) to help prevent hypovolaemia, as ascites reaccumulates at the expense of circulating volume.

GASTROENTEROLOGY

Q 6. **List four complications of liver cirrhosis.**   **4 marks**

A **1 mark each for any from the following list.**

Cirrhosis is irreversible and treatment is directed at its complications:

- **Renal failure (hepatorenal syndrome)**
- **Portal hypertension: causes variceal haemorrhage, hypersplenism**
- **Coagulopathy: treatment involves 10 mg IV vitamin K (± fresh frozen plasma if bleeding)**
- **Hepatocellular carcinoma: screen by regular ultrasound scan and alpha-fetoprotein (αFP)**
- **Hepatic encephalopathy: due to 'toxic metabolites' (eg ammonia) in the blood bypassing the liver by portosystemic collaterals, causing neurotoxicity**
- **Spontaneous bacterial peritonitis**

LEARNING POINTS

ⓘ **Hepatic encephalopathy** can occur acutely or chronically. It is graded as shown in Table 4.3:

Grade	Symptoms and signs
1	Altered mood or behaviour
2	Confusion, drowsy
3	Stupor, incoherence, agitation
4	Coma

Table 4.3: Hepatic encephalopathy grading.

ⓘ Other features include fetor hepaticus (pear-drop breath) and a coarse flapping tremor (when arms outstretched and wrists hyperextended). Acute encephalopathy often has a precipitating factor (eg constipation, infection, drugs (eg CNS depressants), electrolyte disturbance (eg secondary to diuretics or GI bleed)). Management involves correction of the underlying cause (eg lactulose: aim for two to four loose bowel motions a day; also helps by reducing absorption of ammonia from bowel), antibiotics, stopping diuretic therapy.

GASTROENTEROLOGY

❶ **Spontaneous bacterial peritonitis** is a serious complication (25% mortality) affecting approximately 10% of people with cirrhotic ascites. It should be suspected in any patient with clinical deterioration, even in the absence of abdominal pain and pyrexia. It is confirmed by sending ascitic fluid for urgent MC&S; a WCC > $250/mm^3$ in aspirated ascitic fluid is considered diagnostic of bacterial peritonitis. It is treated with intravenous antibiotics (eg cefotaxime); oral ciprofloxacin is used prophylactically.

Total: **15 marks**

GASTROENTEROLOGY CASE 3

Dennis, a 64-year-old man, is admitted to the surgical assessment unit with several hours' history of severe epigastric pain radiating to his back, associated with nausea and vomiting. His serum amylase is reported as 1170 U/ml (normal range 0–180 U/ml), confirming a diagnosis of acute pancreatitis.

Q 1. List eight criteria used to assess the severity of pancreatitis. **4 marks**

A ½ mark each for any of the following:

	Criteria	Positive value	Normal range
P	PO_2	< 8 kPa	> 10.6
A	Age	> 55 years	
N	Neutrophils	WCC > 15 x 10⁹/l	4–11
C	Calcium (adjusted)	<2 mmol/l	2.12–2.65
R	Renal function	Urea > 16 mmol/l	2.5–6.7
E	Enzymes	LDH > 600 IU/l	70–250
		AST > 200 IU/l	3–35
A	Albumin	< 32 g/l	35–50
S	Sugar (blood glucose)	> 10 mmol/l	4–6

LEARNING POINTS

ℹ Acute pancreatitis is diagnosed on the basis of clinical features and confirmed by serum amylase levels more than three times the upper limit of normal. However, amylase levels decline over 2–3 days, so a normal amylase does not exclude pancreatitis in patients with symptoms for more than 3 days (amylase is also elevated in non-pancreatic conditions – eg visceral perforation, small-bowel obstruction or ischaemia, leaking aortic aneurysm, ectopic pregnancy). Lipase is also elevated, remains elevated for longer and is normal in non-pancreatic conditions, so is the preferred investigation, where available.

❶ The Glasgow scoring system is used to predict the severity of acute pancreatitis at 48 hours (use PANCREAS acronym, as above). Three or more positive criteria indicate severe pancreatitis (other scoring systems include APACHE II score). Other predictors of a severe attack include clinical impression of severity, obesity (body mass index > 30), pleural effusion on chest X-ray and raised C-reactive protein (CRP > 150 mg/l).

❶ The purpose of predicting severity is to identify those patients at high risk of complications and who should be managed on intensive care. Early complications include: shock (see below), acute renal failure, acute respiratory distress syndrome (ARDS), disseminated intravascular coagulation (DIC) and metabolic complications (eg hyperglycaemia, hypocalcaemia); late complications include pancreatic necrosis and pseudocyst (fluid in lesser sac).

Q 2. **List six causes of acute pancreatitis.**   3 marks

A **½ mark each for any of the following:**
- **Gallstones (50%)**
- **Alcohol (20%): may represent an exacerbation of chronic pancreatitis as opposed to true acute pancreatitis**
- **Idiopathic (20%)**
- **Drugs (5%), eg steroids, furosemide, azathioprine**
- **Viral infection, eg HIV, mumps**
- **Hypertriglyceridaemia**
- **Endoscopic retrograde cholangiopancreatography (ERCP)**

LEARNING POINTS

❶ GET SMASHED is a commonly used acronym for remembering both common and rare (scorpion bites!) causes of pancreatitis.

❶ Gallstones can cause acute pancreatitis by blocking the hepatopancreatic ampulla, causing reflux back up the main pancreatic duct, leading to pancreatic autodigestion. All patients should have an abdominal ultrasound scan to look for gallstones and dilated bile ducts.

Dennis is given high-flow oxygen therapy and aggressive fluid replacement. A urinary catheter is inserted to monitor his urine output.

Q **3. In fluid replacement, what minimum hourly urinary output do you aim for?** 1 mark

A **Aim for urine flow > 0.5 ml/kg body weight or > 30 ml/h.**

LEARNING POINTS

ⓘ Acute pancreatitis is (initially) managed conservatively with oxygen therapy and fluid resuscitation to replace plasma volume deficit (due to third-space fluid loss, ie extracellular fluid trapped in gut, peritoneum and retroperitoneum) and to maintain urine output (may also require central venous pressure monitoring) so as to prevent multi-organ failure.

ⓘ In severe pancreatitis oral intake is inhibited by nausea and vomiting (due to small-bowel ileus), although early enteral nutrition (eg via a nasojejunal or nasogastric tube) is recommended over parenteral feeding, unless limited by ileus.

ⓘ There is no role for prophylactic antibiotics in preventing pancreatic necrosis (see below).

Dennis undergoes an abdominal ultrasound scan, which shows gallbladder stones with their acoustic shadows (see Figure 4.1).

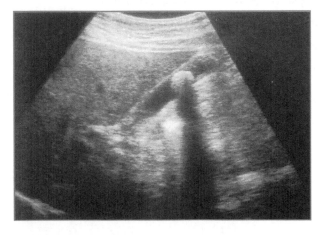

Figure 4.1: Dennis's abdominal ultrasound.

GASTROENTEROLOGY

Q 4. **Name four additional complications of gallstones.** 2 marks

A **½ mark each for any of the following:**

- **Biliary colic: due to bile duct attempting to shift impacted gallstones**
- **Cholecystitis (see below)**
- **Empyema: obstructed gallbladder fills with pus**
- **Obstructive jaundice: due to gallstones obstructing the common bile duct (CBD)**
- **Cholangitis: infection of the bile ducts, causing right upper quadrant pain, jaundice and rigors (Charcot's triad)**
- **Gallbladder perforation and generalised peritonitis**
- **Gallstone ileus: due to gallstones obstructing the small bowel**

LEARNING POINT

ⓘ **Acute cholecystitis** is caused by gallstones obstructing the cystic duct, causing gallbladder distension (which may cause local peritonism) and (sterile) inflammation (raised white cell count, fever). Presenting features include severe right upper quadrant (RUQ) pain with nausea, vomiting and sweating and a positive Murphy's sign. Murphy's sign is arrest of inspiration (due to severe pain) on palpation just below the right subcostal margin, due to the inflamed gallbladder descending to touch your hand (only positive if same test on left-hand side is negative).

Q 5. **What is the recommended procedure within the first 72 hours?** 1 mark

A **Endoscopic retrograde cholangiopancreatography (ERCP) plus sphincterotomy and removal of any stones.**

LEARNING POINTS

ⓘ All patients with severe pancreatitis associated with gallstones (with or without evidence of biliary obstruction) should have ERCP within 72 hours. ERCP involves insertion of an endoscope into the second part of the duodenum, cannulating the ampulla and injecting radio-opaque dye to visualise the biliary tree (an alternative imaging technique is magnetic resonance cholangiopancreatography). Any stone found on X-ray can be removed by sphincterotomy of the biliary sphincter and swept clear.

GASTROENTEROLOGY

❶ Abdominal CT (contrast-enhanced to detect necrosis) is usually performed in patients with severe pancreatitis (or with clinical deterioration) after 7–10 days for detection of pancreatic complications. Fine-needle aspiration of pancreatic tissue may be indicated (eg necrosis associated with signs of sepsis) to diagnose infected necrosis, which is treated by radiological (drainage) or surgical (necrosectomy) intervention. Pseudocysts are only drained if symptomatic.

Dennis undergoes a cholecystectomy before discharge.

Q 6. **List two advantages each of laparoscopic and open cholecystectomy.** 2 marks

A **1 mark each for the following:**
- **Laparoscopic: reduced wound pain, less scar formation, shorter inpatient stay/ quicker recovery**
- **Open: lower risk of bile duct injury, lower risk of damage to adjacent structures, able to simultaneously remove any stones in the common bile duct, technically easier**

LEARNING POINT

❶ Patients with mild gallstone pancreatitis should have cholecystectomy, ideally during the same admission, to prevent risk of a further severe attack of pancreatitis. This will need to be delayed in patients with severe pancreatitis until systemic effects have resolved.

Q 7. **Give four complications of cholecystectomy.** 2 marks

A **½ mark each for any of the following:**
- **Death: less than 1 per 1000**
- **Bile duct injury**
- **Bile leakage**
- **Jaundice due to retained ductal stones (can be removed by ERCP)**
- **General complications of any surgical procedure (eg pulmonary embolism, chest infection, wound infection)**

Total: 15 marks

GASTROENTEROLOGY

GASTROENTEROLOGY CASE 4

Jennifer, a 25-year-old woman, is referred to gastroenterology with several weeks' history of bloody diarrhoea and general malaise.

Q 1. List four causes of bloody diarrhoea.   4 marks

A 1 mark each for any of the following:

- **Ulcerative colitis (UC)**
- **Crohn's disease: rectal bleeding is associated with colonic disease, although is not as severe as UC**
- **Colorectal cancer**
- **Colonic polyps**
- **Ischaemic colitis: due to chronic ischaemia of the bowel**
- **Pseudomembranous colitis: caused by overgrowth of** *Clostridium difficile* **following antibiotic therapy**
- **Infective (dysentery):** *Escherichia coli O157, Shigella, Salmonella, Campylobacter*

LEARNING POINT

ⓘ While UC and Crohn's disease (CD) both cause diarrhoea and abdominal pain, with systemic features such as malaise and weight loss, the hallmark of UC is blood diarrhoea (in an acute setting may be difficult to distinguish from infectious colitis, so always send stool for MC&S).

A flexible sigmoidoscopy is arranged, which reveals a superficial continuous inflammation of the rectum. The mucosa looks reddened and inflamed, consistent with ulcerative colitis (UC) which is confirmed on biopsy.

Q 2. **List four pathological differences between UC and Crohn's disease.**   4 marks

A **1 mark each for any of the following:**

- **UC only involves the bowel mucosa, whereas CD involves all layers of the bowel wall (transmural – this may lead to fistulas)**
- **CD causes skip lesions (normal areas of bowel in between)**
- **CD can affect any part of the gastrointestinal tract (ie mouth to anus), but typically affects the terminal ileum and ascending colon**
- **UC can affect rectum alone (proctitis), but can also extend proximally to involve part or all of the colon (colitis); it rarely spreads proximally beyond the colon (termed 'backwash ileitis'). UC can be classified as either distal disease (only involving rectum and sigmoid colon) or extensive disease**

LEARNING POINT

ⓘ Inflammatory bowel disease (IBD) is investigated by colonoscopy, which allows the extent of disease to be assessed, although in moderate to severe disease (see below) the risk of bowel perforation is high and flexible sigmoidoscopy is safer, with colonoscopy delayed until clinically improved. Additionally, in CD the small bowel is imaged using barium studies (may show strictures, ulceration).

Q 3. **List four extraintestinal manifestations of inflammatory bowel disease (IBD).**   2 marks

A **½ mark each for any of the following:**

Related to disease activity	Unrelated to disease activity
Mouth: aphthous ulcers	**Joints:** sacroiliitis, ankylosing spondylitis
Skin: pyoderma gangrenosum, erythema nodosum	**Liver:** primary sclerosing cholangitis, fatty liver, cirrhosis, cholangiocarcinoma, gallstones
Eyes: conjunctivitis, episcleritis, uveitis	Finger clubbing
Joints: acute arthritis	

LEARNING POINT

ⓘ Extraintestinal manifestations occur in 10–20% of patients, of which only some are related to disease activity. Colectomy does not cure ankylosing spondylitis or primary sclerosing cholangitis.

Jennifer is diagnosed with distal UC and responds well to a combination of oral and topical treatment.

Q 4. **What class of drug is prescribed to maintain remission in UC?** 1 mark

A **Aminosalicylates: the active ingredient is 5-aminosalicylic acid (5-ASA), eg mesalazine, olsalazine, sulfasalazine.**

LEARNING POINTS

❶ Treatment of active UC is discussed below. Maintenance of remission in UC involves oral aminosalicylates; patients with distal disease who have been in remission for > 2 years can stop maintenance therapy. Steroids are ineffective at maintaining remission; azathioprine and mercaptopurine are effective but, owing to their toxicity, are reserved for patients who frequently relapse on aminosalicylates.

❶ Surgery is curative of the intestinal features of UC and typically involves colectomy with an ileostomy or ileo-anal pouch reconstruction. Indications for surgery include: perforation, massive haemorrhage, toxic dilatation and failure to respond to medical treatment. However, surgery is not curative in Crohn's disease, as disease may recur anywhere in the gastrointestinal tract, although patients may require an operation (eg for fistulas, strictures).

Jennifer remains asymptomatic before relapsing, requiring admission to hospital, where she is diagnosed with an attack of her UC.

Q 5. **List six features used to assess the severity of a UC attack.** 3 marks

A **½ mark each for any of the following:**

Features	Mild	Moderate	Severe attack
Motions per day	< 4	4–6	> 6
Rectal bleeding	Little	Moderate	Large amounts
Temperature	Apyrexial	Intermediate	> 37.8 °C
Pulse rate	< 70 bpm	70–90 bpm	>90 bpm
Haemoglobin	> 11 g/dl	10.5–11 g/dl	<10.5 g/dl
Erythrocyte sedimentation rate	Normal	Intermediate	>30 mm/h

LEARNING POINTS

- ❶ UC is a chronic relapsing condition. An attack of UC can be classified according to the above features as mild, moderate or severe, which is used to determine management. Mild and moderate attacks are treated with topical (suppository or enema) and oral aminosalicylates (patients may also require topical/oral corticosteroids).

- ❶ Severe attacks require admission and treatment by intravenous fluids, potassium supplements (also consider total parenteral nutrition), correction of any anaemia, and intravenous corticosteroids. Vital signs, stool frequency and bloods (FBC, U&Es, LFTs, ESR and CRP) should be monitored frequently; intravenous ciclosporin or colectomy may be used in refractory disease. Do not give antidiarrhoeal drugs or opioids, as they increase the risk of perforation.

- ❶ Severity in Crohn's disease (CD) is harder to assess than in UC. Treatment of CD (active disease and maintaining remission) may involve aminosalicylates, corticosteroids (oral budesonide has less systemic absorption than prednisolone), azathioprine, mercaptopurine or methotrexate, elemental diets (which act to rest the bowel), metronidazole (especially if perianal fistulas), and infliximab (anti-TNFα).

Q 6. **Why would you do a plain abdominal X-ray in an acute attack of UC?** 2 marks

A **1 mark for each of the following:**

- **To exclude toxic megacolon**
- **To assess faecal distribution: the distal extent of constipation indicates how far UC extends proximally, as affected bowel will be empty of stool (black with air)**

LEARNING POINT

- ❶ **Toxic megacolon** may occur during an acute severe attack of UC (and CD) and is diagnosed on abdominal X-ray by colon diameter > 5.5 cm. If detected at presentation, patients should have daily abdominal X-rays because if it is not responding to medical management it may require surgery as the risk of perforation is high.

Q 7. **Give four complications of UC.** 4 marks

A **1 mark each for any of the following:**

- **Perforation**
- **Bleeding: massive haemorrhage is rare**
- **Malnutrition**
- **Toxic dilatation of the colon (toxic megacolon)**
- **Primary sclerosing cholangitis**
- **Colon cancer: incidence of colon cancer is increased in UC (and less so in CD). Risk is highest in those with extensive UC for > 10 years or primary sclerosing cholangitis, and such patients require monitoring with regular colonoscopy with multiple biopsies**

LEARNING POINT

ⓘ **Crohn's disease complications** include: strictures (mainly affect small bowel), perianal disease (eg fissures, fistulas and abscesses) and fistulas (ie abnormal communication between bowel and bladder, vagina, and/or skin).

Total: 20 marks

NEUROLOGY
CASES: ANSWERS

NEUROLOGY CASE 1

George, a 67-year-old smoker, presents to his GP following an episode of slurred speech earlier that day, which resolved in less than 30 minutes. On examination he is in sinus rhythm, blood pressure is 154/83 mmHg and he is neurologically intact. Owing to his high risk of stroke, he is admitted for further assessment.

Q 1. **What should be started immediately?** 1 mark

A **300 mg aspirin.**

LEARNING POINTS

ⓘ Following a transient ischaemic attack (TIA) (or stroke, see below), aspirin (300 mg daily) should be started immediately: this is continued for 2 weeks followed by definitive antiplatelet treatment (75 mg aspirin plus dipyridamole; following a stroke, aspirin is replaced by clopidogrel).

ⓘ Modifiable risk factors will also need to be addressed (eg smoking, hypertension, hypercholesterolaemia).

ⓘ Patients with suspected TIA should have their risk of subsequent stroke assessed (eg using the ABCD2 system, shown in Table 5.1).

Symbol	Feature	Criterion	Score
A	Age	≥ 60 years	1
B	Blood pressure	≥ 140/90 mmHg	1
C	Clinical feature of the TIA	Unilateral weakness	2
		Speech disturbance without weakness	1
D	Duration of symptoms	≥ 60 min	2
		10–59 min	1
		< 10 min	0
D2	Diabetes	Diabetic	1

Table 5.1: ABCD2 score.

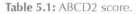

NEUROLOGY

ⓘ Those at high risk (eg ABCD2 score ≥ 4 (as in George's case) or crescendo TIA (≥ 2 TIAs in a week)) should be admitted for further assessment; lower-risk patients are typically assessed in a TIA clinic within a week.

George undergoes a number of inpatient investigations, including carotid Doppler.

Q 2. **What are the criteria for carotid endarterectomy?**   2 marks

A **1 mark for each of the following:**
- **Symptomatic: stroke or TIA in distribution of internal carotid artery**
- **Severe stenosis: 70–99% of luminal diameter: there is no benefit in patients with totally occluded lumen or stenosis < 70%**

LEARNING POINTS

ⓘ All TIA/stroke patients who are surgical candidates for carotid endarterectomy should undergo carotid Doppler within 1 week of the episode, and if they meet above criteria, they should undergo carotid endarterectomy within 2 weeks.

ⓘ Other investigations following a TIA may include:
- Full blood count: polycythaemia and thrombocytosis cause hypercoaguable state
- Glucose and lipids: secondary prevention
- Erythrocyte sedimentation rate: to screen for underlying inflammatory disease (non-specific test)
- Electrocardiogram: exclude atrial fibrillation
- Echocardiogram (eg if recent myocardial infarction, murmur): exclude cardiac sources of emboli (eg atrial fibrillation, aortic or mitral valve disease, intracardiac thrombus)
- Brain imaging (MRI/CT): many patients with a TIA have a cerebral infarct on brain imaging

George's blood pressure and cholesterol are optimised, he is commenced on appropriate antiplatelet medication, although he continues to smoke on discharge. Unfortunately, 3 months later he presents with a stroke.

NEUROLOGY

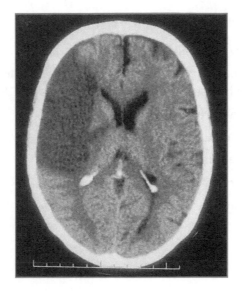

Figure 5.1: George's brain CT scan.

Q 3. What cerebral artery is affected (please refer to Figure 5.1)?   1 mark

A Right middle cerebral artery (MCA).

LEARNING POINT

❶ MCA supplies lateral surfaces of cortex, optic radiation and internal capsule (which contains ascending sensory and descending motor tracts).

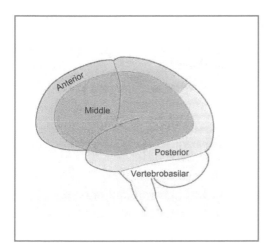

Figure 5.2: Arterial supply to the brain.

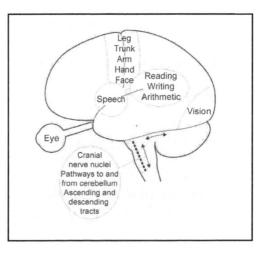

Figure 5.3: Functions of the brain.

Q 4. **What features of a stroke may be present?**   2 marks

A ½ **mark each for any from the following list.**

The middle cerebral artery (MCA) is the largest cerebral artery and most commonly involved in a stroke. The following suggest MCA territory:

- **Loss of use of contralateral face and arm**
- **Loss of feeling in contralateral face and arm**
- **Dysphasia: if dominant hemisphere**
- **Visuospatial disorder: if non-dominant**
- **Contralateral homonymous hemianopia**

LEARNING POINTS

ℹ A lesion to the anterior cerebral artery causes motor and/or sensory loss in contralateral leg.

ℹ **Ischaemic strokes** can be classified into four clinical subtypes based on neurological deficit and vascular territory affected:

- Total anterior circulation infarct (TACI): higher dysfunction (eg dysphasia), motor and/or sensory deficit, and homonymous hemianopia
- Partial anterior circulation infarct (PACI): two of three TACI criteria
- Lacunar infarct (LACI: small penetrating arteries supplying internal capsule, basal ganglia and thalamus): unilateral weakness and/or sensory loss; no evidence of higher cerebral dysfunction
- Posterior circulation infarct (POCI): cerebellar or brainstem syndromes, loss of consciousness, isolated homonymous hemianopia

Q 5. **Is George's stroke due to infarction or haemorrhage?**   1 mark

A **Infarction.**

LEARNING POINTS

ℹ There are two main types of stroke: 15% caused by haemorrhage and 85% owing to infarction (ie as a result of local thrombus formation), atherothromboembolism (eg thrombus associated with atheroma in arterial supply to brain) or a heart embolus (all three cause infarction by occluding the cerebral artery).

NEUROLOGY

ⓘ A stroke due to infarction is visualised as a low-density area (ie black on CT scan) with loss of grey/white-matter differentiation. There is often a surrounding whiter area owing to cerebral oedema. Haemorrhage initially appears as an area of increased density (ie white). Occasionally, infarcted brain can become haemorrhagic, causing a further deterioration in the patient's condition.

ⓘ It is important to differentiate between haemorrhage and infarction (or other pathology), as their management differs. This is not possible clinically, so all patients should have a CT brain within 24 hours: if CT shows infarction, give aspirin (300 mg daily, either orally or rectally).

ⓘ Urgent CT brain is indicated with deteriorating consciousness and known coagulopathy, to exclude potentially reversible causes (eg expanding cerebellar or cerebral haematoma requiring surgical evacuation) or indications for thrombolysis (with alteplase) – patients with confirmed infarction on imaging who present within 4½ hours of definite onset of symptoms and with no contraindications to thrombolysis.

George is thrombolysed and transferred to the stroke ward for rehabilitation, where over the following weeks he makes good progress.

Q 6. **Name six health professionals involved in George's rehabilitation.** 3 marks

A **½ mark each for any from the following list.**

Rehabilitation of stroke patients (in hospital and back in the community) involves a multidisciplinary approach:

- **Physician/GP: to treat modifiable risk factors such as hypertension, hyperlipidaemia**
- **Dietitian: to address any nutritional problems as a result of the stroke (eg dysphagia)**
- **Physiotherapist: to help reduce spasticity, increase mobility**
- **Occupational therapist: to reduce functional disabilities**
- **Speech therapist: to treat any dysphagia, dysphasia, dysarthria**
- **Community nurse: to enable the patient to continue to live at home**
- **Social worker: to ensure the appropriate care package is in place**

NEUROLOGY

LEARNING POINT

ⓘ Initially blood pressure following a stroke may be high owing to disturbance of cerebral autoregulation. It should not be treated in the acute phase, as it may impair cerebral perfusion (unless there is coexisting hypertensive encephalopathy).

Total: **10 marks**

NEUROLOGY

NEUROLOGY CASE 2

Lisa, a 21-year-old student, is brought into the Emergency Department after having a 'black-out' while watching TV at home with one of her flatmates.

Q 1. **What 6 questions would you ask Lisa's flatmate?**　　　　3 marks

A **½ mark each for any of the following:**

- **What was patient doing when episode happened? Watching TV can trigger a seizure**
- **Was there any loss of consciousness?**
- **How long did the episode last? It may last minutes with a seizure**
- **Where there any movements (eg jerky movements of arms and legs suggests seizure; typically flaccid during vasovagal)?**
- **Any injury (eg tongue biting is suggestive of a seizure)?**
- **Any incontinence? Urinary incontinence is non-specific, faecal incontinence is suggestive of a seizure**
- **Any colour change? Pale/green suggests vasovagal syncope (VS)**
- **How soon did patient come around? Rapid recovery with no confusion and amnesia suggests VS or arrhythmias; sleepiness with confusion and amnesia suggests epilepsy**

LEARNING POINT

ⓘ There are a number of causes of a black-out (eg vasovagal syncope, epilepsy, arrhythmias), so it is very important to take a detailed history from both the patient and a witness to help establish the diagnosis (eg it is often possible to diagnose vasovagal syncope or epilepsy on clinical grounds alone).

Lisa's flatmate tells you that she suddenly stopped talking, fell to the floor and then started moving her arms and legs in jerky movements. Lisa has no memory of the attack itself and had no warning of it happening.

Q 2. **List six causes of seizures.**   3 marks

A **½ mark each for any of the following:**

- **Genetic: primary generalised seizure**
- **Alcohol: both intoxication and withdrawal**
- **Drugs (eg tricyclics); also withdrawal of certain drugs (eg benzodiazepines)**
- **Stroke**
- **Pyrexia: in young children (febrile convulsion)**
- **Infection (ie meningitis, encephalitis)**
- **Metabolic abnormalities (eg hyponatraemia, hypoglycaemia – rare in non-diabetics): always check blood glucose when managing a seizure**
- **Space-occupying lesion (eg brain tumour)**
- **Head injury**

LEARNING POINTS

ⓘ Seizures are the result of abnormal electrical activity in part or all of the brain; convulsions are the **motor** signs of a seizure. Epilepsy is defined as a recurrent tendency to spontaneous seizures.

ⓘ Epilepsy can be classified according to whether the seizure is due to electrical activity occurring immediately within both hemispheres (primary generalised seizure) or within a focal part of the brain (partial seizure). Partial seizures may remain focal or may spread to involve both hemispheres, causing secondary generalised seizures (see below).

ⓘ The features associated with a partial seizure (eg temporal lobe epilepsy) depend on the location of the epileptic activity. In *secondary* generalised seizures these focal features may precede the generalised seizure and are termed the aura (ie warning to the patient of an impending seizure); in *primary* generalised seizures there is no warning (as in Lisa's case). However, often the main indications that a seizure has a focal cause are the post-epileptic features (eg unilateral weakness (Todd's palsy) indicates a focal motor cause). When a patient presents with features suggestive of a focal cause for their seizure (or from their electroencephalogram (EEG)), underlying structural disease (eg space-occupying lesion), must be excluded by magnetic resonance imaging (MRI).

Lisa is discharged the next morning following her suspected seizure with a neurology outpatient appointment arranged.

Q 3. **What advice should Lisa receive about driving?** 1 mark

A **Patient should not drive for 1 year.**

LEARNING POINT

ⓘ Following a seizure, patients should not drive for 1 year. This discussion should be clearly documented in the patient's notes. It is the patient's responsibility to notify the DVLA, but if the patient's doctor believes the patient is continuing to drive against advice, they can break patient confidentiality and inform the DVLA.

Q 4. **What is the most useful investigation to confirm the diagnosis of epilepsy?** 1 mark

A **Electroencephalogram (EEG).**

LEARNING POINT

ⓘ During a seizure the EEG is abnormal, showing focal (eg in the temporal lobe) or generalised 3/per second spike and wave activity, confirming the type of epilepsy (partial or generalised). However, in about 60–70% of patients the EEG is normal between seizures (may also get false positives, so should only be performed to support a diagnosis of epilepsy); the chance of detecting epileptic activity can be increased by repeat EEGs during sleep or by specific methods (eg hyperventilating or photic (light) stimulation).

Several weeks later Lisa has a second tonic-clonic seizure, and her neurologist decides to start her on anticonvulsive treatment.

Q 5. **What is first-line treatment for Lisa's type of epilepsy?** 1 mark

A **Sodium valproate.**

LEARNING POINT

ⓘ Sodium valproate is the first-line anti-epileptic drug (AED) for *primary* tonic-clonic seizures. Carbamazepine or lamotrigine are first-line for partial seizures (with or without secondary generalisation).

ⓘ Withdrawal may be considered if seizure-free for more than 2 years. The AED should be withdrawn slowly (over months); patients should not drive from commencement of withdrawal to 6 months after cessation.

NEUROLOGY

Q 6. **How would you treat a prolonged seizure?** 3 marks

A **½ mark each for any from the following list.**

Treatment of prolonged seizures (status epilepticus if seizure > 30 minutes) involves:

- **Secure airway (eg lay in recovery position, suction, remove loose-fitting teeth, consider airway adjuncts)**
- **High-flow oxygen**
- **Check blood glucose (eg fingerprick test)**
- **Intravenous access**
- **Intravenous lorazepam: 4 mg; if unable to obtain IV access, consider rectal diazepam or buccal midazolam**
- **If seizure continues, intravenous phenytoin infusion**
- **Anaesthetic management: paralysis and ventilation**

LEARNING POINTS

ⓘ Patients with a history of prolonged or repeated seizures may be prescribed buccal midazolam or rectal diazepam for treatment in the community while awaiting further care.

ⓘ Investigations in prolonged seizure (and following first seizure) may include: full blood count, coagulation screen (if coagulopathy suspected/known), urea and electrolytes, liver function tests, calcium, glucose, toxicology screen (if indicated from history), anticonvulsant levels (if already on AEDs).

Q 7. **What advice concerning anti-epileptic drugs do you give women of childbearing age?** 3 marks

A **1 mark each for any of the following:**

- **Warn about interactions of AEDs with the oral contraceptive pill (OCP)**
- **Explain about the risk of untreated epilepsy during pregnancy**
- **Explain about the risk of teratogenicity with anti-epileptic drugs**

LEARNING POINT

ⓘ Some AEDs induce hepatic enzymes and therefore increase metabolism of the combined oral contraceptive pill (COC). A higher dose COC is recommended (50 microg of oestrogen as a starting dose) or discuss alternative options (eg intrauterine device).

ℹ The main priority in pregnant women is to control seizures, as the risk of harm to both the mother and fetus during a seizure may outweigh the risk of AEDs.

ℹ AEDs, particularly sodium valproate (often the woman is switched to a less teratogenic AED pre-conception), increase the risk of congenital abnormalities, including neural tube defects (NTDs). To reduce the risk of NTDs the woman should take 5 mg folic acid pre-conception and during pregnancy. They should also be offered alpha-fetoprotein measurements and an ultrasound scan at 18–20 weeks to screen for structural anomalies.

Total: **15 marks**

NEUROLOGY CASE 3

Harold, a 68-year-old man, is referred to neurology outpatients. As he enters the consultation room, you note that he has a very slow, shuffling gait suggestive of Parkinson's disease.

Q 1. What are the three main features of Parkinson's disease?   3 marks

A 1 mark each for the three features.

The three main (motor) features of Parkinson's disease, which may occur in isolation or together, unilaterally or bilaterally, are:

- **Tremor: see below for distinguishing features. May affect hands, tongue, lips and legs**
- **Rigidity: described as lead-pipe rigidity in limbs, trunk and neck. Cogwheel rigidity is due to combined rigidity and tremor. This is best elicited by passively rolling the wrist, feeling for a juddering sensation**
- **Bradykinesia, ie slowness of movement: causes slow shuffling gait, especially when turning (festination refers to difficulty in stopping), expressionless face with reduced blinking, reduced fidgeting, quiet monotonous speech and micrographia (spidery writing). Bradykinesia can be assessed in the hands by asking the patient to simulate playing the piano and in the legs by tapping their heel**

LEARNING POINTS

❶ Parkinson's disease is a clinical diagnosis on the basis of its characteristic features (± resolution of symptoms on an L-dopa trial). Falls (due to postural instability) are also very common in Parkinson's disease and are often considered the fourth characteristic feature.

❶ Typically patients complain of difficulty in rolling over in bed, difficulty in getting out of a chair, progressive slowing down (eg in walking, getting dressed) and deterioration in their handwriting.

Q 2. **List three characteristic features of a parkinsonism tremor.**   **3 marks**

A **1 mark for each from the following list.**

There are several characteristic features of a parkinsonism tremor that allow it to be differentiated from the other forms of tremor (ie intention and postural tremor):

- **The tremor is slow (described as pill-rolling, of thumb over finger)**
- **The tremor is worse at rest**
- **The tremor is reduced (or eliminated) on distraction**
- **The tremor is reduced (or eliminated) on movement**
- **The tremor is often asymmetrical (or even unilateral)**

LEARNING POINTS

ⓘ **Intention tremor** is associated with cerebellar disease (eg multiple sclerosis, cerebellar stroke, alcohol misuse). The tremor is worse on movement (eg finger–nose test). It is associated with other features of cerebellar disease (eg dysdiadokokinesis, gait ataxia).

ⓘ **Postural tremor** is typically rapid and worsened by a particular posture (eg arms outstretched). May be due to exaggerated physiological tremor (eg anxiety, hyperthyroidism), drugs (eg β-agonists), or benign essential tremor (typically a family history, eased by alcohol; propranolol is an effective treatment).

On the basis of the history and examination you diagnose Parkinson's disease.

Q 3. **Other than Parkinson's disease, list two other causes of parkinsonism.**

2 marks

A **1 mark each for any from the following list.**

While Parkinson's disease is the most common cause of parkinsonism, other causes include:

- **Drugs, eg neuroleptics (dopamine receptor antagonists – eg haloperidol), metoclopramide**
- **Stroke**

NEUROLOGY

- **Wilson's disease: toxic accumulation of copper in liver (causing cirrhosis) and brain**
- **Progressive supranuclear palsy: characterised by absent vertical gaze and dementia**
- **Multisystem atrophy (MSA): characterised by autonomic failure (eg postural hypotension)**

LEARNING POINT

ℹ 'Parkinson plus syndromes' (eg MSA, PSP) refers to the neurodegenerative diseases with the classic features of Parkinson's disease and additional features that help distinguish them from Parkinson's disease. These syndromes are usually more rapidly progressive and less likely to respond to Parkinson's disease medication.

Q 4. **What is the underlying pathophysiology of Parkinson's disease?**   1 mark

A **Loss of dopaminergic neurones in the substantia nigra of the midbrain.**

LEARNING POINTS

ℹ The substantia nigra forms part of the basal ganglia (ie extrapyramidal system), which is responsible for the initiation and maintenance of fast, fluid movement. Parkinson's disease is a progressive neurodegenerative disorder due to loss of dopaminergic neurones in the substantia nigra, which normally communicates with the corpus striatum using dopamine as the neurotransmitter. The corpus striatum still receives cholinergic (ACh) stimulation that normally opposes the action of dopamine, but in its absence causes inhibition of the motor cortex, causing parkinsonism symptoms/signs.

ℹ Dopamine itself is synthesised by dopa decarboxylase (DOPA) and inactivated by catechol-O-methyltransferase (COMT) and monoamine oxidase B (MAO_B).

Several months later Harold is started on L-dopa, which greatly improves his motor symptoms.

Q 5. **What class of drug is combined with L-dopa to prevent peripheral side-effects?**   1 mark

A **Dopa decarboxylase (DOPA) inhibitor – ie beneserazide, carbidopa (in combination with L-dopa are called co-beneldopa and co-careldopa, respectively).**

NEUROLOGY

LEARNING POINTS

ⓘ Typically first-line treatment is with a dopamine receptor agonist (eg bromocriptine, ropinirole: these agonists have been associated with impulse control disorders such as pathological gambling), although eventually all patients will require L-dopa.

ⓘ L-dopa is a precursor of dopamine (which cannot cross the blood–brain barrier) that is converted to dopamine by DOPA both peripherally and within the brain. It is given with an extracerebral DOPA inhibitor to prevent peripheral dopamine conversion and its associated side-effects (eg nausea and vomiting, which is treated with domperidone (dopamine antagonist that does not cross the blood–brain barrier)).

Q 6. **Name three limitations of L-dopa therapy.**   3 marks

A **1 mark each for any of the following:**
- **Reduced efficacy over time (even with increasing doses)**
- **L-dopa-induced dyskinesias**
- *On-off* **effect: fluctuations in motor performance between normal function (on) and restricted mobility (off)**
- **Shortening of duration of action of each dose (ie end-of-dose deterioration: dyskinesias often become prominent at the end of the duration of action)**

LEARNING POINTS

ⓘ Due to these limitations, commencement of L-dopa therapy is typically delayed, initially using alternative treatments (eg dopamine agonists) to treat the motor symptoms.

ⓘ Modified-release preparations and/or MAO_B inhibitors (eg selegiline) and/or COMT inhibitors (eg entacaone) may help the end-of-dose deterioration.

ⓘ Surgery (eg deep-brain stimulation) is usually reserved for patients in whom motor symptoms are refractory to medical treatment.

Harold is followed up for his Parkinson's disease by a nurse specialist, who also enquires about common non-motor symptoms.

NEUROLOGY

Q 7. **List two non-motor symptoms of Parkinson's disease.** 2 marks

A **1 mark each for any from the following list.**

Patients with Parkinson's disease are often more disabled by the non-motor symptoms of the disease:

- **Fatigue: very common, due to muscle fatigue from tremor and rigidity and fluctuations in mobility**
- **Dementia**
- **Depression: very common, although it may be difficult to diagnose due to the quiet monotonous voice and difficulties with facial expression, which make patients appear depressed even when they are not**
- **Constipation: due to slowing of bowel motility and reduced mobility**
- **Problems with eating and swallowing: aspiration is common. Referral to speech and language therapist can help**
- **Poor sleep: due to worsening of Parkinson's symptoms during night, as the effectiveness of medication wears off before the morning dose**

Total: 15 marks

NEUROLOGY

OBSTETRICS AND GYNAECOLOGY CASES: ANSWERS

OBSTETRICS AND GYNAECOLOGY CASE 1

Julie, a 24-year-old teacher, visits her GP on Monday requesting emergency contraception. She recently started a new relationship with a colleague called Paul and had unprotected sexual intercourse on Saturday night. She is on the ninth day of her 28-day cycle.

Q 1. **What would you advise Julie?**   2 marks

A **1 mark each for any of the following:**

- **She is at risk of pregnancy and should be offered emergency contraception (EC)**

- **She could have hormonal EC: levonorgestrel (single dose of 1.5 mg within 72 hours of unprotected sexual intercourse (UPSI), or ulipristal (single dose of 30 mg within 5 days of UPSI); the sooner she takes this the more effective it is. Subsequent period may be early or late: if any doubt menstruation has occurred, perform pregnancy test at least 3 weeks following UPSI**

- **She could have a copper IUD fitted. This is more effective than hormonal EC, and she could use it for future contraception as well. This can be fitted up to 5 days after UPSI or up to 5 days after the earliest expected date of ovulation (whichever is the later). In this example, she has a 28-day cycle, therefore the copper IUD could be fitted up until day 19 of her cycle. This is because implantation happens at least 5 days after ovulation. The patient should also be screened for sexually transmitted infections and given prophylactic antibiotics (eg azithromycin) when the IUD is inserted**

- **Discuss the risk of sexually transmitted infections: offer screening or referral to GUM clinic**

- **Discuss regular contraception: offer follow-up consultation**

Julie chooses the pill for future contraception.

Q 2. **Describe two contraceptive mechanisms of the combined oral contraceptive (COC).** 1 mark

A **1 mark for any of the following:**

- **Oestrogen and progesterone exert negative feedback on GnRH, LH and FSH, preventing follicular development and ovulation**
- **Progestogen causes endometrial atrophy, preventing implantation**
- **Progestogen acts on cervical mucus, making it hostile to ascending sperm**

LEARNING POINT

ⓘ The COC contains both oestrogen and progestogen. In general the preparation with the lowest content of both to provide good cycle control is prescribed (to minimise side-effects). The COC is one of the most reliable and popular methods of contraception and, if used properly, less than one in a hundred women will become pregnant in a year.

Q 3. **List six contraindications to the COC.** 3 marks

A **½ mark each for any of the following:**

- **Breastfeeding: impairs lactation**
- **Ischaemic heart disease (IHD) or multiple ($\geq$ 2) risk factors for IHD, including: hypertensive (avoid if > 160/95 mmHg), family history, smoker, age > 35 years (avoid if > 50 years), obesity, diabetes (avoid if complications)**
- **Previous stroke**
- **Focal migraine with aura (causes cerebral ischaemia, increasing the risk of stroke)**
- **Previous deep vein thrombosis/pulmonary embolism (DVT/PE) or multiple risk factors for venous thromboembolism (eg thrombophilia, prolonged immobilisation)**
- **Liver disease: cirrhosis (severe decompensated disease), liver tumour, active viral hepatitis**
- **Breast cancer (as potentially oestrogen-sensitive)**

OBS & GYNAE

LEARNING POINTS

🛈 Blood pressure must be checked when prescribing the COC; stop if
> 160/95 mmHg.

🛈 The contraindications to the COC relate mainly to oestrogen, which induces
a prothrombotic state, thus increasing the risk of IHD, stroke and DVT/PE. If a
woman is contraindicated the COC, she may be prescribed the progestogen-
only pill (POP).

Nothing in Julie's history contraindicates the pill. She is prescribed a
3-month supply of a COC and advised on its side-effects.

Q 4. **Name four *minor* side-effects Julie may experience.**   2 marks

A **½ mark for any of the following:**
- **Depression**
- **Headaches**
- **Loss of libido**
- **Nausea and vomiting**
- **Breast tenderness**
- **Oligomenorrhoea**
- **Breakthrough bleeding/spotting (in first few cycles)**
- **Chloasma (facial pigmentation)**
- **Fluid retention**

LEARNING POINTS

🛈 Weight gain is not associated with the COC.

🛈 More serious (though rare) side-effects include DVT/PE, stroke, IHD, liver
impairment, cervical cancer and breast cancer (any increased risk disappears
10 years after cessation). However, these risks must be weighed against the
reduced risk of ovarian and endometrial cancer.

OBS & GYNAE

Q 5. List four pieces of additional advice you would give Julie.   2 marks

A ½ mark each for any of the following:

- When to start the pill – ie start on first day of period so as to exclude pregnancy. Can be started on the same day as miscarriage or abortion, though should be delayed for 3 weeks after childbirth.

- Limitations of the COC (eg it does not protect against sexually transmitted infections (STIs)).

- Factors that reduce its effectiveness (eg if diarrhoea or vomiting within 2 hours of taking the pill, take another pill as soon as possible, if taking liver enzyme inducing medication (eg rifampicin, certain anticonvulsants), need additional contraceptive precautions during and for 4 weeks after stopping).

- Missed pill: if she forgets the pill, she must take one as soon as she remembers (even if this means taking two pills together). If ≥ 2 pills are missed, needs an additional form of contraception for the next 7 days

- Availability of emergency contraception

- Symptoms requiring immediate consultation (eg focal neurological signs, prolonged headache, sudden severe chest pain, shortness of breath, haemoptysis, calf pain, jaundice)

- Major surgery: owing to risk of DVT/PE, should stop 4 weeks before elective major surgery and only restart 2 weeks after full mobilisation

- When you need to see her again (eg repeat prescription, blood pressure check) (see above)

- Preconception advice (eg folate supplements), to wait for one natural period after stopping the pill before attempting conception (so can accurately date pregnancy using last menstrual period)

Total: 10 marks

OBSTETRICS AND GYNAECOLOGY CASE 2

Paul and Julie (aged 37 and 33 years, respectively) visit their GP following 2 years of being unable to conceive. A full history is taken from both.

Q 1. **What general advice would you give to couples trying to get pregnant?**

2 marks

A **½ mark each for any of the following:**

- **Timing of intercourse: recommend intercourse every 2–3 days. It is not recommended to attempt to time intercourse around ovulation, as this is unreliable and stressful**
- **Stop smoking: smoking is associated with decreased fertility in females and reduced semen quality in males**
- **Reduce alcohol intake: excessive alcohol intake in women carries risks for the fetus (fetal alcohol syndrome); in males excessive alcohol intake reduces semen quality**
- **Optimise weight: a body mass index (BMI) < 19 (with irregular periods) or > 29 is likely to be associated with reduced female fertility. In addition, men with a BMI > 29 are likely to have reduced fertility**
- **Preconception advice: eg folic acid 0.4 mg, rubella screening (if non-immune, offer the rubella vaccination and advise against getting pregnant for at least 1 month following vaccination)**

LEARNING POINT

ⓘ As many as 84% of couples in the general population will have conceived within 1 year of having regular unprotected sexual intercourse; 50% of women who do not conceive in the first year are likely to do so in the second year.

Q 2. **List four points that you might elicit in Julie's history that would be suggestive of tubal dysfunction.** 2 marks

A **½ mark each for any of the following:**

1. **Abdominal or pelvic surgery (eg appendectomy)**
2. **Endometriosis**
3. **Peritonitis (eg as a complication of appendicitis)**
4. **History of pelvic inflammatory disease (PID) or sexually transmitted infection (STI)**
5. **Previous ectopic pregnancy**
6. **Tubal ligation (for sterilisation)**

LEARNING POINT

ⓘ It is estimated that tubal factors are responsible for approximately 14% of infertility cases. Tubal disease includes pelvic adhesions and tubal obstruction: Pelvic adhesions (1–3): may affect tubal motility and ovum pick-up. Laparoscopy with dye is the investigation of choice to assess the pelvis, tubes and ovaries.

Tubal obstruction (4–6): impaired tubal patency is investigated by either hysterosalpingography (HSG) – radiopaque dye is instilled through the cervix and should 'leak out' at the end of the tubes into the peritoneal cavity; or by HyCoSy (hysterosalpingo-contrast-sonography) – fluid is introduced into the uterus and flow along the fallopian tubes is assessed by transvaginal ultrasound.

The results of semen analysis and ovulation assessment must be known before investigating tubal function.

As an initial assessment the GP organises a semen analysis for Paul and requests a day-21 progesterone level from Julie.

Q 3. **List three variables measured in semen analysis.** 3 marks

A **1 mark each for any of the variables listed in the table opposite.**

OBS & GYNAE

Variable	Normal range
Volume	> 2 ml
Liquefacation time	within 60 minutes
Sperm concentration	> 20 million/ml
Total sperm count	> 40 million
Motility	> 50% with normal progression
Morphology	> 30% with normal morphology
Vitality	> 75% live
White cell count	< 1 million/ml

LEARNING POINTS

ⓘ If the initial analysis is abnormal, another semen specimen is evaluated; if the second analysis is normal, there is no need for repeat analysis. The best time for the second sample is at least 3 months after the initial sample because the cycle of spermatozoa formation takes about 3 months to complete (although in practice, to minimise anxiety, it is typically repeated after 1 month).

ⓘ Low sperm count or quality (which is typically idiopathic) is found to be the only cause of infertility in about 20% of couples and is a contributory factor in a further 25% of couples.

ⓘ Azoospermia (ie no sperm) is due to primary testicular failure (eg torsion, chemotherapy), hypogonadotrophic hypogonadism (due to luteinising hormone (LH) and follicle-stimulating hormone (FSH) deficiency) or obstructive azoospermia (eg congenital bilateral absence of vas deferens).

The results come back confirming normal semen analysis. Julie's day-21 progesterone concentration is 8 nmol/l.

Q 4. **What is a normal day-21 progesterone concentration?**　　　　1 mark

A **> 25 nmol/l.**

OBS & GYNAE

255

LEARNING POINT

ⓘ Progesterone level is the most commonly used test to assess whether ovulation occurs. Ovulation refers to the release of an egg from the mature follicle in the ovary, stimulated by LH surge. The mature follicle forms the corpus luteum, which under the influence of LH secretes progesterone, which prepares the endometrium for implantation. In the absence of pregnancy, progesterone levels begin to decline about 7 days after ovulation, and this results in shedding of the endometrial lining (menstruation). In a 28-day cycle ovulation occurs 2 weeks before the next period and progesterone levels peak on day 21 (mid-luteal phase).

Q 5. **Give two explanations for Julie's low progesterone concentration.**   2 marks

A **1 mark for each of the following:**
- **Anovulation, eg due to polycystic ovarian syndrome**
- **Incorrect cycle dates**

LEARNING POINTS

ⓘ Regular menstrual cycles are usually indicative of ovulation. However, in women with regular menstrual cycles and more than 2 years' infertility, measure day-21 (in a 28-day cycle) progesterone to confirm ovulation. Women with irregular cycles may need serial blood tests until the next menstrual cycle begins.

ⓘ Ovulatory disorders are responsible for 20% of infertility cases. The cause of infertility is unexplained in 30% of couples.

Julie is referred to gynaecology, where she is diagnosed with polycystic ovarian syndrome (PCOS).

Q 6. **List three clinical features that Julie might have.**   3 marks

A **1 mark each for any from the following list.**
Typical clinical features of PCOS are:
- **Obesity: approximately 40% of females with PCOS are obese**
- **Acne**

- **Virilisation: development of male secondary sexual characteristics (eg deep voice, clitoromegaly)**
- **Hirsutism: presence of excessive facial and bodily hair in a male pattern (though may be disguised)**
- **Menstrual disturbance: amenorrhoea, oligomenorrhoea**

LEARNING POINTS

🛈 Polycystic ovarian syndrome (PCOS) is associated with irregular cycles, anovulation, raised LH producing a LH:FSH ratio ≥ 2:1 (normally 1:1) and androgen excess. Ultrasound scan can demonstrate polycystic ovaries ('string of pearls' sign, ie peripheral small cysts (follicles) > 12 with increased ovarian volume).

🛈 Polycystic ovarian syndrome is related to hyperinsulinaemia and insulin resistance, causing excessive androgen secretion. Obesity worsens the underlying androgen excess owing to adipose tissue conversion of oestrogens to androgens. Treatment of infertility involves weight loss and ovulation induction with clomifene; may involve adjuvant treatment with ovarian drilling (a laparoscopic procedure which involves puncturing a number of follicles to induce ovulation). Metformin is also used, although it remains unlicensed for the treatment of PCOS.

Julie's infertility is treated with clomifene.

Q 7. **List two complications associated with this treatment.**   2 marks

A **1 mark each for any of the following:**
- **Ovarian hyperstimulation syndrome (OHSS): OHSS causes abdominal distension due to ovarian enlargement and cyst formation. Severe hyperstimulation can cause thromboembolic events, ascites and pulmonary effusions. Prevention requires carefully monitoring via ultrasound scanning and early recognition of the symptoms**
- **Multiple pregnancy: affects approximately 20% of clomifene-treated pregnancies**
- **Ovarian cancer: may increase risk of ovarian cancer and therefore its use is restricted typically to six cycles**

LEARNING POINTS

❶ Clomifene is an oestrogen antagonist that acts by preventing normal negative oestrogen feedback in the hypothalamus, thereby increasing gonadotropin-releasing hormone (GnRH) and hence gonadotropins, which stimulate the ovary to produce more follicles.

❶ Other treatments for infertility include intrauterine insemination (IUI) and in-vitro fertilisation (IVF).

Total: **15 marks**

OBSTETRICS AND GYNAECOLOGY CASE 3

Julie and her husband Paul are both delighted to discover that she is pregnant after many years of trying. Julie is now ten weeks pregnant (her last menstrual period (LMP) was on 15 July and her cycle is normally a regular 28 days) and she attends the antenatal clinic for her booking visit.

Q 1. **When is Julie's expected date of delivery according to Naegele's rule?** 1 mark

A **21 April.**

LEARNING POINT

ℹ The due date is estimated by taking the first day of a woman's last menstrual period, subtracting 3 months, adding 1 week and adjusting the year if necessary. However, this assumes the cycle length is 28 days and is therefore less accurate if ovulation happens early/late or menstrual periods are irregular.

Q 2. **List four blood tests you would offer.** 2 marks

A **½ mark each for any of the following:**

- **Full blood count: to exclude anaemia (< 10.5 g/dl in pregnant women). The most common cause is iron deficiency as iron requirements are increased in pregnancy; it also drops during pregnancy because of haemodilution (due to increase in plasma volume)**
- **ABO group: in case the mother requires an urgent blood transfusion; also required in investigation of neonatal jaundice (due to ABO incompatibility between mother and baby)**
- **Rhesus status**
- **Red cell alloantibodies**
- **Haemoglobinopathies (sickle cell disease and thalassaemia), if considered high risk (eg from family origin questionnaire)**
- **Rubella antibodies: ideally screen preconception and, if negative, immunise**

OBS & GYNAE

259

(MMR vaccine) and practise safe sex for ≥ 3 months. If non-immunity is only discovered at the booking visit, educate on importance of avoiding contact with infected individuals, and immunise postnatally

- **Syphilis serology: need to exclude syphilis, which may cause congenital syphilis**
- **Hepatitis B virus and HIV: measures need to be taken to prevent vertical transmission**

LEARNING POINTS

🛈 Also perform urine dipstick. If a urinary tract infection is suspected, send sample for culture. Asymptomatic bacteriuria during pregnancy can progress to pyelonephritis, which is associated with preterm labour, fetal death and intrauterine growth retardation (IUGR). Proteinuria in conjunction with raised blood pressure may indicate pre-eclampsia (occurs later in pregnancy).

🛈 Rhesus haemolytic disease occurs when a Rhesus negative (Rh−ve) mother gives birth to a Rhesus positive (Rh+ve) baby. If Rh+ve fetal cells cross the placenta the mother may produce anti-Rhesus antibodies (anti-D are the most common antibodies), which in a subsequent pregnancy may cross the placenta into the fetal circulation and cause haemolysis. To prevent isoimmunisation all Rh−ve women are given anti-D antibodies at 28 and 34 weeks and following any potential 'leaks' (eg abortion, ectopic pregnancy, amniocentesis/CVS, ante-partum haemorrhage) and delivery (if infant is Rh+ve).

🛈 The schedule of appointments in routine antenatal care is as follows:
- 10 weeks: booking scan – gestational age should be determined using the crown-rump length
- 16 weeks: discuss blood results, manage anaemia (eg iron supplements) BP + proteinuria
- 18–20 weeks: anomaly scan
- 28 and 34 weeks: includes measurement of BP, proteinuria and symphysis–fundal height. Anti-D prophylaxis, if appropriate. Repeat screen for anaemia and red cell alloantibodies at 28 weeks
- 36, 38, 40, 41 and 42 weeks: offer membrane sweep at 41 weeks.

Q 3. **List four examples of dietary advice you would give Julie.** 2 marks

A ½ mark each for any of the following:
- **Take 400 µg/day folic acid: this should ideally be taken preconception and during the first trimester to reduce risks of neural tube defects (eg anencephaly,**

spina bifida). Women who are diabetic, obese or on anti-epileptic drugs should take 5 mg/day

- **Vitamin D supplements:** 10 μg/day throughout pregnancy
- **Eat plenty of fruit and vegetables**
- **Avoid vitamin A supplementation** (potentially teratogenic) and liver (which contains high vitamin A levels)
- **Prevent** *Listeria* infection (may cause mid-trimester miscarriage, preterm labour, congenital listeriosis) by avoiding drinking unpasteurised milk, soft cheeses (eg brie), pâté and any uncooked/undercooked meals
- **Prevent** *Toxoplasma* infection (may cause congenital abnormalities) by avoiding raw/undercooked meats (eg steaks) and by always washing hands after handling raw meat
- **Prevent** *Salmonella* infection (may cause neonatal septicaemia) by avoiding raw eggs, including mayonnaise and raw/undercooked meats, especially poultry
- **Avoid alcohol in first trimester** (may cause fetal alcohol syndrome) and limit intake to 1 unit/day for 1 or 2 days a week thereafter

Q 4. List four common minor symptoms of pregnancy Julie may experience.   2 marks

A ½ mark each for any of the following:

- **Nausea and vomiting:** affects up to 75% of women. Typically worse during the first trimester
- **Backache:** common in late pregnancy. Felt over the sacroiliac joints, owing to progesterone-mediated relaxation of ligaments and muscles
- **Breathlessness:** caused by progesterone-induced hyperventilation, lowering maternal $PaCO_2$ so as to increase CO_2 exchange across the placenta from fetus to mother
- **Constipation:** caused by progesterone-mediated reduced gut motility, exacerbated in late pregnancy by pressure of enlarged uterus. Ensure adequate fluid and fibre intake
- **Heartburn:** caused by progesterone-mediated relaxation of lower oesophageal sphincter
- **Hypotension:** owing to changes in the cardiovascular system (peripheral resistance falls during pregnancy)
- **Urinary frequency:** due to pressure of fetal head on the bladder (need to exclude urinary tract infection)

OBS & GYNAE

- **Ankle oedema: due to fluid retention and mechanical obstruction preventing venous return**
- **Varicose veins: compression stockings may help symptoms**
- **Haemorrhoids**
- **Itching: pruritus gravidarum begins in the third trimester: treat with aqueous cream. Need to check LFTs to exclude cholestasis of pregnancy (rare condition associated with prematurity and perinatal death)**

Because of her age Julie requests screening for Down syndrome.

Q 5. **Name two markers measured to screen for trisomy 21.**   2 marks

A ½ **mark each for any of the following:**

- **Nuchal translucency (NT): ultrasound measurement of translucent subcutaneous space (due to fluid accumulation) at the back of the fetal neck Increased thickness of fluid is associated with fetal abnormalities (chromosomal and structural)**
- **Alpha fetoprotein (AFP): low levels of AFP are associated with trisomy 21; high levels are associated with structural abnormalities (eg neural tube defects)**
- **Beta-hCG (human chorionic gonadothropin): increased in trisomy 21**
- **Pregnancy-associated plasma protein A (PAPP-A): decreased in trisomy 21**
- **Unconjugated oestriol (uE$_3$): decreased in trisomy 21**
- **Inhibin A: increased in trisomy 21**

LEARNING POINT

ⓘ Various combinations of the above are used in the first or second trimester to screen for trisomy 21 (Down syndrome). The combined test (on the basis of NT, hCG and PAPP-A) is used to screen for Down syndrome between 11 and 14 weeks. The quadruple test (AFP, uE$_3$, β-hCG, inhibin A) is used to screen between 15 and 20 weeks. These tests will estimate the risk of a baby with trisomy 21 (based on maternal age). If the risk is high, the mother is offered a diagnostic test (eg amniocentesis, chorionic villus sampling), although these carry a risk of miscarriage (0.5–2%).

At 34 weeks Julie attends the antenatal clinic for her regular antenatal care. On obstetric examination the midwife finds that the symphysis–fundal height is 30 cm.

OBS & GYNAE

Q 6. **Give two reasons why Julie may be small for dates.** 2 marks

A **1 mark each for any of the following:**
- **Incorrect dates**
- **Intrauterine growth restriction (IUGR)**
- **Constitutionally small baby**
- **Oligohydramnios (ie reduced amniotic fluid – eg due to fetal urinary tract abnormalities, idiopathic)**

LEARNING POINTS

ⓘ Symphysis–fundal height (measured from the fundus to the top of the symphysis pubis in cm) gives a rough estimation of the gestational age of the baby in weeks (eg at 34 weeks the fundal height should be 34 cm ± 3 cm).

ⓘ Causes of large for dates: multiple pregnancy, polyhydramnios, constitutionally large baby, fetal abnormality, maternal diabetes.

Q 7. **List four causes of intrauterine growth restriction (IUGR).** 2 marks

A **½ mark each for any of the following.**

Causes of IUGR can be classified as:
- **Maternal causes: eg malnutrition, smoking, systemic disease (eg renal disease, anaemia)**
- **Placental insufficiency: eg multiple gestation, pre-eclampsia**
- **Fetal causes: eg infections (eg cytomegalovirus), congenital malformations, chromosomal abnormalities (eg Down syndrome, Turner syndrome)**

LEARNING POINTS

ⓘ Intrauterine growth restriction (IUGR) can be divided further into symmetrical and asymmetrical. Asymmetrical IUGR is caused by placental insufficiency – ie the fetus is starved, brain growth (and hence head circumference) is relatively spared at the expense of liver glycogen and fat stores (causing reduced abdominal circumference). Pregnancies at risk of IUGR (eg small for dates) can be monitored, and a decision made whether to continue the pregnancy or deliver the baby on the basis of fetal monitoring, growth charts, gestational age and umbilical artery blood flow (absent or reverse end-diastolic blood flow indicates poor perfusion, causing fetal hypoxia).

ⓘ Babies with IUGR have an increased risk of hypoxia and death (in utero and during labour); hypothermia, hypoglycaemia, jaundice due to polycythaemia (postnatally); and type 2 diabetes, hypertension and cardiovascular disease (in adulthood).

OBS & GYNAE

Julie's blood pressure (BP) is raised at 154/94 mmHg (her booking BP was 116/78 mm Hg) and she has 2+ protein in her urine so she is admitted to the pregnancy assessment unit with pre-eclampsia.

Q 8. List four symptoms associated with pre-eclampsia.   2 marks

A ½ mark each for any of the following:

- **Headaches**
- **Visual disturbance (eg blurring or flashing)**
- **Nausea and vomiting**
- **Swelling of face, hands and feet**
- **Epigastric pain**
- **Irritability**
- **Generalised malaise**

LEARNING POINTS

ℹ️ However, pre-eclampsia may also be asymptomatic, so regular screening is essential. This involves regular antenatal blood pressure checks and urinalysis for proteinuria. Admit the mother if her BP > 30/20 mmHg over booking blood pressure, > 160/100 mmHg or > 140/90 mmHg with proteinuria.

ℹ️ Risk factors for pre-eclampsia include: < 20 or > 35 years of age, BMI > 25, nulliparous, previous pre-eclampsia, family history, multiple gestation, and pre-existing hypertension or renal disease (reduced risk in smokers).

ℹ️ Pre-eclampsia typically develops after 20 weeks (and usually resolves 10 days after delivery) and is a multisystem disorder affecting the placenta (causing IUGR), kidneys, brain (causing eclampsia), liver, blood (causing haemolysis) and coagulation (causing disseminated intravascular coagulation ((DIC)). There is no cure except to terminate the pregnancy and deliver the baby, although in mild to moderate pre-eclampsia BP may be reduced (eg oral labetalol) while awaiting fetal maturation. The timing of birth will depend on the severity of pre-eclampsia and fetal condition (eg from cardiotocography (CTG), ultrasound of fetal growth, umbilical artery Doppler).

ℹ️ HELLP syndrome is a very severe form of pre-eclampsia: **HE**molysis, eleveated **L**iver enzymes (deranged), **L**ow **P**latelet count.

Total: **15 marks**

OBSTETRICS AND GYNAECOLOGY CASE 4

Julie, who is 34^{+5} pregnant, is admitted with pre-eclampsia. Fetal monitoring is reassuring, so her hypertension is treated with labetalol, while her blood pressure and bloods are regularly monitored. At 37 weeks it is decided to induce labour, so her cervix is assessed using the Bishop's score.

Q 1. **List four features used to assess the Bishop's score.**   2 marks

A **½ mark each for any of the following features:**

Feature	Bishop's score			
	0	1	2	3
Dilatation (cm)	< 1	1–2	2–4	> 4
Length of cervix (cm)	> 4	2–4	1–2	< 1
Station (relative to ischial spines)	−3	−2	−1/0	+1/+2
Consistency	Firm	Medium	Soft	Soft
Position	Posterior	Middle	Anterior	Anterior

Q 2. **What Bishop's score is considered favourable for induction?**   1 mark

A **A score of > 5 indicates that the cervix is favourable for induction.**

LEARNING POINT

ⓘ If nulliparous women are induced with an unripe cervix, the risks of prolonged labour, fetal distress and caesarean section are increased.

Q 3. **What is used to make the cervix favourable for induction?**   1 mark

A **Intravaginal prostaglandin: can be administered as pessary, gel or tablet.**

LEARNING POINT

❶ The majority of inductions are started with prostaglandins (PGE$_2$). Once the cervix is favourable, artificial rupture of membranes (ARM or amniotomy) is performed; oxytocin infusion may be used to augment contractions.

Induction of labour is successful. Julie's labour is recorded on her partogram, while her baby is monitored by cardiotocography (CTG) to assess fetal distress.

Q 4. **List six *maternal* observations recorded on the partogram.** 3 marks

A **½ mark each for any of the following.**

The partogram is a graphic record of labour, allowing a visual record of cervical dilatation against the expected norm plus key maternal and fetal observations, thus allowing active management if required:

- **Heart rate, blood pressure and temperature**
- **Strength and frequency of contractions**
- **Cervical dilatation**
- **Urine volume: to exclude maternal dehydration**
- **Urinalysis (eg proteinuria, ketonuria)**
- **Intravenous infusions (eg oxytocin)**
- **Any drugs**
- **Liquor (ie colour of vaginal discharge)**
- **Station: indicating the descent of the presenting part in relation to the ischial spines**

LEARNING POINT

❶ Fetal observations include heart rate (normal range 110–160 bpm), position (displayed graphically), extent of fixing/engagement, moulding or caput.

Q 5. **What four components are used to interpret a CTG?** 2 marks

A **½ mark for each of the following.**

Cardiotocography monitors fetal heart rate alongside uterine contractions and is used in labour to detect fetal hypoxia (supported by passage of fresh meconium and fetal scalp pH < 7.2). The four components used in interpreting a CTG are:

- **Baseline heart rate: should be 110–160 bpm (abnormal if < 100 or > 180)**

- **Baseline variability: baseline heart rate should vary between 6 and 25 bpm (abnormal if it varies < 5 bpm over a 90-minute period)**
- **Accelerations: defined as increase in heart rate of [3] ≥ 15 bpm (from the baseline) for ≥ 15 seconds in response to uterine activity. Reassuring feature**
- **Decelerations: defined as decrease in heart rate of [3] ≥ 15 bpm (from the baseline) for ≥ 15 seconds. The timing of the deceleration in relation to the contractions classifies them into: a) early: trough of deceleration coincides with peak of contraction and are usually considered a normal response to the uterine contraction; b) late: they are considered abnormal; or c) variable: interpretation is more complex**

LEARNING POINT

❶ If CTG is abnormal, lie the mother on her left side (to avoid compression of vena cava, stop any oxytocin infusion and take fetal scalp blood sample; If pH < 7.2 deliver immediately.

Julie's contractions are inefficient, so she is started with an infusion of oxytocin.

Q 6. **List two potential complications of using oxytocin.** 1 mark

A **½ mark for each of the following:**

- **Uterine hyperstimulation: uterus should contract ≤ 4 per 10 minutes. Excessive contractions may cause fetal distress. When labour is induced, the fetus requires regular/continuous CTG monitoring**
- **Water intoxication: oxytocin has antidiuretic hormone- (ADH-) like effects. The risk is reduced by restricting infusion volume**

LEARNING POINTS

❶ In a multiparous woman oxytocin may also cause uterine rupture.

❶ When augmenting labour, oxytocin should be used with care as delay may be due to cephalopelvic disproportion (CPD), as opposed to inefficient uterine contractions.

Julie's contractions become progressively more frequent and painful. Three hours later her cervical dilatation is reassessed (last measurement was 4 cm) and plotted on the partogram, demonstrating that Julie's labour is progressing satisfactorily.

Q 7. **By how many centimetres should the cervix be dilated now?**   1 mark

A **By 7 cm, ie an increase of 3 cm above last recording three hours previously of 4 cm.**

LEARNING POINT

❶ Progress in the active phase (of the first stage of labour) is assessed by cervical dilatation from 3 cm to fully dilated (10 cm) and effaced. Dilatation typically proceeds at 1 cm/h in a primigravida and 2 cm/h in a multigravida.

Q 8. **List four causes of failure to progress in the first stage of labour.**   2 marks

A **½ mark each for any of the following:**
- **Inefficient uterine contractions**
- **Malpresentation (eg face presentation, breech)**
- **Malposition (eg occiput-posterior)**
- **Cephalopelvic disproportion (CPD): disproportion between the fetal head and maternal pelvis**
- **Cervical dystocia: failure of cervical dilatation (eg due to previous trauma, surgery)**

LEARNING POINT

❶ Primary dysfunctional labour is slow progress during the active phase of labour (usually due to inefficient contractions). Secondary arrest is initial satisfactory progress, followed by arrest after 7 cm dilatation (usually caused by CPD or malposition). Causes of delay in the second stage of labour (which should last < 1 hour in a primigravida) include CPD (preventing internal rotation, termed 'deep transverse arrest'), occiput-posterior position, secondary uterine inertia, maternal exhaustion, pain and anxiety.

Q 9. **List four sequential stages in the passage of the fetus through the birth canal, leading up to the delivery of the shoulders.**   4 marks

A **1 mark each for any of the following:**
- **Head engages typically in occiput-transverse position**
- **Head descends further into the pelvis**
- **Head flexes onto chest so that the most favourable (smallest) diameter of the fetal scull presents**

- **Internal rotation (directed by the gutter-shaped pelvic floor) so that the head arrives at the pelvic outlet in the anterior-posterior position**
- **Head extends from underneath the pubic symphysis, starting to distend the vulva, allowing the head to be delivered – this is known as 'crowning'**
- **Restitution of the head so that it aligns with the obliquely placed shoulders**
- **External rotation so that the delivered head rotates to lie in transverse position so that the shoulders lie in anterior-posterior plane**

LEARNING POINT

ℹ This is followed by delivery of the anterior shoulder followed by posterior shoulder and finally by delivery of the rest of body.

Julie delivers a pink and healthy boy called Alex, who cries immediately.

Q 10. **Give two non-pharmacological techniques for reducing postpartum haemorrhage (PPH).** 1 mark

A ½ **mark for each of the following.**

Uterine contraction, which is under hormonal control of oxytocin, can be increased by:

- **Early suckling: stimulates oxytocin release from post-pituitary gland**
- **Rub up a uterine contraction: massage the fundus to stimulate a contraction**

LEARNING POINT

ℹ Postpartum haemorrhage is bleeding from the genital tract, following either vaginal delivery or caesarean section (more common after C-section). Primary PPH is defined as greater than 500 ml bloodloss in the first 24 hours following delivery (secondary PPH refers to any blood loss after 24 hours post-delivery). It is caused either by failure of the uterus to contract (uterine atonia: 70%), damage to the genital tract (20%), retained tissue, inverted uterus or coagulation disorder.

OBS & GYNAE

Q 11. **Name two drugs that are used in the management of postpartum haemorrhage.** 2 marks

A **1 mark for any of the following:**

- **Oxytocin: this is the first-line prophylactic PPH treatment given in the third stage of labour, either as a stat intramuscular dose (for vaginal delivery) or intravenous infusion (following caesarean section)**

- **Ergometrine: careful in hypertensive patients as ergometrine may cause a sudden rise in blood pressure. Syntometrine is combined oxytocin and ergometrine**

- **Prostaglandin analogues: eg carboprost (given IM) and misoprostol (given orally, PV or PR)**

LEARNING POINT

ℹ These drugs increase uterine contraction and cause vasoconstriction, thereby preventing the uterus from becoming atonic.

Total: 20 marks

PAEDIATRICS
CASES: ANSWERS

PAEDIATRICS CASE 1

Nathan, an 11-month-old infant, is referred to the paediatric assessment unit with a history of irritability and inconsolable crying for the last 8 hours. His mother has noted that he will settle down for a few minutes, but then wakes up and cries loudly, drawing his legs up to his abdomen. There is no fever, vomiting or diarrhoea. His bowels were last open yesterday and were normal. Past medical history is unremarkable, except that Nathan is recovering from gastroenteritis and remains off his feed.

Q 1. **List four causes of inconsolable crying in an infant.**　　　2 marks

A ½ **mark each for any of the following:**
- **Constipation**
- **Cow's milk protein intolerance/lactose intolerance**
- **Gastroesophageal reflux**
- **Infantile colic: see below**
- **Volvulus**
- **Intussusception**
- **Infection: eg urinary tract infection, otitis media, meningitis**
- **Rectal fissure**
- **Testicular torsion**
- **Trauma, eg fracture**

LEARNING POINTS

🛈 The differential diagnosis of an inconsolable infant is extensive. Therefore a good history and examination is paramount.

🛈 Infantile colic is excessive and unexplained crying in an otherwise healthy and well-fed infant under the age of 3 months. It is defined as crying for more than three hours per day, occurring more than 3 days per week and persisting for longer than 3 weeks. Infantile colic is common (up to 20% of infants suffer from it at some point) and typically starts at 2 weeks of age and is often resolved by 4 months. Attacks typically happen late afternoon/evening. They are characterised by the infant pulling his legs against his abdomen with paroxysmal episodes of screaming. Associated features may be a flushed face, clenched fists and a furrowed brow. Infantile colic is a diagnosis of exclusion and the aetiology of it remains unclear. Treatment is not usually necessary or effective.

Nathan is alert, pink and well perfused. His abdomen is not distended and is soft, with normal bowel sounds and with a palpable mass in the right upper quadrant.

Q 2. **What is intussusception?**   1 mark

A **Intussusception is the telescoping (folding into itself) of one proximal segment of the bowel into another more distal segment.**

LEARNING POINT

❶ Intussusception is the leading cause of intestinal obstruction in children aged between 3 months and 6 years (most common in 3–12-month-olds). It is more common in boys and is a life-threatening condition. The mortality is about 2% (if treated), but if left untreated it is fatal in nearly all cases.

Q 3. **In which part of the bowel does intussusception most commonly occur?**

1 mark

A **Terminal ileum: the terminal part of the ileum moves into the colon through the ileoceacal valve. This is called ileocolic intussusception.**

LEARNING POINT

❶ Other types of intussusception include: ileo-ileal (small intestines loop into itself) and colo-colic (large bowel moves into itself).

Q 4. **Name four predisposing factors for intussusception.**   2 marks

A **½ mark each for any of the following.**

Intussusception is due to abnormalities in the intestinal wall which cause a degree of obstruction, triggering the process of intussusception:

- **Viral illnesses (eg gastroenteritis): lymph nodes in the intestinal wall (called Peyer's patches) become swollen and cause a thickening of the intestinal wall**
- **Foreign body**

- **Cystic fibrosis: thought to be related to faecal overloading, in which a faecal bolus may adhere to the intestinal wall and thereby obstruct the bowel**
- **Henoch–Schonlein purpura (HSP): may cause small-bowel haematomas (bruises) in the intestinal wall**
- **Other conditions causing abnormalities of the bowel wall (eg Meckel's diverticulum), intestinal polyp (eg Peutz–Jeghers syndrome, familial polyposis coli)**
- **Post-abdominal surgery: trauma to the intestinal wall**

Q 5. **Name four features of intussusception.**   2 marks

A **½ mark each for any of the following:**
- **Paroxysmal severe intermittent abdominal pain (child draws up legs)**
- **Stool mixed with blood and mucus (referred to as 'redcurrant jelly' stool), a late sign**
- **A sausage-shaped mass in the abdomen (typically right upper quadrant).**
- **Distended abdomen**
- **Vomiting that may become bilious**
- **Diarrhoea (loose watery stools)**
- **Shock: due to third-space fluid loss in the gut**

LEARNING POINT

❶ Intussusception causes compression of blood vessels in the involved part of the bowel which reduces the blood supply, leading to venous obstruction and ischaemia. This causes oedema of the bowel wall, bleeding (redcurrant jelly stools) and disrupted peristalsis. If untreated, this will finally result in necrosis and perforation of the bowel wall.

Suspecting that Nathan has intussusception, you request an abdominal ultrasound scan, shown in Figure 7.1.

Q 6. **What does the ultrasound show?**   1 mark

A **Doughnut or target-sign appearance.**

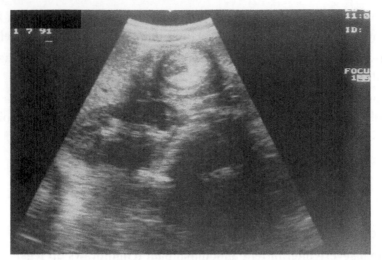

Figure 7.1 Nathan's abdominal ultrasound.

LEARNING POINTS

❶ Ultrasound scan may show a classic doughnut or target-sign appearance, ie alternating hypoechoic and echogenic bowel wall, representing the 'loop within a loop' characteristic of intussusception.

❶ Abdominal X-ray may show distended small bowel and absence of gas in the distal colon. X-rays though are usually reserved for when perforation is suspected.

Q 7. **How would you treat intussusception in Nathan?** 1 mark

A **Radiological reduction via an air or barium enema. The air increases the pressure within the bowel, which may unfold the affected part of the intestine.**

LEARNING POINT

❶ This is successful in over 75% of patients (if done early enough), although it should only be performed in the absence of peritonitis. After successful reduction, admission to the ward is usually necessary due to the high recurrence rate. Surgical reduction (manual unfolding out of the looped parts of bowel) is indicated when peritonitis is suspected, when the enema has failed and/or the intussusception is present for more than 24 hours, as other treatment options are less effective after this time.

Total: **10 marks**

PAEDIATRICS CASE 2

Rebecca is born at 40 weeks' gestation by normal vaginal delivery weighing 3.2 kg. Her mother (gravida 1, para 1) went into labour spontaneously, and labour was not prolonged. Rebecca's APGAR scores were 9 and 10 at 1 and 5 minutes, respectively, and she was transferred to the postnatal ward together with her mother. At the postnatal check the next day, the midwife notices that Rebecca's skin and sclerae are yellow. Apart from that she appears very well and is breastfeeding satisfactorily.

Q 1. **Are you concerned about Rebecca's jaundice? Briefly explain your reasoning.**   2 marks

A **1 mark each for the following:**

- **Yes**
- **Jaundice < 24 hours after birth is always pathological**

LEARNING POINTS

🛈 Jaundice within 24 hours is pathological and may be due to haemolysis or congenital infection. Bilirubin levels can rise rapidly and, if unconjugated (as in haemolysis), may need aggressive treatment. Jaundice after 24 hours may either be pathological or physiological (see below).

🛈 When examining for jaundice, place the (naked) baby in bright (preferably natural) light. Inspect the sclerae and all of the body. Blanch the skin on the chest or on the top of the nose; if the child is jaundiced, the blanched skin will look yellow. Jaundice is visible when bilirubin levels reach > 40 µmol/l.

Q 2. **Give three reasons why jaundice is common in neonates.**   3 marks

A **1 mark each for any of the following:**

- **Bilirubin is a breakdown product of red blood cells. Neonates have a higher concentration of red blood cells in their circulation; in the first few days of life these red cells are broken down and haemoglobin levels fall**
- **Half-life of red blood cells in neonates (70 days) is shorter than in adults (120 days)**

- **Immaturity of hepatic bilirubin metabolism: resulting in less efficient bilirubin uptake, conjugation and excretion**
- **Breastfeeding: cause of jaundice in breastfed infants is unknown, although it may be related to reduced fluid intake**

LEARNING POINT

❶ Babies who are at increased risk of developing significant hyperbilirubinaemia include:

- Gestational age under 38 weeks
- Previous sibling with neonatal jaundice requiring phototherapy
- Babies who are being exclusively breastfed
- Visible jaundice within the first 24 hours of life

Rebecca's jaundice is investigated. Her blood results are shown below.

Hb	12.2 g/dl (14.5–21.5)	Rebecca's blood group	A, Rh −ve
Platelets	220 x 10⁹/l (150–400)	Maternal blood group	O, Rh −ve
MCV	112 fl (100–135)	Total serum bilirubin	140 µmol/l (3–17) (unconjugated)
WCC	14 x 10⁹/l (10–26)	CRP	< 10 mg/l
Film	Normal RBCs	Direct Coombs' test (DCT)	+ (mildly +ve)

Q 3. **Give three causes of elevated *conjugated* bilirubin in neonates.**   3 marks

A **1 mark each for any of the following:**
- **Bile duct obstruction, eg biliary atresia.**
- **Congenital infections, eg TORCH (Toxoplasmosis, Other (eg syphilis, HIV), Rubella, CMV, Herpes)**
- **Sepsis**
- **Neonatal hepatitis**
- **Inborn error of metabolism (galactosaemia, tyrosinosis)**

LEARNING POINTS

ⓘ Bilirubin is lipid-soluble and must be converted into a water-soluble conjugate to be eliminated from the body. Once conjugated (with glucuronic acid in the liver) bilirubin is excreted through the bile into the small intestine and eliminated into the stool. Conjugated hyperbilirubinaemia is due to conditions/illnesses that reduce the rate of secretion of bilirubin into bile or that slow down the flow of bile into the intestines.

ⓘ Biliary atresia is a serious cause of conjugated hyperbilirubinaemia. It is due to inflammation of the large bile duct outside the liver, impairing the flow of bile from the liver to the small intestine. It typically presents with prolonged (conjugated) jaundice, pale stools and dark urine. The cause of biliary atresia is unknown. It is estimated that biliary atresia affects one in 8000–15,000 live births worldwide. Early diagnosis is vital, as surgical correction by 8 weeks of age greatly improves the outcome. Biliary atresia is the main cause of chronic cholestatic liver disease in children, and a common reason for liver transplantation in children.

ⓘ Unconjugated hyperbilirubinaemia occurs when there is:
- Too much bilirubin production, as in haemolysis (Rhesus and ABO incompatibility, spherocytosis, G6PD deficiency)
- Failure of bilirubin uptake (eg Gilbert syndrome)
- Impaired conjugation of bilirubin (eg Crigler–Najjar syndrome)
- Other causes, such as physiological or breast milk jaundice (see above)

Q 4. **What does the Direct Coombs' Test (DCT) detect and what does it indicate?**   2 marks

A **1 mark each for the following:**
- **The direct Coombs' test (also called direct antiglobulin test) detects the presence of antibody-coated red blood cells**
- **This indicates immune-mediated haemolysis (eg Rhesus or ABO incompatibility)**

Q 5. **From the blood results, what is the cause of her jaundice?**   2 marks

A **ABO incompatibility.**

PAEDIATRICS

LEARNING POINTS

❶ A moderately reduced haemoglobin, elevated unconjugated bilirubin and a (mildly) positive Coombs' test are typically seen in ABO incompatibility. This is confirmed by maternal blood group O and neonatal blood group A. The mother will have circulating anti-A (and anti-B) IgG antibodies which can cross the placenta and cause immune-mediated haemolysis.

❶ Rhesus incompatibility is not possible, as both Rebecca and her mum are Rhesus negative. Blood film is normal, making spherocytosis unlikely.

Q 6. How do you record bilirubin measurements? 1 mark

A On a 'bili chart' (officially called 'treatment threshold graphs').

LEARNING POINTS

❶ Take serial measurements of bilirubin (every 4–6 hours, depending on how steeply levels are rising) and plot on this chart (see Figure 7.2 below).

❶ Bilirubin levels tend to increase linearly. Therefore, plotting serial concentrations on a chart can be used to predict when phototherapy or exchange transfusion may be required. The decision to start phototherapy depends on level of serum bilirubin, gestational age of the baby and rate of rise of bilirubin.

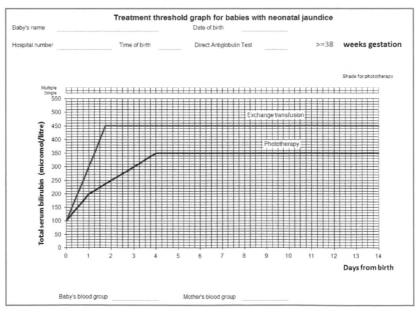

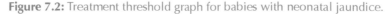

Figure 7.2: Treatment threshold graph for babies with neonatal jaundice.

PAEDIATRICS

Q 7. **How does phototherapy work?**   1 mark

A **Light (blue and white light) converts unconjugated bilirubin by photodegradation into harmless water-soluble metabolites, which are excreted in bile and urine.**

If unconjugated bilirubin reaches high levels it can become neurotoxic, termed 'kernicterus'.

Q 8. **Give three clinical features of kernicterus.**   3 marks

A **1 mark each for any of the following:**
- **Sleepiness**
- **Poor feeding**
- **Low muscle tone**
- **Poor Moro response**
- **High-pitched cry**
- **Irritability**
- **Seizures**
- **Arched back (opisthotonus)**

LEARNING POINTS

ⓘ Unconjugated bilirubin is lipid-soluble and when levels exceed the binding capacity of albumin, unconjugated bilirubin can cross the blood–brain barrier. Deposition of bilirubin in the basal ganglia and brainstem has severe neurological consequences (kernicterus), which can even be permanent.

ⓘ Risk factors for kernicterus are:
- Serum bilirubin levels > 340 μmol/l
- A rapidly rising bilirubin level (greater than 8.5 μmol/l/h).

ⓘ Early signs of kernicterus typically happen 3–4 days after birth.

PAEDIATRICS

Q 9. Give three long-term complications of kernicterus.   3 marks

A **1 mark each for any of the following:**

- **Learning difficulties**
- **Enamel dysplasia**
- **Cerebral palsy, eg dyskinesia cerebral palsy due to bilirubin deposition in the basal ganglia (typically causing ataxia and choreoathetosis)**
- **Sensorineural deafness: all babies treated for jaundice undergo hearing tests (brainstem evoked audiometry) before discharge**

LEARNING POINT

ⓘ These complications appear around 18–24 months of age.

Fortunately for Rebecca, phototherapy is successful, and she joins her new family at home 4 days later on oral folic acid. She is followed up 2 weeks later in outpatients for a repeat full blood count to ensure late haemolysis is not occurring.

Total: 20 marks

PAEDIATRICS CASE 3

Chelsea, a 3-month old baby girl, is referred to paediatrics with a 2-day history of feeding difficulties and a cough. On examination, she has a runny nose and looks dehydrated. Furthermore she has signs of respiratory distress, with a widespread expiratory wheeze; SaO$_2$ (on air) 90%.

Q 1. **List six signs of respiratory distress in an infant.** 3 marks

A **½ mark each for any of the following:**
- **Tachypnoea (respiratory rate > 50/min)**
- **Nasal flaring (enlargement of the opening of the nostril during breathing)**
- **Subcostal recession**
- **Intercostal recession**
- **Tracheal tug**
- **Chest hyperinflation**
- **Liver displaced inferiorly**
- **Cyanosis or pallor**
- **Use of accessory muscles (eg causing head bobbing)**
- **Expiratory grunting: caused by closure of epiglottis in order to try to create positive airway pressure during expiration**
- **Tachycardia**
- **Feeding difficulties**

LEARNING POINT

ⓘ Wheeze is a whistling sound caused by turbulent airflow. It is a sign of a lower airway narrowing, usually due to inflammation. It is typically heard in the expiratory phase of respiration. Causes of wheezing in an infant include viral-induced wheeze, asthma, bronchiolitis, inhalation of a foreign body and cardiac failure.

Q 2. What is the normal heart rate and respiratory rate in infants?　　　2 marks

A 1 mark each of the following:

Age	Respiratory rate (/min)	Heart rate (/min)
Infant (< 1 year)	30–40	110–160
Young child (2–5 years)	20–30	95–140
Older child (5–12 years)	20–25	80–120

LEARNING POINT

❶ Normal systolic blood pressure in infants is 70–90 mmHg.

Chelsea's mum tells you that she is not taking her bottle and her nappies are much drier than normal.

Q 3. List four signs indicating dehydration in an infant.　　　2 marks

A ½ mark each for any of the following:

1. **Dry tongue (< 5%)**
2. **Dull, dry eyes (< 5%)**
3. **Sunken anterior fontanelle (5–10%)**
4. **Reduced skin turgor (5–10%)**
5. **Delayed (ie > 2 s) capillary refill time (5–10%)**
6. **Irritability (5–10%)**
7. **Dry nappy, ie oliguria/anuria (>10%)**
8. **Weak pulse (>10%)**
9. **Reduced blood pressure: normal systolic blood pressure in the infant is 90/70 (> 10%)**

LEARNING POINT

❶ Signs 1–2 indicate mild dehydration, ie < 5% loss of body weight. Signs 3–6 (plus earlier signs) indicate moderate dehydration, ie 5–10% loss of body weight. Signs 7–9 (plus earlier signs) indicate severe dehydration, ie > 10% loss of body weight. This percentage classification is used to calculate fluid replacement requirements.

Q 4. How is the maintenance fluid requirement of a child calculated?   1 mark

A **It is calculated per kg of body weight (100–50–20 rule):**

- **0–10 kg: 100 ml/kg/day**
- **11–20 kg: 1000 ml + 50 ml/kg/day**
- **Above 20 kg: 1500 ml + 20 ml/kg/day for each additional kg over 20 kg**

LEARNING POINT

🛈 So for example, the maintenance fluid requirement per day of a 25-kg child is:

1000 ml (100 x 10 kg) + 500 ml (50 x 10 kg) + 100 ml (20 x 5 kg) = 1600 ml/day

that is 1580/24 = 65 ml/h.

Fluid deficit can be calculated using the following formula:

% dehydration x weight (kg) x 10

that is, for a 25 kg child who is 10% dehydrated: 10 x 25 x 10 = 2500.

This should be added to the maintenance fluid requirements to make total fluid requirements/day.

You diagnose Chelsea with bronchiolitis and admit her to the ward, where she is barrier-nursed to prevent spread.

Q 5. List four clinical features of bronchiolitis.   2 marks

A **½ mark each for any of the following:**

- **Dry cough**
- **Runny nose**
- **High-pitched expiratory wheeze**
- **Signs of respiratory distress (see above)**
- **Fine inspiratory crackles**
- **Tachycardia**
- **Poor feeding (secondary to increased work of breathing, nasal secretions and exhaustion)**
- **Apnoea: common in the very young babies and may be a presenting feature in premature or low-birth-weight babies)**

PAEDIATRICS

LEARNING POINT

ℹ️ Bronchiolitis is typically preceded by a coryzal illness for 2–3 days. It mainly affects children < 2 years of age (peak incidence is at 3–6 months) and is more common in the winter.

Q 6. **List four types of patients at risk of bronchiolitis.** 2 marks

A **½ mark each for any of the following:**
- **Premature babies**
- **Chronic lung disease: defined as O_2 therapy beyond 36 weeks of gestation**
- **Congenital heart disease**
- **Down syndrome**
- **Cystic fibrosis**
- **Immune deficiency, eg severe combined immune deficiency (SCID)**
- **Parental smoking**

Q 7. **What is the most common cause of bronchiolitis and how is it detected?**

2 marks

A **1 mark each for the following:**
- **Respiratory syncytial virus (RSV): causative agent in approximately 70% of cases**
- **Nasopharyngeal aspirate (NPA) for RSV confirmation by immunofluorescent-labelled antibody detection**

LEARNING POINTS

ℹ️ Respiratory syncytial virus (RSV) is very common and is a highly contagious virus. It spreads from respiratory secretions by coughing/sneezing. By 1 year of age 70% of children will have been infected with RSV, of whom 20% develop symptomatic disease.

ℹ️ Other causes of bronchiolitis include adenovirus, influenza virus and parainfluenza virus.

Q 8. **How would you manage Chelsea?** 3 marks

A **1 mark each for any of the following:**
- **Give oxygen: initially via nasal cannula or head box**
- **Continuous SaO$_2$ monitoring: bronchiolitic infants are at risk of apnoeas**
- **Monitor feeds: if the infant is unable to feed orally consider NG tube or IV fluids**
- **Consider nasal suction to clear secretions if there are signs of nasal blockage**

LEARNING POINTS

ⓘ In most infections the illness is self-limiting, usually lasting 3–7 days; typically symptoms peak at day 4–5. Risk factors for severe bronchiolitis (requiring admission) are: poor feeding (less than 50% of usual intake), apnoeas, lethargy, grunting, cyanosis, respiratory rate more than 70 breaths per minute, oxygen saturations below 94% and severe chest wall recession. The threshold for hospital admission is lower in premature infants and infants with co-morbidities.

ⓘ There is no evidence to support the use of inhaled/nebulised bronchodilators and steroids. Antibiotics are not indicated, unless secondary bacterial pneumonia is suspected.

ⓘ Bronchiolitis is a clinical diagnosis. There is no place for blood tests or X-rays to diagnose acute bronchiolitis. In cases of severe acute bronchiolitis a blood gas can be helpful to identify babies who are in respiratory failure and may need respiratory support.

Q 9. **What is the prophylactic antibody for RSV?** 1 mark

A **Palivizumab.**

LEARNING POINT

ⓘ This is a humanised monoclonal RSV antibody. It is not recommended for routine use but should be considered prophylactically in children < 1 year with significant co-morbidity (ie immune deficiency, extreme prematurity, chronic lung disease and acyanotic congenital heart disease). It does not prevent infection but reduces the severity of complications of RSV disease.

PAEDIATRICS

Q 10. **How would you monitor the effectiveness of treatment?**   2 marks

A **½ mark each for any of the following:**

- **Respiratory rate**
- **Heart rate**
- **Temperature**
- **SaO$_2$**
- **Tolerating oral feeds**

LEARNING POINT

🛈 Discharge criteria for bronchiolitis are: temperature $< 38\,^{\circ}\text{C}$; feeding adequately (more than 75% of usual intake); SaO$_2$ $> 94\%$ in air; respiratory rate < 50/min; and heart rate < 140/min. On discharge (or babies not requiring admission) parents and/or carers should receive information about bronchiolitis – namely, the duration of symptoms, its treatment and prognosis.

Total: **20 marks**

PAEDIATRICS CASE 4

James, a 3-year-old boy, is referred to the paediatric outpatient clinic because of poor weight gain over the past 6 months. He was born at full term weighing 3.2 kg. However, over the past 6 months his Mum says he has become irritable, his abdomen seem distended, and he has lots of liquid stools that are foul-smelling and difficult to flush. On examination, James is pale and his abdomen is protruded. There is wasting of his muscles (especially buttocks) and his ankles seem swollen.

Q 1. **Define failure to thrive.**   1 mark

A **Failure to thrive (FTT) is defined as poor weight gain in infants (< 1 year old) and toddlers (1–3 years), with a fall across two or more weight centile lines.**

LEARNING POINTS

ⓘ A less strict definition is 'rate of growth that does not meet the expected potential for a child of that age'. Nowadays a more parent-friendly term for failure to thrive is 'faltering growth pattern'.

ⓘ In order to diagnose FTT the child's weight, height and head circumference should be accurately plotted on a growth chart to assess the trend.

Q 2. **List four non-organic causes of failure to thrive.**   2 marks

A **½ mark each for any of the following:**
- **Inadequate food intake (eg due to insufficient food offered)**
- **Inappropriate foods offered (eg too much milk or juice)**
- **Low socioeconomic status (eg unable to afford a good diet)**
- **Mechanical feeding problems (eg poor breastfeeding technique)**
- **Emotional deprivation: disturbed parent–child relationship resulting in infant not demanding food, often accompanied by delays in development dependent on stimulation (eg speech)**
- **Child abuse or neglect**

LEARNING POINT

❶ Causes of FTT can be classified as organic (underlying pathology) or non-organic (psychosocial and environmental causes). Non-organic causes account for > 95% cases of FTT. Organic causes include gastro-oesophageal reflux disease (leading to poor retention of food), coeliac disease, cystic fibrosis and Crohn's disease (all causing malabsorption), and kidney and heart disease (illness-induced anorexia).

Q 3. **What is the likely mechanism of James's diarrhoea?**　　　　1 mark

A **Malabsorption.**

LEARNING POINTS

❶ Liquid, pale, foul-smelling and difficult to flush stools (called steatorrhoea) are typically caused by malabsorption. Malabsorption is due to a defect in the digestive process. This can be: (1) failure to produce enzymes needed to digest certain foods (lack of pancreatic enzymes in cystic fibrosis, lack of lactase in lactose intolerance); (2) failure to produce bile salt to emulsify fats as in cirrhosis and gallstone disease; (3) due to inflammation or injury to part of the intestine, as in coeliac disease, radiation-induced injury (radiation enteritis) or inflammatory bowel disease; or (4) due to abnormal gut flora caused by bacterial overgrowth or parasite infestation.

❶ Other symptoms of malabsorption include abdominal pain, bloating and distension, which are caused by bacterial fermentation of undigested food substances producing gaseous products.

Q 4. **Why does James have ankle oedema?**　　　　1 mark

A **Hypoproteinaemia (hypoalbuminaemia).**

LEARNING POINTS

❶ Malabsorption causes failure to absorb nutrients from the diet – fats, carbohydrates, protein, vitamins and/or minerals. Failure to absorb protein causes oedema due to the reduction in plasma oncotic pressure, which caused a shift of fluid from the intravascular to the interstitial space. Reduced protein is also the cause of the muscle wasting and atrophy found in malabsorption syndromes.

ⓘ Other manifestations of malabsorption are: (1) anaemia, due to iron, folate and/ or B_{12} deficiency; (2) osteoporosis or rickets, due to calcium and vitamin D deficiency; (3) weight loss and fatigue due to carbohydrate, protein and fat malabsorption; and (4) bleeding disorders due to vitamin K deficiency.

As part of his investigations, James is screened for coeliac disease.

Q 5. **What is the serological screening test for coeliac disease?** 1 mark

A **Anti-tissue transglutaminase (tTG) antibodies: this is an IgA antibody, so IgA deficiency (which has a higher prevalence in coeliac disease) is also screened for to avoid false negatives.**

LEARNING POINTS

ⓘ If it is equivocal, screen for IgA anti-endomysial antibodies. A positive screening test requires a duodenal biopsy to confirm the diagnosis. To avoid false negatives the child needs to be on a gluten-containing diet prior to any serological testing and/or duodenal biopsy.

ⓘ Screening for coeliac disease is recommended if a child presents with any of the following signs and symptoms: chronic or intermittent diarrhoea; failure to thrive; persistent nausea and vomiting; prolonged fatigue; recurrent abdominal pain; abdominal distension; unexplained weight loss; unexplained iron deficiency anaemia.

ⓘ Screening is also recommended in the following conditions: autoimmune thyroid disease; dermatitis herpetiformis; type 1 diabetes; and a first-degree relative with coeliac disease.

James's serological screening test is positive, and he is referred for a duodenal biopsy, which subsequently confirms coeliac disease.

Q 6. **List two histological changes on biopsy seen in coeliac disease.** 2 marks

A **1 mark each for any of the following:**
- **Flat jejunal mucosa (reducing the area available for intestinal absorption)**
- **Villous atrophy**
- **Crypt hyperplasia due to inflammatory cell infiltrate in the lamina propria**

LEARNING POINTS

ⓘ Coeliac disease is an immune disorder triggered by an environmental agent (gluten). Gluten causes a T-cell-mediated inflammatory response in the proximal small bowel that damages the mucosa and leads to malabsorption. It is more common in people with autoimmune diseases (eg type 1 diabetes), those who have family members with coeliac disease, those with genetic conditions (Down, Williams and Turner syndromes) and in those with the *HLA DQ2/DQ8* gene.

ⓘ Prevalence of coeliac disease is approximately one in a hundred. Symptoms in children may occur around weaning (following the introduction of gluten into the diet), and the child typically presents between 1 and 3 years of age (though be aware that it can present at any age!).

Q 7. **Which rash is associated with coeliac disease?**   1 mark

A **Dermatitis herpetiformis.**

LEARNING POINT

ⓘ This presents as erythematous raised patches, typically on the elbows, knees and buttocks. These lesions may blister and cause pruritus. Treatment is by gluten-free diet and dapsone, but it may take months for the rash to clear.

Q 8. **List three food groups James will now have to avoid.**   3 marks

A **1 mark each for any of the following:**

Need to avoid the following food groups, which all contain gluten:

- **Wheat**
- **Rye**
- **Barley**
- **Oats: this is more controversial but as most commercially available oats are contaminated with gluten, they should also be avoided**

LEARNING POINTS

ℹ Children should only be started on a gluten-free diet if they have their diagnosis confirmed by biopsy, and never on the basis of a positive antibody test alone. Current practice is that a gluten-free diet should be adhered to for life, and the child should receive regular dietetic advice. Gluten-free foods can be obtained on prescription, and membership of the Coeliac Society should be encouraged.

ℹ In addition to dietary restrictions, nutritional deficiencies should be identified (including iron, folate, vitamin D and calcium) and corrected. Pneumococcal vaccine is also recommended in all children with coeliac disease, as most patients will have some degree of hyposplenism.

Q 9. **Give three complications of coeliac disease.** 3 marks

A **1 mark each for any of the following:**
- **Anaemia: folate, B$_{12}$ or iron deficiency due to malabsorption**
- **Small-bowel non-Hodgkin lymphoma**
- **Intestinal malignancies: oesophageal and large-bowel squamous carcinoma, small-bowel adenocarcinoma**
- **Osteoporosis: due to calcium and vitamin D malabsorption**
- **Infertility**
- **Hyposplenism: increased risk of infections**

LEARNING POINT

ℹ Benefits of a gluten-free diet include: resolution of GI symptoms (this can be spectacular); normalisation of antibody tests and small-bowel histology; reversal of bone demineralisation and infertility; and return of level of risk for intestinal malignancy to that of normal population level.

Total: **15 marks**

PAEDIATRICS

PAEDIATRICS CASE 5

Marie, a 17-month-old toddler, is referred by her GP after Mum has noticed that, ever since she started walking, she appears to be limping. Marie appears unaware of this and does not complain of any pain. She was born by elective caesarean section due to breech presentation.

Q 1. **With regards to her motor milestones, at what ages would you expect Marie to do the following?**   7 marks

A 1 mark for each of the following:

1. **Crawl:**   8–9 months

2. **Walk:**   12–18 months

3. **Run:**   1.5–2 years

4. **Kick a ball:**   2–2.5 years

5. **Ride a tricycle:**   3 years

6. **Hop on one foot:**   4 years

7. **Climbs stairs adult fashion:**   5 years

ⓘ Developmental milestones are divided into four areas: (1) gross motor; (2) fine motor and vision; (3) speech, language and hearing; and (4) social, emotional and behaviour. There is variation in the rate in which children develop but there are limit ages by which a child should have acquired certain skills. Further assessment is indicated if the child falls outside these limit ages. Most common causes of developmental delay are cerebral palsy, primary muscle disorders and global developmental delay.

Q 2. **Name two pathological gaits in children.**   1 mark

A ½ mark for any of the following:

1. **Trendelenburg (or waddling gait): caused by weakness of abductor muscles causing downward tilting of the hip on the opposite side, with the patient having to swing that leg round to make a step. Causes include developmental dysplasia of the hip, Legg–Calvé–Perthes disease (see below) and slipped capital femoral epiphysis**

2. **Antalgic gait:** adopted because of (hip) pain. Patient leans to side of pain in the hip and takes short, heavy, quick steps on that side and longer steps on the unaffected side. Causes include infection, trauma, slipped femoral epiphysis, limb deformity, arthritis

3. **Ataxic gait:** wide-based gait due to loss of proprioception or cerebellar disturbance, eg in ataxic cerebral palsy

4. **Foot drop:** difficulty with dorsiflexion of the foot. The knee is raised high to lift foot off the ground, which otherwise scrapes the floor, eg in cerebral palsy or peroneal muscle atrophy

5. **Spastic gait:** stiff legs with unbalanced coordination of different muscle groups, eg knees and thighs are crossed (scissoring), foot is often dragged along the floor. Due to CNS lesions, eg cerebral palsy

Q 3. **What is your differential diagnosis?**   2 marks

A **½ mark for any of the following:**

1. **Developmental dysplasia of the hip (DDH)**

2. **Trauma: fractures, sprain, contusion**

3. **Infectious: osteomyelitis, septic arthritis**

4. **Neoplastic: osteogenic sarcoma**

5. **Neuromuscular: cerebral palsy (in males also consider Duchenne's muscular dystrophy)**

6. **Rheumatological disorders**

LEARNING POINTS

ⓘ Your history should include: (1) How long has she been limping, eg acute onset in trauma and septic arthritis? (2) Any history of trauma (also be aware of non-accidental injury)? (3) Can she weight-bear, eg not weight-bearing is seen in septic arthritis? (4) Does she appear to be in pain; if so when is the pain worst (pain in morning may suggest rheumatoid conditions, night pain (especially if it wakes the child from sleep) points more towards a neoplastic process)? (5) Any weakness in the leg, eg neuromuscular conditions? Are any other joints affected: may suggest a viral illness, rheumatological conditions? (6) Any associated features: fever or weight loss? Is she able to do her normal activities?

ⓘ Be aware of referred pain, eg hip pathology causing knee pain, so therefore always examine the whole limb.

PAEDIATRICS

Q 4. **Which non-traumatic cause of a limp needs immediate intervention?** 1 mark

A **Septic arthritis.**

LEARNING POINTS

ⓘ Septic arthritis typically affects the hip joint in young children and knees in older children and adults. In the majority of cases of septic arthritis in children the child is less than 3 years old.

ⓘ Clinical manifestations include fever, joint effusion, raised inflammatory markers, and refusal to move the affected limb or weight-bear.

ⓘ If an effusion is present, which can be confirmed with ultrasound scan, the key investigation is joint aspiration for microscopy, culture and sensitivities. Common causative organisms include *Staphylococcus aureus*, *Haemophilus influenzae* and Group B *Streptococcus*. Intravenous antibiotics should be started immediately after joint aspiration as joint destruction can be very rapid and lead to permanent loss of function.

Q 5. **What two manoeuvres can you do to test for congenital hip problems in neonates?** 1 mark

A **½ mark for the following:**
- **Barlow test: Attempt to dislocate an unstable hip. The thigh is taken between examiner's thumb and fingers (middle finger over greater trochanter) and is adducted and pressed posteriorly. If positive, dislocation is felt as the femoral head slips out of the acetabulum**
- **Ortolani test: This is the opposite of the Barlow test as it attempts to reduce a dislocated hip. The neonate's thigh is taken between thumb and fingers and abducted and pulled anteriorly. If positive the examiner will feel a 'clunk' as the femoral head is reduced into the acetabulum**

LEARNING POINTS

ⓘ 1 in 100 newborns has an unstable hip, ie developmental dysplasia of the hip (DDH), which if untreated may lead to pain, stiffness (causing problems with gait) and osteoarthritis. Risk factors include positive family history, multiple pregnancy and prematurity, primigravida, breech presentation and oligohydramnios (restricting intrauterine movement). In addition to the above Barlow or Ortolani tests, look for discrepancy in leg length and asymmetry of leg creases on examination. The signs in older infants and young children are leg length discrepancy, reduced abduction of the affected leg and standing or walking with external rotation.

ⓘ If DDH is suspected, an ultrasound scan of the hip is recommended to assess hip stability and acetabular development; X-rays are more useful in older infants and children. Treatment depends on the child's age at diagnosis: the aim is to reduce dislocation and maintain reduction of the hip. Rarely, reduction may cause avascular necrosis of the capital femoral epiphysis secondary to compression of the cartilage.

On examination Marie's left leg is externally rotated and shorter than her right leg. Subsequent X-ray confirms developmental dysplasia of the hip and she is referred to orthopaedics for further management.

Your next patient also presents with a limp, a 12-year-old boy whose weight lies on the 90th centile and who has been complaining for several weeks of an intermittent limp and knee pain, making cycling painful.

Q 6. **What is the most likely diagnosis from this history?** 1 mark

A **Slipped upper femoral epiphysis (SUFE).**

ⓘ A limp (antalgic gait) together with thigh, knee or groin pain (though not hip pain) for several weeks in a pubescent, **obese** male (three times as common in males) is most likely to be due to SUFE. It is defined as inferior and posterior slippage of the proximal femoral epiphysis through the growth plate. It can be classified into stable (chronic symptoms) and unstable (acute presentation) depending on the degree of disruption between capital femoral epiphysis and femoral neck.

Q 7. **What is the typical finding on examination of the hip?** 1 mark

A **Decreased internal rotation.**

LEARNING POINTS

ⓘ The first sign is decreased internal rotation of the hip, followed by increased external rotation and flexion and abduction of the hip (sometimes to a fixed position). With time a discrepancy in leg length may develop and atrophy of the muscles of the thigh.

ⓘ Treatment depends on the severity of the slippage but in unstable and acute cases of SUFE internal fixation is necessary. Complications of SUFE include avascular necrosis and chondrolysis (destruction of the articular cartilage of the hip joint).

PAEDIATRICS

Q 8. **Which other hip pathology in a child is associated with avascular necrosis?**   **1 mark**

A **Legg–Calvé–Perthes disease (LCPD).**

LEARNING POINT

🛈 LCPD is idiopathic avascular necrosis of the capital femoral epiphysis (CFE). It is caused by interruption of the blood supply to the CFE, leading to osteonecrosis of the ossification centre of the femoral epiphysis. In some children revascularisation and subsequent normal bone growth occur while in others LCPD develops. It is more common in boys (2–12 yrs old). Clinical presentation is with a limp, hip or groin pain, muscle spasm and decreased range of movement (internal rotation and abduction). X-rays are necessary to determine the extent of damage to the CFE. Treatment is conservative with the aim of limiting the deformity of the femoral head. The main complication is development of osteoarthritis in adulthood.

Total: **15 marks**

PALLIATIVE CARE
CASE: ANSWERS

PALLIATIVE CARE CASE 1

Margaret, with known inoperable squamous cell bronchial carcinoma, is reviewed by her oncologist with worsening back pain that is no longer eased by paracetamol.

Q 1. **List six 'red flag' back pain features.**   3 marks

A ½ mark each for any of the following:

1. **Young (< 20 years) or old (> 55 years)**

2. **Non-mechanical back pain**

3. **Thoracic spine tenderness/pain**

4. **Systemic features (eg weight loss, unwell)**

5. **Taking steroids: increased risk of infection and osteoporosis**

6. **History of malignancy**

7. **Disturbance of bladder and/or bowel function**

8. **Saddle anaesthesia**

9. **Weak legs/gait disturbance**

LEARNING POINT

❶ These features may indicate a sinister underlying cause for the back pain, requiring further investigation (see below). Symptoms 7–9 indicate cord compression/cauda equina syndrome, requiring urgent referral (see below).

Q 2. **Name four primary cancers that metastasise to bone.**   2 marks

A ½ mark each for any of the following:

• **Lung**

• **Breast**

• **Prostate**

• **Thyroid**

• **Kidney**

LEARNING POINT

❶ When investigating metastatic bone disease, alkaline phosphatase (ALP) (a marker of new bone formation) is raised, erythrocyte sedimentation rate (ESR) is raised, calcium may be raised (see below), skeletal X-rays may show osteolytic (or osteosclerotic with prostate metastases) lesions, while radio-labelled bone scans will detect bony metastases as areas of increased bone activity (often before radiological changes become evident).

A bone scan confirms secondary deposits in the thoracic vertebrae, and she is referred for palliative radiotherapy and commenced on morphine.

Q 3. **Describe the three steps of the analgaesic ladder.** 3 marks

A **1 mark each for the following:**
- **Step 1: non-opioid (eg paracetamol, NSAID) ± adjuvant**
- **Step 2: weak opioid (eg codeine) + non-opioid ± adjuvant**
- **Step 3: strong opioid (eg morphine) + non-opioid ± adjuvant**

LEARNING POINTS

❶ Analgesics should be given regularly, as persistent pain requires preventive therapy. If the optimal dose of an analgesic fails to control the pain, move up the ladder, not sideways (ie don't simply swap to a different drug from the same class).

❶ Adjuvants include corticosteroids (used to reduce peritumour oedema), antispasmodics (eg used to treat muscle spasm, bowel colic), bisphosphonates (used to treat bony metastases), and anti-epileptics/antidepressants (used to treat neuropathic pain).

Q 4. **List four side-effects of morphine.** 2 marks

A **½ mark each for any of the following:**
- **Nausea and vomiting: prescribe concomitant anti-emetics (eg cyclizine)**
- **Constipation: due to decreased peristalsis. Prescribe concomitant laxatives (eg senna, a stimulant laxative)**
- **Drowsiness/sedation: tends to resolve after 5 days**
- **Dry mouth**

- **Hypotension: due to vasodilatation**
- **Respiratory depression (rarely a problem if titrated against pain)**
- **Addiction (again, rarely a problem in palliative care)**
- **Pruritus**

LEARNING POINTS

ℹ Typical starting dose for morphine is 5–10 mg four times daily, titrating upwards by 30–50% each time. Once pain is controlled, convert to a modified-release preparation – eg morphine sulphate tablets (MST), which is prescribed bd (Σdaily morphine/2).

ℹ Because pain is a physiological antagonist to the CNS depressant effects of opioids, morphine rarely causes respiratory depression.

Q 5. **Why should morphine be used with caution in renal failure?** 1 mark

A **½ mark each for the following:**
- **May cause an overdose: reverse with naloxone (though this also reverses all of their pain control)**
- **May cause myoclonus**

LEARNING POINT

ℹ Morphine is metabolised to morphine-3-glucuronide (M3G) and M6G. Both metabolites are excreted via the kidneys; morphine should be used with caution in renal failure, as it may cause an overdose (owing to an accumulation of M6G) and myoclonus (owing to an accumulation of M3G). Fentanyl is the drug of choice in renal failure.

Margaret's bone profile is shown below:

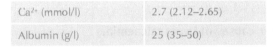

Ca^{2+} (mmol/l)	2.7 (2.12–2.65)
Albumin (g/l)	25 (35–50)

Q 6. **Calculate Margaret's adjusted calcium.** 1 mark

A **3.0 mmol/l, ie 2.7 + 0.3 ([40–25] x 0.02)**

LEARNING POINT

ⓘ Approximately 40% of calcium is bound to albumin. Normally total calcium is measured, which reflects both bound and unbound calcium, although only the latter is physiologically relevant. Total calcium can be adjusted for changes in albumin concentration (affecting levels of unbound calcium) by adding 0.02 mmol/l to the Ca^{2+} concentration for every 1g/l that albumin is < 40 g/l.

Q 7. **Give four symptoms of hypercalcaemia.**   2 marks

A **½ mark each for any of the following:**
- **Abdominal pain**
- **Nausea and vomiting**
- **Anorexia**
- **Constipation**
- **Polyuria**
- **Polydipsia**
- **Confusion**
- **Tiredness**
- **Depression**

LEARNING POINTS

ⓘ Calcium may be raised owing to bony metastases or tumour secretion of parathyroid hormone- (PTH-) related protein (a paraneoplastic phenomenon).

ⓘ Acute hypercalcaemia often presents with dehydration as a result of vomiting and polyuria, abdominal pain and constipation, and confusion. In the acute setting it is treated by rehydration with intravenous saline and intravenous bisphosphonates, which inhibit osteoclast activity, thereby reducing bone resorption.

Q 8. **List two further causes of hypercalcaemia.**   1 mark

A **½ mark each for any of the following:**
- **Excessive parathyroid hormone (PTH) secretion: may be due to primary or tertiary hyperparathyroidism. Primary is due to parathyroid hyperplasia, adenoma or carcinoma and usually causes mild hypercalcaemia; secondary is compensatory parathyroid hypertrophy in response to chronic hypocalcaemia**

(eg in renal failure); calcium levels are low or normal; tertiary is due to prolonged stimulation of the parathyroid in long-standing hypocalcaemia so that PTH release is no longer under feedback control of calcium

- **Hyperthyroidism**
- **Excessive calcium intake**
- **Excessive vitamin D intake**
- **Drugs (eg thiazides, calcium-sparing diuretics)**
- **Sarcoidosis (producing excess vitamin D)**

LEARNING POINT

ⓘ More than 90% of cases of hypercalcaemia are caused by malignancy or hyperparathyroidism.

Q 9. **Name two other palliative care emergencies.**   1 mark

A **½ mark each for any of the following:**
- **Spinal cord compression (SCC)**
- **Major haemorrhage:, eg erosion of an artery by tumour**
- **Superior vena caval obstruction (SVCO)**
- **Raised intracranial pressure (ICP)**

LEARNING POINTS

ⓘ Spinal cord compression (SCC) should be considered in any cancer patient with severe back pain or 'off legs'. Limb weakness, and urinary and bowel disturbance are late signs. Patients should be commenced on dexamethasone while awaiting urgent whole-spine MRI, while treatment may involve radiotherapy and spinal surgery. Early detection improves the prognosis: 95% of patients who are mobilising at diagnosis will continue to do so, whereas only 5% of patients 'off legs' at diagnosis will regain mobility.

ⓘ Superior vena caval obstruction (SVCO) is typically caused by either lung cancer or lymphoma, obstructing venous return from the head, arms and upper trunk. Features include facial swelling, headache, arm swelling, and prominent distended veins on the neck and chest wall. Treatment includes dexamethasone, stenting, radiotherapy and chemotherapy.

Margaret has had two recent hospital admissions for hypercalcaemia and is now on monthly pamidronate infusions. She takes diclofenac 75 mg bd and morphine sulphate tablets (MST) 120 mg bd for bone pain. Unfortunately, her condition has deteriorated rapidly over the last week, and she is admitted to St John's Hospice. She is nauseous with occasional vomiting, in obvious pain and unable to take oral medications.

Q 10. **Convert her oral morphine to 24-hour diamorphine subcutaneous infusion.** 1 mark

A **80 mg diamorphine, ie 240 mg/3 = 80 mg.**

LEARNING POINTS

❶ Diamorphine is more soluble than morphine and is the preferred choice for parenteral administration (eg via a syringe driver). To convert oral morphine to parenteral diamorphine, divide 24-hour total dose of oral morphine by 3 and prescribe this over 24 hours via a syringe driver (prescribe one sixth diamorphine dose for breakthrough pain).

❶ Another possible form of analgesia in patients unable to take oral medicines is to use fentanyl patches.

Q 11. **Give four potential causes of Margaret's nausea and vomiting.** 2 marks

A **½ mark each for the following:**
- **Drugs (eg morphine, chemotherapy)**
- **Metabolic (eg hypercalcaemia, uraemia)**
- **Raised intracranial pressure (ICP) due to brain metastases**
- **Gastrointestinal causes (eg gastric stasis, ie delayed gastric emptying), intestinal obstruction (eg constipation, tumour)**

LEARNING POINTS

❶ Vomiting is controlled by the vomiting centre (VC) in the brainstem, which receives input from the cortex (eg ICP), GI tract (eg obstruction), chemotactic trigger zone (CTZ) (eg drugs, metabolic) and vestibular apparatus (eg Ménière's disease).

❶ It is important to determine the cause of the vomiting, as this will determine which anti-emetic to prescribe (see below).

Margaret is prescribed metoclopramide for her nausea and vomiting.

Q 12. **Where does metoclopramide exert its anti-emetic effect?** 1 mark

A **GI tract: prokinetic anti-emetic used to treat nausea and vomiting because of gastric stasis and functional bowel obstruction (contraindicated in mechanical obstruction).**

LEARNING POINT

❶ Other commonly used anti-emetics include:

- Haloperidol (acts on CTZ): for nausea and vomiting caused by drugs or toxins
- Cyclizine (acts on VC): for vagally mediated nausea and vomiting caused by distension or compression of organs in thorax, abdomen or pelvis
- Hyoscine (anticholinergic that acts as an antisecretory/antispasmodic on the GI tract): used to control bowel colic and GI secretions (reducing volume of vomit in obstruction)
- Ondansetron (serotonin (5HT) receptor antagonist that acts on the GI tract and CNS): used for nausea and vomiting of chemotherapy/radiotherapy
- Levomepromazine: broad-spectrum anti-emetic
- Dexamethasone: used in raised ICP and as an adjuvant anti-emetic in chemotherapy.

Total: **20 marks**

PSYCHIATRY
CASE: ANSWERS

PSYCHIATRY CASE 1

Ethel is 74 and lives alone. She has a fall at home and is admitted to hospital with a fractured neck of femur. Postoperatively she is disoriented and has become increasingly restless and agitated with nursing staff. At times she believes she is being poisoned. She is diagnosed with delirium (acute confusional state).

Q 1. **List six possible causes of delirium.** 3 marks

A ½ mark each for any from the list below.

Delirium presents with disturbance of cognition and difficulties in focusing attention. It has an acute onset and fluctuating course with symptoms typically worse at night. There are two main types of delirium. In hypoactive delirium people can appear withdrawn, drowsy and quiet. This can be harder to spot than in those with hyperactive delirium, who can be restless and agitated. The cause of delirium is often multifactorial:

- **Infection: in particular urinary tract infection and pneumonia. Rarely meningitis and encephalitis**
- **Medication: prescribed medications are an important factor in delirium (eg benzodiazepines, opiates). Also consider drug and alcohol intoxication or withdrawal**
- **Patient factors: pre-existing cognitive impairment (ie acute or chronic confusion)**
- **Health-related factors: hip fracture, severe illness or multiple co-morbidities**
- **Metabolic: hypoxia, dehydration, renal failure, liver failure, electrolyte imbalances, hypo- or hyperglycaemia**
- **Vascular: myocardial infarction, stroke**
- **Intracranial lesions (eg raised intracranial pressure, head injury)**
- **Others: constipation and urinary retention**

LEARNING POINTS

ⓘ Delirium is associated with poor outcomes, such as increased duration of stay and mortality. Management involves treatment of the underlying cause(s) and a reduction of associated risks and distress.

❶ Patient-specific measures include: treatment of infection, constipation, hypoxia, ensuring adequate hydration and nutrition, early mobilisation, sufficient pain relief and avoidance of drugs that can affect cognition (eg medication with antimuscarinic side-effects and hypnotics). All medication should be reviewed.

❶ Environmental measures include nursing by same members of staff, repeated orientation, provision of a clock, appropriate lighting levels and encouraging visits from family and friends. Noise levels on the ward should be limited, particularly at night-time. Items with which the patient could harm themselves or others should be removed where possible.

❶ As a last resort medication (eg haloperidol) can be used if the symptoms of delirium pose a significant risk to the patient or others.

Ethel recovers from the episode of delirium and makes a good recovery from her hip fracture before discharge back to her own home. However, her GP is concerned about her increasing forgetfulness and organises a minimental state examination (MMSE) in which she scores 18.

Q 2. **What MMSE score supports a diagnosis of dementia?**　　　　1 mark

A **MMSE < 25 supports a diagnosis of dementia.**

LEARNING POINTS

❶ The MMSE is the most commonly used assessment of cognitive function. MMSE is scored out of 30. A score of 25–30 is considered normal; < 25 supports a diagnosis of dementia in the absence of acute confusion and depression. Dementia can be classified as: 21–24 mild; 10–20 moderate; < 10 severe.

❶ Acetylcholinesterase-inhibiting drugs (ie donepezil, galantamine, rivastigmine) are used to treat mild to moderate dementia in Alzheimer's disease (not recommended in vascular dementia); benefit is assessed by repeating the MMSE at around 3 months, and may be continued if this demonstrates an improvement or no further deterioration in the patient's MMSE score (or global, functional or behavioural symptoms).

Q 3. **What is the commonest cause of dementia?**　　　　1 mark

A **Alzheimer's disease: this is the commonest cause of dementia in all age groups.**

LEARNING POINTS

❶ In adults over 65 years of age the second most common forms of dementia are:

- Vascular dementia: includes small-vessel disease, multi-infarct dementia and post-stroke dementia

- Dementia with Lewy bodies.

❶ In those under 65 years of age, Alzheimer's disease is still the most common cause of dementia. However, other causes such as frontotemporal dementias and alcohol-related dementia are more commonly seen.

Q **4. List four blood tests you would request to exclude treatable causes of dementia.** **2 marks**

A **½ mark each for any in the following list.**

Dementia is a clinical diagnosis but secondary causes must be excluded, as some causes are potentially reversible. First-line investigations include:

- **Full blood count: macrocytosis may indicate unsuspected alcohol abuse (common), vitamin B$_{12}$ or folate deficiency and thyroid disorder**

- **Urea and electrolytes (hyponatraemia, uraemia)**

- **Liver function (alcohol abuse may be suggested)**

- **Bone profile (hypercalcaemia)**

- **Vitamin B$_{12}$ and folate (deficiency)**

- **Thyroid function (hypothyroidism)**

- **Glucose**

LEARNING POINTS

❶ Syphilis serology or HIV testing is not indicated unless there are specific risk factors.

❶ Neuroimaging is recommended to help establish the subtype of dementia and to exclude other pathology (eg subdural haematoma). Magnetic resonance imaging (MRI) is preferred, but CT is most commonly used, as more widely available.

❶ Potentially treatable causes of dementia include: hypothyroidism, vitamin B$_{12}$, thiamine and folate deficiency, chronic alcohol abuse, normal-pressure hydrocephalus, AIDS and syphilis, brain tumours (eg frontal meningiomas) and subdural haematoma. Depression can also present as dementia (pseudodementia).

Ethel is referred to the local memory assessment service.

Q 5. **List six potential risks that should be considered in people with dementia.** 3 marks

A **½ mark each for any of the following:**
- **Risk of self-neglect (eg diet, self-care)**
- **Risk of wandering**
- **Risk of falls**
- **Risk of abuse (eg emotional, financial, physical and sexual)**
- **Fire risk**
- **Risks of self-harm**
- **Risks of aggression towards others (occurs in most at some stage, most often verbal)**
- **Risks from continued driving: patients/carers should be reminded of need to inform DVLA**
- **Carer strain and care breakdown (eg due to increasing dependence, non-concordance, behavioural symptoms)**

LEARNING POINT

ⓘ Memory assessment services encompass the diagnosis, treatment and rehabilitation of patients with dementia and involve shared care between health and social care. The aim is to promote and maintain independence; identifying and managing risks is an integral part of this process.

Total: 10 marks

PSYCHIATRY

RENAL CASES: ANSWERS

RENAL CASE 1

Sheila, a 49-year-old type 1 diabetic, is under the care of the nephrologist. Her current medications include insulin, angiotensin-converting enzyme (ACE) inhibitor (for hypertension) and a non-steroidal anti-inflammatory drug (NSAID) (for chronic back pain). At her annual review her blood pressure is 174/98 mmHg; her blood results are shown in Table 10.1 below.

Hb	8.6 g/dl	Na$^+$	136 mmol/l
MCV	86 fl	K$^+$	5.2 mmol/l
WCC	5.2 x 10⁹/l	Urea	22.9 mmol/l
Platelets	280 x 10⁹/l	Creatinine	246 µmol/l
		eGFR	23 ml/min
HbA$_{1c}$	11.2%	Adj Ca^{2+}	1.82 mmol/l
		PO$_4^{3-}$	2.72 mmol/l

Table 10.1: Sheila's blood results.

Q 1. Outline four functions of the kidney.   4 marks

A 1 mark each for any of the following:

• **Excretion of waste products, including drugs by glomerular filtration and active tubular secretion**

• **Fluid and electrolyte balance**

• **Acid:base balance: secrete hydrogen ions and reabsorb/synthesise bicarbonate (HCO$_3^-$)**

• **Gluconeogenesis: during fasting state**

• **Endocrine functions:**

  - **production of erythropoietin (see below)**

  - **conversion of 25-hydroxy (OH) vitamin D to 1,25-hydroxy (OH)$_2$ vitamin D (calcitriol), the active form of vitamin D (see below)**

  - **control of blood pressure: secretion of renin, which activates the renin-angiotensin pathway**

Q 2. **List three blood test results suggestive of chronic (as opposed to acute) renal failure.** 3 marks

A **1 mark for each of the following.**

The following blood tests suggest chronic, as opposed to acute, renal failure:

- **Normochromic normocytic anaemia, see below**
- **Hypocalcaemia: reduced adjusted calcium (2.12–2.65 mmol/l)**
- **Hyperphosphataemia: raised phosphate (0.8–1.45 mmol/l)**

LEARNING POINTS

ⓘ Previous abnormal urea and electrolytes (U&Es) and small kidneys on ultrasound scan also suggest chronic renal failure (CRF). However, it should be recognised that hypocalcaemia and hyperphosphataemia may also occur in acute renal failure (ARF), and anaemia may be associated with conditions causing ARF.

ⓘ Chronic renal failure, defined as progressive and usually irreversible impairment in renal function, is classified according to the reduction in glomerular filtration rate (GFR) (see Table 10.2 for stages).

Stage	eGFR(ml/min)	Description
1	> 90	Normal
2	60–89	Mild
3	30–59	Moderate
4	15–29	Severe
5	< 15	End-stage

Table 10.2: Stages in chronic renal failure according to eGFR.

Q 3. **Name two factors that might be contributing to her renal failure.** 1 mark

A **½ mark each for any of the following:**

- **Poorly controlled diabetes (as indicated by $HbA_{1c} > 7\%$), causing diabetic nephropathy**
- **Hypertension: poorly controlled blood pressure causing hypertensive nephropathy**
- **NSAIDs: analgaesic nephropathy**

LEARNING POINTS

🛈 Hypertension and diabetes are the two most common causes of chronic renal failure, the risk of which is reduced by tight control (other causes of chronic renal failure include glomerulonephritis, obstructive uropathy and polycystic kidneys).

🛈 While ACE inhibitors may cause acute renal failure, they have been shown to reduce the rate of progression of renal failure in patients with diabetes (and should be commenced in all diabetic patients with microalbuminuria, even if normotensive).

Sheila complains of fatigue, which her nephrologist attributes to her anaemia.

Q 4. **What is the likely cause of her anaemia?**   1 mark

A **Erythropoietin (EPO) deficiency.**

LEARNING POINTS

🛈 The kidneys release EPO to stimulate erythropoiesis in the bone marrow. Chronic renal failure causes a deficiency in EPO, resulting in anaemia.

🛈 This is corrected by excluding other causes (eg iron and folate deficiency) and by giving EPO (given parenterally). Blood transfusions should be avoided in patients in whom kidney transplant is a treatment option, as it increases the risk of HLA sensitisation and hence tissue rejection in renal transplantation.

🛈 The aim is to keep haemoglobin (Hb) levels between 10 g/dl and 12 g/dl. Failure to respond to EPO may be due to:

- Iron deficiency: patients should receive iron supplements to keep their ferritin levels between 200 µg/l and 500 µg/l (may require intravenous iron)

- Chronic infection

- Pure red cell aplasia

- Aluminium toxicity: may occur in haemodialysis patients, as it is a contaminant in the dialysate fluid.

As well as correcting her anaemia, Sheila is commenced on treatment for renal bone disease.

Q 5. **List two treatments to prevent renal bone disease.** 2 marks

A **1 mark each for any of the following.**

Renal bone disease (osteodystrophy) is prevented by aggressively treating hypocalcaemia and hyperphosphataemia by:

- **Dietary phosphate restriction (eg less milk, cheese, eggs)**
- **Phosphate binders (eg calcium-containing phosphate binders, sevelamer, lanthanum)**
- **Alphacalcidol to correct 'activated' vitamin D deficiency plus calcium supplements**

LEARNING POINTS

ⓘ Renal bone disease is caused by reduced renal phosphate excretion resulting in hyperphosphataemia, which in turn stimulates parathyroid hormone (PTH) release. There is also reduced vitamin D activation, resulting in reduced dietary calcium absorption (causing hypocalcaemia) and increased PTH release. Parathyroid hormone acts to promote bone calcium resorption (also causes resorption of phosphate), as well as promoting renal calcium reabsorption (and renal phosphate excretion) so as to oppose any hypocalcaemia, ultimately causing bone disease.

ⓘ Treatment of other complications of chronic renal failure includes low dietary potassium – eg avoid bananas (in treatment of hyperkalaemia), bicarbonate supplements (in severe metabolic acidosis), sodium/fluid restriction (in treatment of fluid overload and hypertension) – and low-protein diet to reduce rate of urea production (in treatment of severe uraemic symptoms).

Q 6. **How would you monitor the effectiveness of such treatment?** 1 mark

A **Monitor parathyroid hormone (PTH) levels.**

LEARNING POINT

ⓘ Parathyroid hormone is measured regularly to assess whether hyperparathyroidism is being effectively suppressed by treating hypocalcaemia and hyperphosphataemia. Parathyroidectomy or cinacalcet (which reduces PTH levels by mimicking actions of calcium on parathyroid receptors) may be used in refractory disease.

RENAL

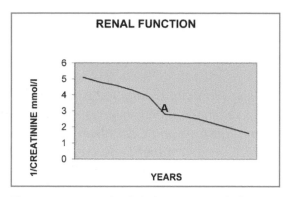

Figure 10.1: A graph of Shelia's reciprocal plasma creatinine against time.

Q 7. Give three possible generic causes for the sharp decline at time A (please refer to Figure 10.1). 3 marks

A **1 mark each for any of the following.**

The decline in renal function can be monitored by reciprocal plots of plasma creatinine, as often the decline is linear, so any rapid decline needs investigating to slow down the ultimate progression to end-stage renal failure (ESRF) and dialysis. Causes of rapid decline include the following:

- **Uncontrolled hypertension**
- **Uncontrolled diabetes**
- **Infection**
- **Dehydration.**
- **Nephrotoxic drugs (eg NSAIDs)**
- **Urinary tract obstruction**
- **Hypercalcaemia**

LEARNING POINT

🛈 The decision to start dialysis depends on eGFR, complications (eg refractory hyperkalaemia) and/or presence of severe uraemic symptoms. The two forms of dialysis are haemodialysis and peritoneal dialysis. In haemodialysis blood is pumped through a semipermeable membrane that allows molecules to diffuse across into the dialysis fluid, down their concentration gradient. Peritoneal dialysis is more simple; dialysis fluid is introduced into the peritoneal cavity using the peritoneal membrane as the semipermeable membrane. The fluid is changed regularly to repeat the process.

Total: **15 marks**

RENAL CASE 2

Christopher, an 84-year-old man, is admitted with a 2-day history of general malaise. On examination, he is hypotensive, pyrexial and clinically dehydrated. His admission urea and electrolytes (U&Es) are: Na⁺133 mmol/l, K⁺ 6.7 mmol/l, urea 41 mmol/l and creatinine 312 micromol/l, and an estimated glomerular filtration rate (eGFR) of 14 (his eGFR the previous month was 66).

Q 1. **List two causes each of prerenal, renal and postrenal causes of renal failure.** 3 marks

A **Prerenal causes (½ mark each for any of the following):**
- **Any cause of hypovolaemia (eg haemorrhage)**
- **Sepsis**
- **Decreased cardiac output (eg heart failure)**
- **Renal artery stenosis**
- **Drugs (eg ACE inhibitors decrease renal blood flow (see below))**

LEARNING POINT

ⓘ Prerenal causes are due to impaired renal perfusion as a result of hypotension or hypovolaemia.

A **Renal causes (½ mark each for any of the following):**
- **Acute tubular necrosis (ATN)**
- **Nephrotoxins (eg NSAIDs, gentamicin)**
- **Pyelonephritis**
- **Glomerulonephritis: immune complex-mediated damage to the glomerulus**
- **Rhabdomyolysis (causing myoglobinuria) (eg following crush injury, drug overdose)**
- **Myeloma**
- **Urate nephropathy: tumour lysis syndrome complicating chemotherapy in haematological malignancies**
- **Hepatorenal syndrome: renal failure secondary to liver failure**
- **Malignant hypertension**

LEARNING POINT

ⓘ Acute tubular necrosis (ATN) is a result of prerenal failure sufficient to cause ischaemic injury to renal tubules (ATN and prerenal failure account for > 80% cases of acute renal failure).

A **Postrenal causes (½ mark each for any of the following):**

- **Urinary stone disease**
- **Benign prostatic hypertrophy**
- **Prostatic carcinoma**
- **Pelvic (eg bladder) or abdominal tumours**
- **Retroperitoneal fibrosis (eg methyldopa, β-blockers)**

LEARNING POINT

ⓘ Postrenal causes (obstructive nephropathy) are due to obstruction to the renal tract anywhere from the calyces to the external urethral orifice. Though typically subacute or chronic, it is treated as acute renal failure as it is (partially) reversible on relief of obstruction (eg by catheterisation, nephrostomy).

Appropriate investigations are undertaken, including an electrocardiogram (ECG), shown in Figure 10.2 below:

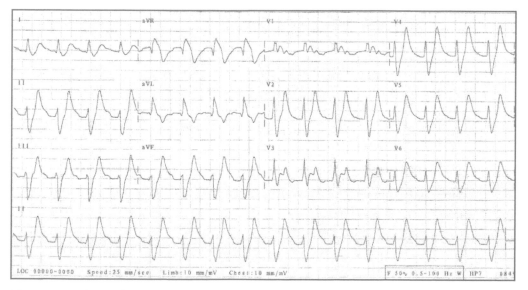

Figure 10.2: Christopher's ECG.

Q 2. **Give two ECG changes associated with hyperkalaemia.**   2 marks

A **1 mark each for any of the following:**

- **Tall-tented T waves**
- **Small (or absent) P waves**
- **Widened QRS complex**

LEARNING POINTS

ⓘ Hyperkalaemia causes hyperpolarisation of cell membranes, causing reduced cardiac excitability, predisposing to arrhythmias. It requires urgent treatment if > 6.5 mmol/l or if associated with the above ECG changes.

ⓘ Other investigations in acute renal failure include (depending on clinical indication):

- Urine dipstick, microscopy and culture: (eg nitrites/leucocytes indicates urinary tract infection (UTI)); haematuria/proteinuria/red blood cell casts may indicate glomerulonephritis

- U&Es, full blood count, liver function tests

- Urate

- Creatinine kinase: markedly raised in rhabdomyolysis

- Myeloma screen: serum/urinary electrophoresis

- Immunology screen (if suggestive of glomerulonephritis): ANA, ANCA, complement (reduced in SLE), anti-GBM antibodies (Goodpasture's syndrome)

- Arterial blood gases: to assess degree of acidosis (see below)

- Blood cultures

- Urgent urological ultrasound scan: to exclude postrenal failure

- Chest X-ray: pneumonia (source of infection), pulmonary oedema (complication of acute renal failure)

Q 3. List four causes of hyperkalaemia.   2 marks

A ½ mark each for any of the following.

Hyperkalaemia is either caused by increased cellular release or failure of excretion:

- Increased cellular release may occur in:
  - metabolic acidosis (eg diabetic ketoacidosis (DKA))
  - cell lysis (eg rhabdomyolysis, blood transfusion)
  - digoxin toxicity: due to inhibition of Na^+/K^+ pump
  - artefactual: haemolysis of blood sample
- Failure of excretion may occur in:
  - renal failure: both acute and chronic renal failure
  - potassium-sparing diuretics (eg spironolactone)
  - ACE inhibitors: inhibit aldosterone-mediated potassium excretion
  - Addison's disease (ie aldosterone deficiency)
  - metabolic acidosis: hydrogen competes with potassium for excretion in the distal convoluted tubule. Thus, in metabolic acidosis, increased hydrogen will compete with potassium for renal excretion, causing hyperkalaemia

Q 4. How would you treat life-threatening hyperkalaemia?   3 marks

A 1 mark each for any of the following:

- Intravenous calcium gluconate (10 ml 10%) if ECG changes: cardioprotective (stabilises the cardiac membranes), although it does not reduce serum potassium concentrations
- Intravenous glucose (50 ml 50% dextrose) and insulin (10–16 units Actrapid): insulin promotes cellular uptake of K^+ by stimulating the $Na^+K^+ATPase$ (glucose to counteract the effects of insulin); nebulised β_2-agonists also drive potassium into cells
- Intravenous bicarbonate if severe metabolic acidosis (see above)
- Calcium resonium (oral or rectal): only treatment that actually removes potassium from body

LEARNING POINT

ⓘ If refractory hyperkalaemia consider renal replacement therapy (see below).

Christopher is diagnosed with acute renal failure secondary to urinary sepsis. His hyperkalaemia is treated appropriately, he is resuscitated with intravenous fluids, commenced on broad-spectrum antibiotics and his nephrotoxic drugs stopped.

Q 5. **Outline how ACE inhibitors and NSAIDs cause acute renal failure.**   2 marks

A **1 mark each for any of the following:**

- **ACE inhibitors: cause prerenal failure (particularly in presence of renal artery stenosis) due to efferent arteriole vasodilation, thereby reducing glomerular filtration pressure**
- **NSAIDs are both a prerenal and renal cause of renal failure:**
- **prerenal cause: reduced glomerular filtration pressure due to inhibition of prostaglandin-mediated afferent arteriole vasodilation**
- **renal cause: direct nephrotoxin**

LEARNING POINT

❶ The management of acute renal failure involves:
- Monitoring of fluid balance, ie fluid balance charts, insertion of urinary catheter ± insertion of central venous pressure (CVP) line
- Fluid resuscitation if hypovolaemic and hypotensive; if hypotensive despite adequate fluid resuscitation may require inotropic support
- Treating the underlying cause (eg antibiotics if septic, stopping nephrotoxic drugs)
- Management of potential complications (see below).

Christopher's blood pressure and urine output respond to fluid resuscitation and his U&Es subsequently indicate recovery of his renal function.

Q 6. **List four indications for renal replacement therapy.**   2 marks

A **½ mark each for any of the following:**
- **Severe uraemic symptoms (eg uraemic encephalopathy)**
- **Uraemic complications (eg pericarditis)**
- **Refractory hyperkalaemia**
- **Severe metabolic acidosis**

- **Refractory pulmonary oedema: if fluid-overloaded, give intravenous furosemide (250 mg over 1 hour)**
- **Removal of drugs causing acute renal failure**

LEARNING POINT

❶ If the above complications of acute renal failure are refractory to medical treatment, the patient may require renal replacement therapy (eg dialysis) while awaiting recovery of renal function.

Q 7. **Name two early complications following recovery from acute tubular necrosis (ATN).**   1 mark

A **1 mark each for any of the following.**

While prerenal failure is rapidly reversed by correction of the underlying cause (as in Christopher's case), recovery of ATN typically takes days to weeks. In the early stages of recovery a diuretic phase may occur where, due to earlier recovery of glomerular function, the glomerular filtration rate (GFR) exceeds renal tubular reabsorption causing:

- **Hyponatraemia**
- **Hypokalaemia**
- **Hypovolaemia**

❶ As a consequence, in these patients careful monitoring of fluid and electrolyte balance is required.

Total: **15 marks**

RESPIRATORY
CASES: ANSWERS

RESPIRATORY CASE 1

Lucy, a 21-year-old asthmatic, presents to the Emergency Department with a 2-day history of increased shortness of breath, wheeze and cough. On examination her pulse is 125 bpm, respiratory rate is 30/min, there is widespread bilateral expiratory wheeze and air entry is reduced throughout.

Q 1. **What three brief questions would you ask?**   3 marks

A **1 mark each for the following:**

- **Ask about usual treatments**
- **Best peak expiratory flow (PEF): used to assess severity severity/effect of treatment**
- **Previous admissions to hospital for acute attacks, including transfer to ICU (this may give an indication of the potential severity of her asthma)**

LEARNING POINT

❶ The only investigations needed before **immediate treatment** are PEF (though may be too ill) and pulse oximetry (SpO_2).

Q 2. **List three criteria used to indicate a severe asthma attack.**   3 marks

A **1 mark each for any of the following:**

- **Severe breathlessness/can't complete sentences**
- **Respiratory rate ≥ 25/min**
- **Pulse rate ≥ 110 bpm**
- **PEF 33–50% of predicted or best**

Q 3. **List three criteria used to indicate a life-threatening asthma attack.**   3 marks

A **1 mark each for any of the following:**

- **Silent chest, cyanosis or poor respiratory effort**
- **Exhaustion, confusion or coma**
- **PEF < 33% of predicted or best**

- **SpO$_2$ < 92%**
- **PaO$_2$ < 8 kPa; normal PaCO$_2$ (see below)**
- **Arrhythmia, including bradycardia**

LEARNING POINT

ℹ️ If there are any life-threatening features, warn ICU, as the patient may require transfer to ICU for respiratory support, including intubation (similarly warn ICU if the patient has been admitted to ICU with previous asthma attacks).

Q 4. List two arterial blood gas (ABG) markers of a *life-threatening* attack.   1 mark

A ½ **mark each for any of the following:**

- **Normal or high PaCO$_2$: PaCO$_2$ should normally be low secondary to hyperventilation**
- **Respiratory failure (ie PaO$_2$ < 8 kPa irrespective of O$_2$ therapy)**
- **Acidosis: either respiratory or metabolic (due to lactic acid build-up caused by increased respiratory effort)**

LEARNING POINT

ℹ️ Patients with SpO$_2$ < 92% or other features of life-threatening asthma should have ABG measurement.

Lucy is diagnosed with a severe asthma attack and is treated appropriately.

Q 5. What is your immediate management in *severe* asthma?   3 marks

A 1 mark for each of the following:

- **Sit patient upright and give high-flow (40–60%) O$_2$: CO$_2$ retention is not usually aggravated by O$_2$ therapy in asthma. Aim to maintain SpO$_2$ at 94–98%**
- **Nebulised salbutamol (5 mg) and ipratropium bromide (500 mcg): ideally bronchodilators should be driven by oxygen; may need continuous nebulisation**
- **Oral prednisolone (40–50 mg) or IV hydrocortisone (200 mg): continue prednisolone 40–50 mg daily for at least 5 days**

LEARNING POINTS

ℹ️ Admit patients with any feature of a life-threatening attack or features of a

RESPIRATORY

severe attack persisting after initial treatment.

ⓘ Patients whose PEF is > 75% best or predicted 1 hour after initial treatment may be discharged.

Q 6. What additional treatment may be used in life-threatening asthma? 1 mark

A **Magnesium sulphate: 1.2–2 g IV infusion over 20 minutes.**

LEARNING POINTS

ⓘ Single dose of IV magnesium sulphate should be considered in life-threatening asthma or severe asthma not responding to inhaled bronchodilator therapy.

ⓘ Intravenous magnesium sulphate is also used in the treatment of eclamptic seizures and ventricular arrhythmias, in particular torsade de pointes.

Q 7. When would you request a chest X-ray in an asthma attack? 1 mark

A **1 mark for any of the following:**

- **Suspected pneumothorax: may be a cause of sudden deterioration in patients with asthma**
- **Suspected pneumonia**
- **Life-threatening asthma**
- **Failure to respond to treatment satisfactorily**
- **Requiring ventilation**

LEARNING POINT

ⓘ A chest X-ray is not routinely recommended in the absence of the above.

Lucy's breathing improves and she is transferred to the wards.

Q 8. List two ways in which the effects of treatment can be assessed non-invasively. 1 mark

A **½ mark each for any of the following:**

- **Clinically (eg respiratory rate, wheeze, ability to complete sentences)**
- **Pulse oximetry (SpO$_2$)**
- **Peak expiratory flow (PEF)**

LEARNING POINT

ⓘ Discharge may safely take place as soon as clinical improvement is apparent.

Lucy continues to improve, and discharge is planned for the following day.

Q 9. **What four things should Lucy have before discharge?**   4 marks

A **1 mark each for any of the following:**
- **Been on discharge medications for 24 hours**
- **Treatment with oral and inhaled steroids in addition to bronchodilators**
- **PEF > 75% best or predicted and < 25% variability**
- **Inhaler technique checked**
- **Management plan agreed using PEF monitoring and symptoms: eg when to double-up on daily dose of inhaled steroids, use of rescue oral steroids**
- **GP follow-up appointment within 2 working days**
- **Appointment at respiratory clinic within 1 month**

LEARNING POINT

ⓘ All patients attending hospital with an asthma attack should be reviewed by a respiratory physician, preferably within 30 days. Furthermore, patients admitted with severe/life-threatening asthma should be followed up for at least 1 year after the admission.

Total: 20 marks

RESPIRATORY CASE 2

Tom, a 63-year-old lifelong smoker, attends his GP with increasing breathlessness, a chronic cough and regular sputum production. His notes reveal frequent winter chest infections requiring antibiotics. Suspecting a diagnosis of chronic obstructive pulmonary disease (COPD), his GP requests spirometry: FEV₁ 54%, FEV₁/FVC < 0.7.

Q 1. **On the basis of Tom's spirometry what is the severity of COPD?**　　1 mark

A **Moderate COPD.**

LEARNING POINTS

FEV_1/FVC	FEV_1 % predicted	COPD severity
< 0.7	≥ 80%	Mild
< 0.7	50–79%	Moderate
< 0.7	30–49%	Severe
< 0.7	< 30%	Very severe

🛈 When diagnosing COPD, alongside spirometry, also request a chest X-ray (to exclude other diagnoses) and FBC (to identify anaemia or polycythaemia). If there is evidence of cor pulmonale, also request an electrocardiogram (ECG) and echocardiogram.

🛈 Asthma and COPD rarely coexist (and can usually be distinguished on the basis of history and examination). Asthma may be present if there is a large (> 400 ml) increase in FEV_1 to bronchodilators or following a 2-week course of oral prednisolone; in asthma (unlike COPD), there is usually a significant (≥ 20%) diurnal or day-to-day variability in peak expiratory flow rate (PEFR).

Q 2. **What advice would you offer?**　　1 mark

A **Stop smoking.**

LEARNING POINT

❶ All COPD patients who still smoke, regardless of age, should be encouraged to stop smoking and offered help (eg nicotine replacement therapy or varenicline as part of a smoking cessation programme).

Tom is started on an ipratropium bromide inhaler by his GP.

Q 3. When are inhaled corticosteroids indicated in COPD? 1 mark

A ½ mark each for the following:
- **FEV_1 < 50% predicted**
- **In patients who have frequent exacerbations (≥ 2 year), irrespective of FEV_1**

LEARNING POINTS

❶ First-line treatment in COPD is either a short-acting β-agonist (SABA, eg salbutamol) or short-acting muscarinic antagonist (SAMA, eg ipratropium bromide), as required. In patients who remain breathless or have exacerbations, maintenance therapy with a long-acting β-agonist (LABA, eg salmeterol) and/or long-acting muscarinic antagonist (LAMA, eg tiotropium) can be offered. If frequent exacerbations and/or FEV_1 < 50% predicted, can add in an inhaled corticosteroid.

❶ Mucolytic therapy (eg carbocisteine) may help symptoms in patients with a chronic cough.

❶ All patients should have the pneumococcal vaccination and annual influenza vaccination.

❶ Patients at risk of exacerbations should have a rescue course of antibiotics and corticosteroids at home with advice when to start (eg sputum becomes purulent).

❶ Maintenance therapy with oral steroids is not recommended. However, some patients may be difficult to wean following a COPD exacerbation; such patients should be managed on the lowest dose possible, with osteoporosis prophylaxis.

Q 4. **List two qualifying criteria for home O$_2$ therapy.** 1 mark

A **½ mark each for the following:**

• **pO$_2$ < 7.3 kPa (on two separate occasions when COPD is stable at least 3 weeks apart)**

• **pO$_2$ < 8 kPa with evidence of secondary polycythaemia, nocturnal hypoxaemia or evidence of cor pulmonale**

LEARNING POINTS

❶ To achieve improved survival (50% improvement in 3-year survival) O$_2$ therapy (1–3 litre/min) must be given > 15 h/day.

❶ Cor pulmonale is right heart failure secondary to chronic pulmonary hypertension (of which COPD is the most common cause). Characteristics of cor pulmonale include peripheral oedema, raised jugular venous pressure (JVP), right ventricular heave, and loud pulmonary second heart sound. The ECG may show signs of right heart strain (eg right axis deviation).

The following winter Tom is admitted to the Emergency Department with severe dyspnoea and cough productive of green sputum. On examination his temperature is 37°C, pulse is 95 bpm, respiratory rate 35/min, he has widespread expiratory wheeze, reduced air entry throughout and is cyanosed.

Q 5. **What four brief questions would you ask regarding his COPD?** 2 marks

A **½ mark each for asking about any of the following:**

• **Usual treatments, including home nebulisers and oxygen therapy**

• **Previous acute episodes and their treatment**

• **Normal exercise tolerance**

• **Smoking history**

• **Any allergies to any medications (eg penicillin)**

RESPIRATORY

Q 6. **What is your immediate medical management (including doses, where appropriate)?** 3 marks

A **1 mark each for the following:**

- **Controlled O_2 therapy: aim is to keep SaO_2 > 90% without worsening respiratory acidosis/hypercapnia (see below)**

- **Nebulised bronchodilators – ie salbutamol (2.5–5 mg qds) and ipratropium bromide (500 µg qds)**

- **Oral steroids: 30 mg prednisolone for 7–14 days (after which it can be stopped abruptly or tapered, if previous difficulty coming off steroids; if prolonged treatment, will require dose reduction on cessation to avoid a potential addisonian crisis)**

LEARNING POINTS

❶ Intravenous aminophylline may be used if response to nebulised bronchodilators is poor: it has a narrow therapeutic range, causing arrhythmias and seizures in toxic range, so it requires monitoring of plasma levels.

❶ Investigations include: chest X-ray; ECG; bloods, including FBC, arterial blood gases (ABGs); sputum microscopy; and culture if purulent and blood cultures if pyrexial.

The arterial blood gases (ABG) results (on air) are shown below:

pH	**7.37**	**(7.35–7.45)**
pO_2	**6.9 kPa**	**(>10.6)**
pCO_2	**4.2 kPa**	**(4.7–6)**
HCO_3^-	**25 mmol/l**	**(22-28)**
BE	**–1.2**	**(±2)**

Q 7. **What type of respiratory failure do the ABGs show?** 1 mark

A **Type I respiratory failure.**

LEARNING POINT

❶ pH and bicarbonate are within normal limits: pO_2 is < 8kPa, ie respiratory failure, without pCO_2 retention, ie type I as opposed to type II.

Q 8. **How will these ABGs influence your immediate management?** 1 mark

A **Since ABGs do not indicate CO_2 retention, increase O_2, aiming for $SaO_2 > 92\%$.**

LEARNING POINTS

- In the presence of type II respiratory failure (ie $pCO_2 > 6$ kPa), O_2 therapy should be limited to 24–28% as the respiratory centre is insensitive to CO_2 and respiration is driven by hypoxia. Excessive O_2 therapy may cause life-threatening hypercapnia.

- To prevent precipitating or worsening respiratory acidosis, ABGs should be repeated approximately 20 minutes after each change in O_2 treatment until the patient is stable.

Q 9. **List four signs of hypercapnia.** 2 marks

A **½ mark each for any of the following:**
- **Tachycardia**
- **Bounding pulse**
- **Peripheral vasodilatation**
- **Hand flap**
- **Papilloedema**
- **Confusion**
- **Coma**

LEARNING POINT

- Non-invasive ventilation (NIV) (eg bi-level positive airway pressure (BiPAP)), should be considered for any patient with respiratory acidosis/hypercapnia. Worsening respiratory acidosis on treatment is a sensitive indicator of a deteriorating patient and may require admission to ICU for invasive ventilation (although patients should always have agreed ceilings of therapy in the event of a deterioration).

The diagnosis is made of infective COPD exacerbation, which is successfully treated with amoxicillin.

Q 10. What two organisms are commonly responsible for COPD exacerbations?   2 marks

A 1 mark each for any of the following:

- *Streptococcus pneumoniae*
- *Haemophilus influenzae*
- *Moraxella catarrhalis*

LEARNING POINT

❶ Oral antibiotics should only be prescribed if purulent sputum or sputum volume has increased with worsening dyspnoea; typically amoxicillin, a macrolide, or a tetracycline, are prescribed. Also consider physiotherapy to help clear sputum.

Total: 15 marks

RESPIRATORY CASE 3

As the surgical FY1, you are bleeped to review Derek, a 76-year-old man 4 days postop hemicolectomy, who is complaining of right-sided pleuretic chest pain with associated breathlessness. On examination, you find signs of a deep vein in thrombosis (DVT) in his left leg.

Q 1. List three signs of a DVT on examination. 3 marks

A 1 mark each for any of the following:

- **Swollen leg**
- **Distended veins**
- **Tenderness**
- **Increased warmth**

LEARNING POINTS

❶ However, none of the signs of a DVT are unique to a DVT (eg also seen in cellulitis), which can only be reliably confirmed by Doppler ultrasound examination (if negative, but clinical suspicion remains high, may need repeating 1 week later).

❶ The Wells' score, as shown in Table 11.1, is used to assess the probability of a DVT.

Clinical feature	Score
Active cancer	1
Bedridden > 3 days or major surgery last 4 weeks	1
Paralysis, paresis or recent plaster immobilisation of leg	1
Collateral superficial veins (non-varicose)	1
Entire leg swollen	1
Local tenderness along distribution of deep venous system	1
Pitting oedema (greater in symptomatic leg)	1
Calf swelling > 3cm compared with asymptomatic leg	1
Alternative diagnosis to DVT as likely or more likely	−2

Table 11.1: Wells' score.

ⓘ If intermediate (1–2 points) and high (≥ 3 points) probability, do Doppler; if low risk (0 points) measure D-dimer: if negative, it excludes DVT.

ⓘ While a negative D-dimer can exclude venous thromboembolism (VTE), it is also raised in infection, malignancy and pregnancy, so it has a low sensitivity.

Q 2. **List six risk factors for pulmonary embolism (PE).** 3 marks

A **½ mark each for any of the following.**

Risk factors are any cause of immobility or hypercoagulability:

- **Recent surgery (eg major abdominal or pelvic surgery, hip or knee replacement)**
- **Prolonged immobilisation (eg plaster cast, bed rest, recent air travel)**
- **Malignancy (eg abdominal, pelvic, advanced metastatic)**
- **Pregnancy and puerperium**
- **Drugs: combined oral contraceptive pill, hormone replacement therapy (HRT)**
- **Hypercoagulability disorders (ie thrombocytosis, polycythaemia, thrombophilia)**
- **Family history of VTE**
- **Previous VTE**

LEARNING POINT

ⓘ Examples of thrombophilia include: antiphospholipid syndrome (lupus anticoagulant and/or anticardiolipin antibody); factor V Leiden (activated protein C resistance); antithrombin III deficiency; protein C or S deficiency; and prothrombin gene mutation.

Derek undergoes a number of investigations, including an electrocardiogram (ECG). Suspecting a PE, he is commenced on low-molecular-weight heparin (LMWH), while awaiting a CT pulmonary angiogram.

Q 3. **What does this ECG show (see Figure 11.1)?** 1 mark

A **Right bundle branch block (RBBB).**

LEARNING POINTS

ⓘ In PE the ECG is often normal, although it may show sinus tachycardia, RBBB (eg widened QRS complex, RSR (M) pattern in V1), right heart strain (eg inverted T waves in V1-4), right axis deviation (+ve in III, -ve in I); the classical $S_IQ_{III}T_{III}$ (ie deep S waves in I, pathological Q waves and inverted T waves in III) is rare.

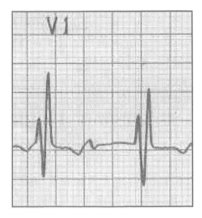

Figure 11.1: Derek's ECG

❶ Other investigations include:

- Full blood count (FBC): polycythaemia, thrombocytosis

- Baseline clotting screen: in preparation for anticoagulation

- D-dimer (see above)

- Chest X-ray: often normal in PE or small effusion; used to exclude pneumothorax

- Arterial blood gases (ABGs): may show reduced pO_2 and reduced pCO_2 (due to hyperventilation)

- CT pulmonary angiogram (CTPA): this is very sensitive for detecting PE. Echo can also be used to diagnose a massive PE.

❶ Thrombophilia screen is reserved for younger patients with recurrent VTEs or strong family history of VTE. Investigations for occult malignancy are only indicated when it is suspected on clinical examination, chest X-ray or routine blood tests.

The diagnosis of PE secondary to a DVT is made. Derek is anticoagulated with warfarin with a target international normalised ratio (INR) of 2–3.

Q 4. **What is the mechanism of action of warfarin?** 1 mark

A **Vitamin K antagonist.**

LEARNING POINTS

🛈 Warfarin inhibits the reductase enzyme responsible for regenerating the active form of vitamin K (needed for the synthesis of factors II, VII, IX and X). Heparin enhances the effects of antithrombin III and deactivates factor X (as does low-molecular-weight heparin (LMWH)).

🛈 The treatment of PE involves O_2, analgesia, anti-embolism stockings, LMWH, and addressing any underlying cause. Thrombolysis is reserved for patients with massive PE causing shock. Once PE has been confirmed, start warfarin; LMWH should be continued until INR is in therapeutic range (2–3). This is because initially warfarin has a prothrombotic effect (protein C and S are also vitamin K-dependent), so the patient needs to be adequately anticoagulated when commencing warfarin.

🛈 Duration of anticoagulation in VTE:

- 4–6 weeks if temporary risk factor
- 3 months for first idiopathic VTE
- 6 months for all others
- Indefinite/lifelong treatment in recurrent VTE.

Q 5. How can you reduce the risk of VTE in hospitalised patients?   2 marks

A 1 mark each for any of the following.

Hospital-acquired VTE is a significant cause of morbidity/mortality that can be significantly reduced by the following measures:

- **Ensure adequate hydration**
- **Anti-embolism stockings: knee- or thigh- length. Contraindications include peripheral vascular disease**
- **Anticoagulate (eg LMWH: continue until patient is no longer at increased risk)**
- **Encourage patients to mobilise as soon as possible**

LEARNING POINTS

🛈 Do not regard aspirin or other antiplatelet agents as adequate VTE prophylaxis.

🛈 Advise women to stop combined oral contraception or HRT 4 weeks before elective surgery.

Total: **10 marks**

RESPIRATORY CASE 4

*Margaret, a 64-year-old heavy smoker, visits her GP complaining of a
3-month history of cough associated with haemoptysis.*

Q 1. **List three respiratory causes of haemoptysis.**   3 marks

A **1 mark each for any of the following:**

- **Acute lower respiratory tract infections**
- **Lung cancer**
- **Tuberculosis (TB)**
- **Bronchiectasis: may be a cause of massive haemoptysis**
- **Trauma (eg inhalation of a foreign body)**
- **Pulmonary embolism**

LEARNING POINT

ⓘ Patients who present with haemoptysis should have an urgent chest X-ray to
exclude underlying lung cancer.

Q 2. **List two other common presenting lung cancer symptoms.**   2 marks

- **Dyspnoea**
- **Chest pain**
- **Weight loss**
- **Non-resolving pneumonia: patients treated for pneumonia who have persistent
  chest symptoms/signs or at risk of lung cancer should have a follow-up chest
  X-ray at 6 weeks**

LEARNING POINT

ⓘ Any patient presenting with unexplained or persistent (> 3 weeks) cough,
chest/shoulder pain, dyspnoea, weight loss, chest signs, hoarseness (due
to involvement of recurrent laryngeal nerve), finger clubbing, or cervical/
supraclavicular lymphadenopathy and signs of metastases (see below) should
also have an urgent chest X-ray.

On examination the only abnormal finding is that she is clubbed.

Q 3. **List two cardiac, two respiratory and two gastrointestinal causes of clubbing.** 3 marks

A **½ mark each for any of the following:**

- **Cardiac: cyanotic congenital heart disease, subacute bacterial endocarditis**
- **Gastrointestinal: inflammatory bowel disease (IBD), cirrhosis, malabsorption (eg coeliacs), gastrointestinal lymphoma**
- **Respiratory: lung cancer, chronic lung suppuration (eg cystic fibrosis, bronchiectasis, empyema, abscess), fibrotic lung disease**

LEARNING POINT

ⓘ Clubbing is an example of a paraneoplastic syndrome. It occurs in approximately 30% of cases (lung cancer is the most common cause of clubbing).

The GP arranges an urgent chest X-ray (see Figure 11.2). The radiological report notes opacification of the right apex with destruction of the second rib, consistent with bronchial carcinoma.

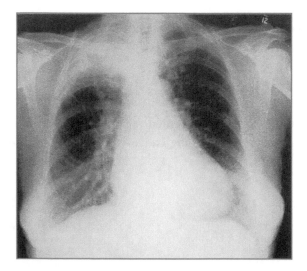

Figure 11.2: Margaret's chest X-ray.

Q 4. **What is this type of lung tumour called?**   1 mark

A **Pancoast tumour.**

LEARNING POINTS

🛈 Pancoast tumour refers to a lung tumour in the apex of the lung. It may cause rib erosion, involve the brachial plexus, causing pain down the medial aspect of the arm, or involve the sympathetic chain, causing Horner syndrome.

🛈 Lung cancer complications can be classified as local (eg Horner syndrome), metastatic and paraneoplastic syndromes (due to tumour secretory products).

🛈 Another local complication is superior vena cava obstruction, causing early-morning headache; puffy face and neck (collar feels tight); distended, non-pulsatile jugular vein; dilated veins on chest wall. The obstruction may be relieved by radiotherapy ± stenting of the vein.

🛈 Examples of paraneoplastic syndromes include: syndrome of inappropriate secretion of antidiuretic hormone (SIADH); Eaton–Lambert syndrome (proximal myopathy); ectopic adrenocorticotropic hormone (ACTH); and hypertrophic pulmonary osteoarthropathy (HPOA), causing joint stiffness and severe pain in wrists and ankles. X-rays show subperiosteal new bone formation often described as an 'onion-skin' appearance. Symptoms improve when the primary tumour is removed.

Q 5. **List four causes of round lesions on the lung on chest X-ray.**   2 marks

A ½ mark each for any of the following:

- **Primary lung tumours: most lung tumours are bronchial carcinomas, which can be classified as small-cell carcinoma and non-small cell carcinoma (further divided into squamous-cell, large-cell and adenocarcinoma). Rarer forms of lung tumours include bronchiolar-alveolar cell carcinoma**
- **Secondary lung tumours: eg spread from kidney, testis, breast, bone, choriocarcinoma or gastrointestinal tract (usually multiple)**
- **'Round pneumonia'**
- **Abscess (usually with air–fluid level)**
- **Cyst, eg hydatid**
- **Foreign body**
- **Granuloma, ie nodular accumulation of macrophages (eg tuberculosis, sarcoidosis)**
- **Rheumatoid nodule**

RESPIRATORY

Q 6. **Where does lung cancer metastasise to?** 2 marks

A **½ mark each for any of the following:**

- **Bone: causing pain and pathological fractures. Treatment includes: NSAIDs, IV bisphosphonates and radiotherapy**
- **Liver**
- **Adrenal glands**
- **Brain: may present with headache, seizures, focal neurological deficit, change in personality. Treatment includes dexamethasone and cranial radiotherapy**

Margaret is seen the following week as an outpatient at the respiratory clinic.

Q 7. **What two investigations would you arrange to confirm lung cancer?** 2 marks

A **1 mark each for any of the following:**

- **Contrast-enhanced CT scan of chest, liver and adrenals: this is the first investigation in suspected lung cancer**
- **Bronchoscopy: to obtain biopsy for histological diagnosis. Patients require pulmonary function tests and lateral chest X-ray in preparation**
- **CT- or ultrasound- (including endoscopic) guided biopsy**
- **Positron-emission tomography (PET) scan: detects increased uptake of labelled glucose by cancer cells**

LEARNING POINTS

🛈 Sputum for cytology is an insensitive test and reserved for patients with central tumours who are unable to tolerate bronchoscopy.

🛈 Staging is important for treatment and prognosis. Non-small-cell carcinoma is staged using the TNM (tumour, node, metastasis) system; small-cell carcinoma, which has usually metastasised at presentation, is staged as limited or extensive.

🛈 Blood tests include liver function tests (bronchial carcinoma may metastasise to the liver), bone profile (may metastasise to bone, causing Ca^{2+} and ALP), and urea and electrolytes (U&Es) (eg hyponatraemia due to syndrome of inappropriate antidiuretic hormone secretion (SIADH) – an example of a paraneoplastic syndrome).

ⓘ The treatment of lung cancer includes surgery (wedge resection, lobectomy or pneumonectomy), radiotherapy and chemotherapy. Patients with small-cell lung cancer may also be offered prophylactic cranial radiotherapy due to its propensity to metastasise to the brain.

Total: **15 marks**

RESPIRATORY CASE 5

John, a 72-year-old insulin-dependent diabetic, visits his GP with a 3-day history of cough, dyspnoea and general malaise. He is prescribed amoxicillin but continues to deteriorate and is admitted to hospital the following day.

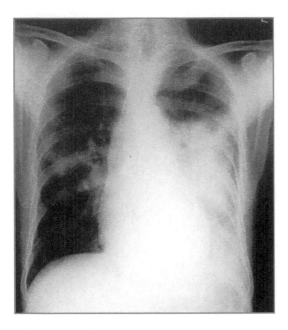

Figure 11.3: John's chest X-ray.

Q 1. **What is your diagnosis (see Figure 11.3)?**   2 marks

A **Left lower lobe (1 mark) pneumonia (1 mark).**

LEARNING POINTS

ⓘ Loss of the left hemidiaphragm and preservation of the left heart border indicate the pneumonia is in the left lower lobe. In right lower lobe pneumonia there is loss of the right hemidiaphragm; in right middle lobe pneumonia there is loss of the right heart border.

❶ Involvement of only one lobe is a good prognostic indicator; conversely, bilateral or multilobe pneumonia on chest X-ray indicates severe pneumonia (see below).

❶ Appropriate investigations include full blood count (FBC), C-reactive protein (CRP), urea and electrolytes (U&Es), liver function tests (LFTs), blood cultures, arterial blood gases (ABGs) (if SaO_2 < 92%) and sputum for microbial culture and sensitivity (MC&S); in severe cases screen for atypical organisms (see below).

Q 2. **List two poor prognostic features in the history.**   **2 marks**

A **1 mark each for the following:**
- **72 years old**
- **Diabetes**

LEARNING POINTS

❶ Age > 65 years and coexisting chronic disease are associated with a poor prognosis. Failure to respond to treatment would also represent a poor prognostic sign, although in this case John has only received a short course of oral antibiotics.

❶ The **CURB-65** score (in association with clinical judgement) is a simple tool for assessing severity, ie ≥ 3 of the following indicates severe pneumonia: (1) **C**onfusion, eg < 8/10 on abbreviated mental test score; (2) **U**rea > 7 mmol/l; (3) **R**espiratory rate > 30/min; (4) **B**lood pressure: systolic < 90 mmHg or diastolic < 60 mmHg; and (5) age > **65** years.

❶ Management of pneumonia is based on its severity. If not severe, treat with oral antibiotics, eg amoxicllin (500 mg tds) and/or clarithromycin (500 mg bd); doxycycline (100 mg od) is an alternative. If severe, treat with intravenous antibiotics, eg either co-amoxiclav (1.2 g tds) or cefuroxime (1.5 g tds) with clarithromycin (500 mg bd). Fluoroquinolones (eg levofloxacin) are first line in *Legionella* pneumonia.

John is diagnosed with severe pneumonia and treated with intravenous co-amoxiclav and clarithromycin (to cover atypical organisms).

RESPIRATORY

Q 3. **List three causes of 'atypical' pneumonia.** 3 marks

A **1 mark each for any of the following:**

- *Mycoplasma pneumoniae*: **tends to affect young adults; it occurs in epidemics every 3–4 years**
- *Legionella pneumophila*: **outbreaks are usually associated with contaminated showers, water-cooling or air-conditioning systems**
- *Coxiella burnetii* **(Q fever)**
- *Chlamydia* **species (eg** *Chlamydia psittaci*, *Chlamydia pneumoniae*)

LEARNING POINTS

❶ It is important in the history to enquire about any pet birds (*C. psittaci*) or recent stay in a hotel (*Legionella*).

❶ Atypical infections are 'atypical' because they do not respond to penicillin and cause general (eg diarrhoea) as well as respiratory symptoms.

❶ In patients with severe pneumonia (or suspicion of atypical pneumonia) blood should be sent for atypical serology (ie specific antibodies against atypical organisms) and urine screened for *Legionella* antigen (can also screen for pneumococcal antigen).

Microbiology call the ward to report Gram-positive cocci in John's blood, while awaiting culture and sensitivity.

Q 4. **What is the most likely cause of John's pneumonia and how can this be prevented?** 2 marks

A **1 mark each for the following:**

- *Streptococcus pneumoniae* **is a Gram-positive (ie stains purple) coccus and is the most common cause of pneumonia, accounting for 60–75% of cases; it responds to penicillins.**
- **Pneumococcal vaccination: should be offered to all those with a chronic illness (eg diabetic patients)**

LEARNING POINTS

❶ Other common causes of community-acquired pneumonia include *Mycoplasma pneumoniae* (5–15%: intracellular organism that does not Gram-stain) and *Haemophilus influenzae* (5%: Gram-negative).

ⓘ Panton–Valentine leucocidin-producing *Staphylococcus aureus* (PVL-SA) is also a Gram-positive coccus, but is not a common cause of pneumonia; it is associated with lung cavitation and multi-organ failure.

Q 5. List six parameters used to assess treatment progress.　　　3 marks

A ½ mark each for any of the following:

- **Heart rate**
- **Respiratory rate**
- **Blood pressure**
- **Temperature**
- **SaO$_2$ (or O$_2$ requirements necessary to maintain adequate SaO$_2$)**
- **Mental status**
- **C-reactive protein (CRP): this is a sensitive marker of treatment progress**
- **White cell count**

LEARNING POINT

ⓘ In patients not progressing satisfactorily the chest X-ray should be repeated to look for complications.

John fails to make good progress and clinical examination reveals reduced breath sounds at the right base. His chest X-ray is repeated, which shows a right pleural effusion.

Q 6. What is the most likely complication?　　　1 mark

A Empyema.

LEARNING POINTS

ⓘ Empyema refers to pus in the pleural space. The fluid should be tapped and sent for pH analysis. If the pH < 7.2, the effusion should be treated as an empyema (see below). The presence of frank pus is diagnostic of an empyema, so the appearance of pleural aspirate should also be recorded. Untreated, extensive fibrosis occurs in the pleural cavity, weight loss and clubbing develop, and the mortality rate is high.

RESPIRATORY

❶ Other complications of pneumonia that may be seen on chest X-ray include pleural effusion and lung abscess (cavitating area of localised suppurative (pus-forming) infection – appears as a fluid-filled cavity).

Q 7. **How should this be treated?**   2 marks

A **1 mark each for the following:**

- **Tube drainage: ideally this should be performed under ultrasound guidance**
- **High-dose intravenous antibiotics: the pleural fluid should be sent for culture to ensure appropriate antibiotics are given**

LEARNING POINT

❶ Patients should be considered for thoracic surgery if they have ongoing signs of sepsis in association with a persistent pleural collection despite drainage and antibiotics.

Total: 15 marks

RHEUMATOLOGY
CASES: ANSWERS

RHEUMATOLOGY CASE 1

Hayley, a 36-year-old woman, is referred to rheumatology with a two-month history of stiff, painful, swollen hands associated with general malaise.

Q 1. **List four *inflammatory* causes of polyarthropathy.** 2 marks

A **½ mark each for any of the following:**
- **Rheumatoid arthritis**
- **Crystal arthropathies (eg gout)**
- **Arthritis associated with viral illness (eg parvovirus or mumps)**
- **Seronegative arthropathy (arthritis associated with psoriasis, inflammatory bowel disease and ankylosing spondylitis)**
- **Reactive arthritis: arthritis following infection (eg post-dysentery or post-non-gonococcal urethritis (NGU))**
- **Connective tissue disorders (eg systemic lupus erythematosus)**

LEARNING POINTS

🛈 Rheumatoid arthritis is a systemic inflammatory disorder that affects predominantly women (3:1) and can occur at any age. It typically presents with pain, stiffness and swelling of the proximal small joints of the hands and feet.

🛈 Other less common presentations include monoarthritis (a single swollen joint) or palindromic arthritis (joint swelling that occurs intermittently, lasting just a few days at a time).

You examine Hayley's hands and wrists.

Q 2. **Give four features of rheumatoid arthritis on examination of the hands and wrists.** 4 marks

A **1 mark each for any of the following:**
- **Boggy swelling (synovitis) of proximal small joints of hands (metacarpophalangeal (MCP), proximal interphalangeal (PIP))**

- **Sausage-shaped fingers (spindling): due to soft-tissue swelling**
- **Wasting of small muscles of the hand**
- **Swan-neck deformity: fixed hyperextension of PIP joint and flexion of distal interphalangeal (DIP) joint**
- **Boutonnière (or button-hole) deformity: fixed flexion of PIP joint**
- **Z-deformity of the thumb**
- **Finger drop: due to rupture of finger extensor tendons**
- **Subluxation of the wrist**
- **Prominent radial head (piano key)**
- **Symmetrical changes**

LEARNING POINTS

❶ Initially there is often just swollen fingers and MCP joint swelling. The other changes occur later, if the disease remains unchecked.

❶ Rheumatoid arthritis is a systemic disease affecting many organs. Extra-articular features include: haematological (anaemia); eyes (Sjögren syndrome (dry eyes), scleritis); cardiovascular system (pericarditis, pericardial effusions); respiratory system (lung fibrosis); skin (ulcers, nodules, vasculitis, pyoderma grangrenosum); nervous system (carpal tunnel syndrome, peripheral neuropathy, mononeuritis multiplex, cervical myelopathy); Felty syndrome (splenomegaly and neutropenia that is associated with infections); and renal (renal failure).

You organise some blood tests and send Hayley for an X-ray of her hands and feet.

Q 3. Give four X-ray changes in the hands in rheumatoid arthritis.   2 marks

A ½ mark each for any of the following:

Early changes:
- **Soft-tissue swelling**
- **Periarticular osteopenia**
- **Loss of joint space**

Late changes:
- **Bony erosions at the joint margins**
- **Subluxation and dislocation of joints**
- **Carpal bone destruction**

LEARNING POINTS

ⓘ Increasingly, ultrasound scan is being used to detect erosions before they become evident on X-ray.

ⓘ Rheumatoid factor (RF) are autoantibodies directed at antibodies (eg anti-IgG IgM). Although often negative at the start of rheumatoid arthritis, they are eventually positive in 70–80% of patients. However, RFs are not diagnostic of rheumatoid arthritis, as they are present in up to 10% of the normal population, although they are prognostic; patients with a positive RF usually follow a more aggressive disease course. 'Seronegative' rheumatoid arthritis refers to patients with arthropathy but without detectable RF: these individuals tend to have milder joint disease.

ⓘ Anti-CCP (cyclic citrullinated peptide) are also autoantibodies, rarely positive in the absence of rheumatoid arthritis and often positive at the outset, thereby aiding early diagnosis and treatment (see below).

You clinically diagnose Hayley with rheumatoid arthritis. You give her an intramuscular glucocorticoid injection, while commencing her on methotrexate.

Q 4. **List two side-effects of methotrexate.**   2 marks

A **1 mark each for any of the following:**
- **Liver toxicity: need to monitor liver functions tests (LFTs), initially weekly then 3-monthly, once dose stabilised**
- **Pneumonitis**
- **Bone marrow suppression: patients should be advised to report all signs and symptoms of infection, especially a sore throat**
- **Gastrointestinal toxicity, eg stomatitis (inflammation of mucous lining of mouth)**

LEARNING POINTS

ⓘ Methotrexate, which is given weekly, inhibits dihydrofolate reductase, which utilises folate for DNA synthesis. As a consequence, it is cytotoxic, particularly in rapidly dividing cells (malignant cells but also cells lining the gastrointestinal tract and in bone marrow). This toxicity is minimised by folate supplementation, typically 5 mg the following day. Folinic acid is used to treat methotrexate overdose, as it allows DNA synthesis in the presence of dihydrofolate reductase inhibition.

❶ Rheumatoid arthritis is treated with disease-modifying antirheumatic drugs (DMARDs) earlier and more aggressively than in the past to prevent erosive disease and deformities. Methotrexate is the first-line DMARD; alternatives include sulfsalazine, leflunomide and hydroxychloroquine (which may be given in combination). Glucocorticoids (oral, intramuscular, intra-articular) are often used to achieve symptom control in newly diagnosed rheumatoid arthritis and in flare-ups.

❶ The tumour necrosis factor alpha inhibitors (anti-TNF) (ie adalimumab, etanercept, infliximab) are usually reserved for patients who have failed to respond to at least two DMARDs, including methotrexate (and ideally should be given in combination with methotrexate, although this is influenced by the anti-TNF prescribed). Complications include infections, blood disorders and reactivation of latent tuberculosis: patients need to be assessed for TB before treatment (eg history of previous TB, chest X-ray).

❶ Alongside medication, treatment of rheumatoid arthritis also includes patient education, physical therapy, splints and surgery.

Q 5. **Give four complications of long-term oral steroid treatment.**　　　2 marks

A **½ mark each for any of the following:**
- **Impaired glucose tolerance (may progress to diabetes mellitus)**
- **Mental disturbance, eg euphoria, agitation or depression**
- **Osteoporosis (especially a risk in postmenopausal women)**
- **Avascular necrosis of the femoral neck**
- **Cushing syndrome: easy bruising, moon face, buffalo hump, striae**
- **Wasting and thinning of the skin**
- **Muscle wasting (proximal myopathy)**
- **Hypertension**
- **Dyspepsia (may also cause peptic ulcer disease)**
- **Cataracts**
- **Immune suppression, increasing risk of infections**

LEARNING POINT

❶ Prolonged use of corticosteroids may also cause suppression of the hypothalamus-pituitary-adrenal (HPA) axis. Acute adrenal insufficiency (addisonian crisis) may develop if steroids are withdrawn too quickly or during physiological stress (eg surgery, trauma or illness). Therefore, in prolonged steroid treatment, ie > 3 weeks, steroids should be withdrawn slowly (to allow the HPA axis to recover) and patients should carry a steroid treatment warning card.

Hayley is followed up by the rheumatology nurse specialist who monitors her response to treatment.

Q 5. **What score is used to monitor disease progression?** 1 mark

A **Disease activity score of 28 joints (DAS28): widely used indicator of disease activity and response to treatment.**

LEARNING POINT

❶ The joints in DAS28 are (bilaterally): PIPJ (10 joints), MCPJ (10), wrists (2), elbows (2), shoulders (2) and knees (2), and are assessed for tenderness and swelling. In addition, the ESR is measured, as well as a subjective assessment by the patient of global health (not just disease activity) during the preceding week (on a scale between 0 and 100) so as to calculate DAS28 score: score > 5.1: very active disease; 3.2–5.1: moderate activity; 3.1–2.6: mild; < 2.6: remission. Furthermore, a decrease in DAS28 score of < 0.6 indicates a poor response to treatment.

Q 6. **List four features associated with a poor prognosis.** 2 marks

A **½ mark each for any of the following:**
- **Female sex**
- **Multiple joint involvement**
- **Early functional disability**
- **Early X-ray changes, see above**
- **Extra-articular features, see above**
- **Insidious onset**
- **HLA DR4 positive**
- **Positive RF/anti-CCP**

Total: 15 marks

RHEUMATOLOGY

RHEUMATOLOGY CASE 2

Julie, a 28-year-old woman, presents with arthralgia and fatigue. On examination, she has a typical butterfly rash. Suspecting a diagnosis of systemic lupus erythematosus (SLE), you request a number of investigations.

Q 1. **List six investigations you would request to help establish the diagnosis.** 3 marks

A ½ **mark each for any of the following:**

- **Full blood count (FBC): leucopenia, lymphopenia, thrombocytopenia**
- **Urea and electrolytes (U&Es): renal nephritis, see below**
- **Erythrocyte sedimentation rate (ESR): elevated**
- **Autoantibody screen: eg ANA, anti-dsDNA, anti-Sm and other extractable nuclear antigens (ENA) (eg anti-Ro, anti-La)**
- **Serum complement levels: reduced C3 and C4 levels (due to complement consumption by circulating immune complexes)**
- **Urinalysis: proteinuria, red blood cell casts**
- **Electrocardiogram (ECG): pericarditis**
- **Chest radiograph, eg pleural effusion**
- **Joint radiographs: erosive changes are not seen in SLE, and would be more suggestive of rheumatoid arthritis**

LEARNING POINTS

ⓘ Systemic lupus erythematosus is diagnosed on the basis of ≥ 4 (serially or simultaneously) of the following **clinical** and **laboratory** criteria:

- Malar (butterfly) rash
- Discoid rash: erythematous raised patches that eventually progress to areas of scarring. Discoid lupus is restricted to the skin with no systemic involvement
- Skin photosensitivity
- Oral ulcers (oral or nasopharyngeal)

- Arthritis: radiologically the joints appear normal, ie non-erosive
- Serositis: pleuritis (eg pleuritic chest pain, pleural effusion), pericarditis
- Renal involvement, see below
- Neurological disorder: seizures, psychosis
- Haematological disorder: anaemia, leucopenia, thrombocytopenia, lymphopenia
- Immunological disorder: anti-double-stranded (ds) DNA antibody; anti-Smith (anti-Sm) antibody, antiphospholipid antibodies, false-positive syphilis test (due to anticardiolipin antibodies)
- Antinuclear antibody (ANA) positive.

❶ SLE is a non-organ-specific autoimmune disease. It occurs more commonly in females (particularly Afro-Caribbeans), typically presenting in early adult life (although can present at any age – neonates or the very elderly). Its presenting symptoms are highly variable and mild cases may only present with arthralgia and fatigue. Therefore always consider SLE in your differential in any female who presents with inflammatory arthritis.

❶ Numerous drugs are associated with causing a lupus-like syndrome (eg isoniazid, hydralazine). Drug lupus typically affects the skin and lungs; kidney and CNS involvement is rare. The symptoms resolve once the drug is stopped.

❶ The clinical features of SLE are caused by autoantibodies against a range of antigens. For example, ANA antibodies occur in 95% of SLE cases, although they are also present in other autoimmune diseases (eg RA, scleroderma) so are not diagnostic. Anti-dsDNA and anti-Sm are the SLE-specific antibodies, occurring in approximately 80% and 30% of cases, respectively.

Julie's urinalysis shows 3+ proteinuria.

Q 2. **What is the likely cause of Julie's proteinuria?**   1 mark

A **Lupus nephritis: SLE is a cause of glomerulonephritis (confirmed on renal biopsy).**

LEARNING POINTS

❶ Clinical manifestations of lupus nephritis vary from proteinuria (may progress to nephrotic syndrome), hypertension and haematuria through to end-stage renal failure (ESRF).

RHEUMATOLOGY

❶ Renal disease is the leading cause of early mortality in patients with SLE. While mild disease is typically treated with corticosteroids, severe renal disease is treated with immunosuppressants (eg mycophenolate or cyclophosphamide). In long-standing SLE the main cause of mortality is cardiovascular disease due to accelerated atherosclerosis.

Q 3. **List three treatment options for Julie's joint symptoms.**   3 marks

A **1 mark each for any of the following:**

- **Non-steroidal anti-inflammatory drugs (NSAIDs): use with caution if there is renal disease**
- **Antimalarials (hydroxychloroquine): also used for skin disease**
- **Corticosteroids: flares are typically treated with corticosteroids**
- **Disease-modifying antirheumatic drugs (DMARDs), eg methotrexate, azathioprine – used as either steroid-sparing agents or for refractory disease**

LEARNING POINTS

❶ Systemic lupus erythematosus (SLE) is a relapsing and remitting disease. Typically the nature of the disease becomes established in the first 5 years or so; if no significant problems have occurred during this time, they are unlikely to do so. The treatment of non-major organ involvement SLE is listed above; cyclophosphamide is reserved for major organ involvement (ie CNS, kidneys, blood dyscrasias).

❶ Complement levels (reduced), erythrocyte sedimentation rate (ESR) (raised) and anti-ds DNA antibodies (raised) can be used to monitor disease activity. C-reactive protein (CRP) is very useful in differentiating an SLE flare-up from infection, as CRP is usually normal in a flare but raised in infection. Susceptibility to infection, due to both the disease itself and immuno-suppressants, is a major cause of early mortality.

Two years later Julie speaks to her GP about the possibility of becoming pregnant.

RHEUMATOLOGY

Q 4. What are the potential problems Julie might face during her pregnancy? 3 marks

A **1 mark each for any of the following:**

- **Flare-up of her SLE: typically joints and skin**
- **Pre-eclampsia**
- **Miscarriage**
- **Preterm birth**
- **Intrauterine growth restriction (IUGR)**
- **Congenital heart block.**
- **Neonatal lupus: causes transient discoid lupus rash: due to placental transfer of maternal antibodies and resolves with clearance of these antibodies**

LEARNING POINTS

ⓘ A proportion of SLE patients (30%) have antiphospholipid (APL) syndrome, which is caused by antiphospholipid antibodies (lupus anticoagulant and anticardiolipin antibodies). APL is characterised by venous and arterial thromboembolism (causing both pulmonary emboli and strokes). Paradoxically the activated partial thromboplastin time (APTT) is often elevated (which would normally suggest tendency towards bleeding rather than clotting); this occurs because these antibodies, which in vivo cause a thrombotic tendency, interfere with the in-vitro APTT test.

ⓘ In pregnancy APL can cause miscarriage, preterm birth, IUGR and pre-eclampsia. These complications are prevented by the use of low-dose aspirin throughout pregnancy (heparin is also used to prevent recurrent miscarriage).

ⓘ In patients with SLE the presence of anti-Ro and anti-La antibodies that cross the placenta can lead to congenital heart block, including complete heart block, which requires pacing. It is therefore important to screen for these antibodies in women with known SLE who are considering pregnancy; positive women undergo fetal echocardiography to identify fetal bradycardia.

Total: **10 marks**

SURGICAL CASES: ANSWERS

SURGICAL CASE 1

Q 1. **From what age are women invited to attend the NHS breast screening programme?**   1 mark

A **From 50 years old.**

LEARNING POINT

ⓘ The NHS breast screening programme was started in 1988. The aim of screening is to detect early, non-palpable non-invasive disease which can be treated with breast conservation. All women aged between 50 and 70 are invited 3-yearly for single oblique view mammography (two-view mammogram at first screening) with the option of self-referral for older women (mammography is not considered effective in premenopausal women due to the lower incidence of breast cancer and the increased density of breast tissue).

Q 2. **List six criteria used in deciding whether to screen for a disease.**   6 marks

A **1 mark each for any of the following.**

The Wilson criteria for screening:

- *Is the disease to be screened an important health problem:* **breast cancer affects 1 in 12 women and is a leading cause of cancer death in women.**
- *Is there a recognisable early stage of the disease:* **compared with symptomatic cancers, screen-detected cancers are smaller, more likely to be non-invasive (20% of screen-detected cancers are non-invasive), while any invasive cancers are more likely to be better differentiated, of special type and node-negative, all of which confer a better prognosis (half of the invasive cancers are clinically undetectable)**
- *Is there a sensitive and specific (valid) test available for the early detection of the disease:* **mammography is approximately 85% sensitive (detects cancer when it is present) and 90% specific (identifies healthy women as cancer-free)**
- *The test must be acceptable with a high participation rate:* **1.8 million women are screened annually (77% of those invited)**
- *There should be suitable facilities for the diagnosis and treatment of detected abnormalities.* **Any woman with mammographic abnormalities is referred for triple assessment: 8% of women are referred at initial screen and 3% on subsequent screening**

- *Does screening result in reduced morbidity/mortality?* **It is estimated that since the programme began, screening has resulted in a 10% reduction in the breast cancer death rate (although this is an area of continuing controversy)**

- *There should be appropriate treatment options*

- *The benefits of screening must be of an acceptable financial cost:* **the annual screening programme costs £96 million and detects 14,000 cancers (approximately a third of all breast cancers)**

LEARNING POINT

ⓘ Other English screening programmes include bowel cancer (faecal occult blood is screened every 2 years in patients aged 60–69 years old) and cervical cancer (women aged between 25 and 64 years are invited every 3 years until aged 49 and then every 5 years for a cervical smear test).

Elizabeth's mammogram (see Figure 13.1) demonstrates an irregular mass in the central part of the left breast, which has spicules radiating from it, and she is urgently referred for triple assessment.

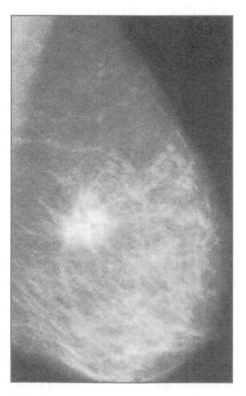

Figure 13.1: Elizabeth's mammogram.

Q 3. **What are the three components of the triple assessment?** 3 marks

A **1 mark each for the following:**
- **Clinical examination, see below**
- **Imaging – mammogram and/or ultrasound scan: in women < 35 years, owing to increased tissue density, ultrasound scan is used to image the breast**
- **Cytological assessment: fine-needle aspiration (FNA) or needle core biopsy (or occasionally open biopsy)**

LEARNING POINT

ℹ On mammography (specialised X-ray image of the breast) fat appears grey, while denser glandular tissue appears white. Breast cancers have an irregular margin, are ill-defined and dense (whiter than surrounding breast).

Q 4. **List four signs of breast cancer on breast examination.** 2 marks

A **½ mark each for any of the following:**
- **Lump: hard, irregular, fixed, usually painless**
- **Breast asymmetry: this can be accentuated by extending her arms above her head and then placing them on her hips**
- **Skin dimpling: tethering of skin to underlying cancer**
- **Eczema/ulceration of the areola: Paget's disease (ductal cancer involving the nipple)**
- **Peau d'orange: oedema of the skin**
- **Nipple deviated or inverted**
- **Bloody nipple discharge**
- **Palpable axillary lymph nodes**

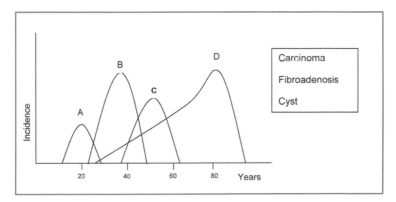

Figure 13.2: Age incidence of common breast lumps.

Q 5. **From the graph shown in Figure 13.2 identify which breast lump corresponds to which peak in incidence.** 2 marks

A **½ mark each for the following**

A: Fibroadenoma: most common cause of a breast lump in a young woman

B: Fibroadenosis: tender or painful diffuse lumpiness prior to menstruation

C: Cyst

D: Carcinoma

LEARNING POINT

❶ Breast cancer (adenocarcinoma arising from the glandular epithelium) is classified as **non-invasive** (ie ductal and lobular carcinoma in situ, not all cases of which progress to invasive cancer) or **invasive** (penetrates basement membrane of ducts and lobules into surrounding normal tissue). The most common invasive subtype is ductal carcinoma (85%).

Unfortunately, the results of Elizabeth's triple assessment confirm a diagnosis of breast cancer.

Q 6. **Name four metastatic sites for breast cancer.** 2 marks

A **½ mark each for the following:**

• **Bone: most common site; bisphosphonates reduce pain and complications of skeletal metastases (eg pathological fractures)**

• **Lung**

• **Liver**

• **Brain**

LEARNING POINT

❶ Breast cancer is typically staged using the TNM system: tumour size (T), whether spread to lymph nodes (N) and whether evidence of metastases (M).

SURGICAL

Q 7. List four potential treatment options for Elizabeth's breast cancer.   2 marks

A ½ mark each for any of the following:

The management of patients with breast cancer involves: surgery, radiotherapy and drug therapy or a combination of these, and is determined by stage, general health (performance status) menopause and receptor status.

- Surgery: quadrantectomy, wide local excision (or lumpectomy), mastectomy
- Radiotherapy: used after surgery to prevent local recurrence
- Hormonal treatment: tamoxifen is an oestrogen-receptor (ER) antagonist and is typically used in ER-positive premenopausal women. Aromatase inhibitors (eg anastrozole and letrozole) block conversion of androgens to oestrogens in peripheral tissue; they do not inhibit ovarian oestrogen synthesis and therefore are used in postmenopausal women
- Chemotherapy is used for ER-negative tumours to help shrink operable tumours (neoadjuvant therapy) and prevent relapse following surgery (adjuvant therapy) and also for metastatic disease
- Trastuzumab (Herceptin), a monoclonal antibody, is used in those breast cancers (approximately 20%) which over-express human epidermal growth factor receptor 2 (HER2)

LEARNING POINT

❶ Breast-conserving surgery (BCS) includes lumpectomy and quadrantectomy.

Q 8. What is a sentinel node?   1 mark

A The sentinel node is the first lymph node that drains an area of tissue (or tumour).

LEARNING POINT

❶ The lymphatic system is a network that returns interstitial fluid back into the systemic circulation. As an area of tissue is drained, the lymphatic fluid flows in an orderly way; the first lymph node it flows through is termed the 'sentinel node' (and hence breast cancers that metastasise via the axillary lymphatic system will follow a similar course).

SURGICAL

Q 9. What is the advantage of performing a sentinel node biopsy? 1 mark

A It allows axillary nodal status to be assessed without the need for axillary clearance.

LEARNING POINTS

ⓘ Axillary clearance (to both stage the disease and treat the axilla) is considered in all women with invasive breast cancer. However, it is associated with significant morbidity (lymphoedema, shoulder stiffness, reduced range of movement) and in women with clinically early breast cancer and no palpable nodes clearance often reveals negative nodes.

ⓘ The sentinel node status is highly predictive of axillary status; only if positive would axillary clearance be performed. The sentinel node can be identified (and hence sampled) by injection of dye and/or isotope into the peritumoural site and tracing its course into the axilla.

Total: **20 marks**

SURGICAL CASE 2

Ethel, a frail 82-year-old in sheltered accommodation, is brought into the Emergency Department after being found by her carers lying at the side of her bed. On examination, you suspect that she has suffered a fractured hip.

Q 1. **What findings would be consistent with a hip fracture?**　　　　**2 marks**

A ½ **mark each for any of the following:**
- **Leg shortened**
- **Leg externally rotated**
- **Patient unable to weight-bear: although patients with undisplaced or incomplete fractures may be able to weight-bear**
- **Bruising: may not be present with intracapsular fractures, as bleeding confined to within the capsule**
- **Swelling in the hip region**
- **Tenderness over the hip joint (felt in the groin) and greater trochanter**
- **Pain on movement of affected leg**
- **Crepitus on movement of affected leg**

LEARNING POINTS

❶ In patients with suspected hip fracture, pain needs to be assessed at presentation and treated appropriately. Increasingly, femoral nerve blocks are being used in emergency departments for effective analaesia and to limit opioid dosage.

❶ Approximately 70,000 hip fractures occur each year and the annual cost (including medical and subsequent social care) is £2 bn. Hip fractures are a significant cause of mortality – 10% die within 1 month (typically due to underlying co-morbidities) – and morbidity: 25% of patients require a higher level of care on discharge.

You request anteroposterior (AP) (shown in Figure 13.3) and lateral X-rays to confirm your diagnosis.

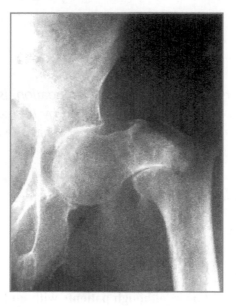

Figure 13.3: Ethel's anteroposterior X-ray.

Q 2. **Is this fracture intra- or extracapsular?**   1 mark

A **Extracapsular: displaced trochanteric fracture.**

LEARNING POINT

❶ Hip fractures are classified as **intracapsular** or **extracapsular** (see figure below) depending on the site of the fracture in relation to the insertion of the capsule of the hip joint (indicated with arrows) onto the proximal femur. The classification is important in determining their management.

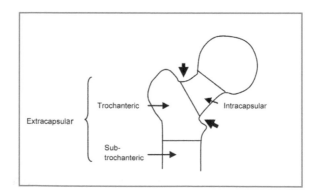

Classification of hip fractures

The orthopaedic surgeon elects to fix Ethel's hip fracture with a dynamic hip screw (DHS), and she is scheduled for surgery on the trauma list.

Q 3. **Name a late complication of treating intracapsular fractures by internal fixation as opposed to hemiarthroplasty.** 2 marks

A **1 mark each for the following:**
- **Non-union**
- **Avascular necrosis (AVN) of the femoral head**

LEARNING POINTS

ⓘ Intracapsular fractures can disrupt the blood supply to the head of the femur, causing non-union or avascular necrosis (extracapsular fractures are less likely to disrupt the blood supply).

ⓘ Intracapsular fractures are treated by either internal fixation (eg cancellous screws) or arthroplasty (hemiarthroplasty or total hip replacement). The choice of treatment depends on the patient's age, mobility and degree of displacement. Internal fixation is indicated in undisplaced fractures or displaced fractures in younger patients (aim is to try and preserve the head due to the functional deterioration of a hemiarthroplasty). Arthroplasty is indicated in displaced fractures. If internally fixed, intracapsular fractures are followed up to exclude AVN or non-union, treatment of which is arthroplasty.

Q 4. **As the FY1 doctor what eight things should you ensure are done before surgery?** 2 marks

A **¼ mark each for any of the following:**
- **Full blood count (FBC): anaemia (may require a transfusion prior to surgery if Hb < 8 g/dl)**
- **Urea & electrolytes (U&Es): electrolyte imbalance**
- **Glucose: uncontrolled diabetes**
- **Group and save (or cross-match if Hb < 8 g/dl)**
- **Electrocardiogram: identify any cardiac arrhythmia or ischaemia**
- **Chest X-ray: if you suspect acute chest infection or exacerbation of chronic chest condition**
- **Deep vein thrombosis (DVT) prophylaxis**
- **Patient is nil by mouth (NBM), ie is on IV fluids:** *no drip, no hip*

SURGICAL

- **Consent**
- **Limb is marked: ensures correct hip is operated on**
- **Drug chart with appropriate regular and 'as required' analgesia**

LEARNING POINT

ⓘ Surgery should ideally be performed on the day of, or the day after, admission. Because the occurrence of fall and fracture often signals underlying ill health, co-morbidities should be identified and corrected immediately so as not to delay surgery.

Surgery is successful, and Ethel is encouraged to start partially weight-bearing the following day.

Q 5. **Give four reasons why Ethel should start weight-bearing as soon as possible.**
2 marks

A **½ mark each for any of the following:**
- **Avoids the complications of bed rest (eg DVT, pressure sores)**
- **Prevents joint stiffness**
- **Restores muscle strength**
- **Helps regain balance and increases confidence in walking**
- **Promotes fracture healing**

LEARNING POINT

ⓘ The management of any fracture involves: (a) reduction, (b) fixation and (c) rehabilitation. Weight-bearing (which may require a check X-ray beforehand) is an important part of the rehabilitation process following a hip fracture.

You note from Ethel's extensive medical history that she has several risk factors for a hip fracture, including osteoporosis and a history of falls.

Q 6. **Give three pieces of *general* advice to help prevent osteoporosis.** 3 marks

A **1 mark each for any of the following:**

The following advice should be given to all patients, especially those at increased risk of osteoporosis:

- **Increased level of physical exercise**
- **Stop smoking**
- **Increased dietary calcium intake (eg milk)**
- **Adequate, safe sunshine exposure**

LEARNING POINTS

- Risk factors for osteoporosis include: age; immobility; family history; low BMI (< 18.5). Secondary causes: gastrointestinal (eg coeliac disease, inflammatory bowel disease, chronic liver disease), endocrine (premature menopause, ie < 45 years, male hypogonadism, thyrotoxicosis, oral corticosteroids (> 3 months)); rheumatoid arthritis; and chronic renal failure.

- Osteoporosis is defined as bone mineral density (BMD), expressed as a T-score, ≥ 2.5 standard deviations (SD) below the BMD of a healthy young adult (osteopenia is bone density –1 to –2.5 SD below). When it involves the trabecular bone, it increases the risk of crush fractures of the vertebrae; involvement of cortical bone increases the risk of fractures of the long bone. BMD can be assessed (at the spine and proximal femur) by a dual-energy X-ray absorptiometry (DEXA) scan, although patients > 65 years on long-term steroids or > 75 years following a fractured hip should be treated empirically.

Before discharge, you commence Ethel on a bisphosphonate with calcium and vitamin D supplementation.

Q 7. **How do bisphosphonates prevent osteoporosis?** 1 mark

A **Bisphosphonates inhibit osteoclast activity, thereby preventing bone resorption.**

SURGICAL

LEARNING POINTS

❶ **Bisphosphonates** (eg alendronate) (with calcium and vitamin D supplementation) are first-line treatment (both primary and secondary prevention) of osteoporosis. Other treatments include strontium ranelate and hormone replacement therapy (HRT). Intravenous bisphosphonates are also used to treat hypercalcaemia of malignancy and bone metastases in breast cancer and multiple myeloma.

❶ **Common side-effects** include oesophageal reactions (eg gastro-oesophageal reflux disease, oesophagitis). These are minimised by instructing patients to take tablets while sitting or standing and to remain upright for at least 30 minutes to prevent oesophageal reflux. Osteonecrosis of the jaw is associated with intravenous bisphosphonates; it is minimised by maintaining good oral hygiene and ensuring any dental work is performed **prior** to commencing treatment.

During her inpatient stay Ethel is assessed by the falls intervention team.

Q 8. List four risk factors for falls in the elderly. 2 marks

A ½ mark each for any of the following.

The majority of osteoporosis-related fractures result from low-trauma falls, the causes of which are multifactorial and often modifiable:

- **Gait and balance disorders (eg stroke, Parkinson's disease)**
- **Sensory impairment (eg peripheral neuropathy, visual impairment)**
- **Cognitive or mood impairment (eg dementia, depression)**
- **Orthostatic hypotension**
- **Cardiac arrhythmias**
- **Polypharmacy, sedatives (eg benzodiazepines)**
- **Environmental factors (eg poor lighting, loose rugs)**

LEARNING POINT

❶ The assessment and prevention of falls involves a multidisciplinary approach (eg doctors, physiotherapists, occupational therapists). Interventions include strength and balance training, home hazard assessment and medication review/withdrawal.

Total: **15 marks**

SURGICAL

SURGICAL CASE 3

Doris, a 69-year-old woman, is urgently referred to the lower GI surgeons with suspected colorectal cancer.

Q 1. **List four signs, symptoms or investigations that would warrant urgent referral of patients for suspected colorectal cancer.**

4 marks

A **1 mark each for any of the following:**

- **Increased frequency of defecation or looser stools (≥ 6 weeks)**
- **Rectal bleeding**
- **Iron-deficient anaemia without an obvious cause**
- **Palpable rectal mass**
- **Palpable abdominal mass**

LEARNING POINTS

❶ The National Institute for Health and Clinical Excellence (NICE) referral guidelines are:

- Rectal bleeding WITH a change in bowel habit to looser stools and/or increased frequency of defecation ≥ 6 weeks in those aged > 40 years (decreased frequency of defaecation is low risk of cancer)

- Change in bowel habit to looser stools and/or increased frequency of defecation ≥ 6 weeks WITHOUT rectal bleeding in those aged > 60 years

- A definite palpable right-sided abdominal mass in ALL ages

- A definite palpable rectal (not pelvic) mass in ALL ages

- Rectal bleeding ≥ 6 weeks WITHOUT anal symptoms (eg soreness, itching) in those aged > 60 years

- Iron-deficient anaemia (< 11 g/dl in men, < 10 g/dl in non-menstruating women).

- ❶ Approximately 80% of patients with colorectal cancer present with these symptoms and should be urgently referred (under a 2-week wait) for further investigation. Approximately 20% of patients at presentation are admitted as surgical emergencies (eg large-bowel obstruction, abdominal pain – see below).

- ❶ Initial investigations (all of which require bowel cleansing) may involve: (1) colonoscopy (first line in patients without significant co-morbidities), (2) flexible sigmoidoscopy + barium enema, and (3) CT colonography (virtual colonoscopy).

Doris undergoes colonoscopy, which identifies a suspicious lesion in the sigmoid colon which on biopsy is diagnosed as cancer. She is scheduled for surgery and is counselled about the likelihood of a stoma.

Q 2. **Name three complications of a stoma.** 3 marks

A **1 mark each for any of the following.**

Before surgery all patients should be counselled about the likelihood of having a stoma, why it may be necessary and how long it may be needed for:

- **Psychosocial problems: eg body image problems, relationship problems, decreased ability to work, restriction on social activities**
- **Physical problems: eg stenosis of the stoma, prolapse (protrusion) of the stoma, obstruction, parastomal hernia, dehydration and electrolyte disturbance (especially if high-output), skin problems (eg infection, ulceration, physical damage due to frequent removal)**

LEARNING POINTS

- ❶ A stoma is a surgically created opening (eg of the bowel) to the body surface, (eg colostomy opens out into left iliac fossa (and ileostomy) opens out into right iliac fossa). The stoma care nurse is expert at helping patients managing their stoma (eg good skin care, fitting secure odorless bags) and advising patients on the physical and psychosocial problems associated with stomas.

- ❶ Mainstay of treatment of colorectal cancer involves resection (open or laparoscopic) of the tumour, although this may be palliative rather than curative. Sometimes this involves the formation of a stoma, although this is typically temporary so as to allow the bowel to heal before safe anastomosis at a later date.

SURGICAL

Doris undergoes a sigmoid colectomy. The histopathology findings report that the cancer has extended through the bowel wall, with regional lymph node involvement.

Q 3. **What is the Dukes' classification of Doris's colon cancer?** 1 mark

A **Initial staging involves CT scan of chest, abdomen and pelvis to assess local spread and presence or absence of distant metastases, although it may not be properly staged until resected.**

- **Dukes' stage C**

LEARNING POINTS

❶ Colorectal cancer is staged as follows:
Dukes' A: confined to bowel wall; 95% 5-year survival
Dukes' B: extension through bowel wall; 75% 5-year survival
Dukes' C: involvement of regional lymph nodes; 50% 5-year survival
Dukes' D: distant metastases (typically the liver); 5% 5-year survival.

❶ The TNM (tumour, node, metastases) system is also increasingly used to stage colorectal cancer.

❶ Additional treatments for colorectal cancer (depending on the stage) include: radiotherapy (typically for rectal cancer), chemotherapy and biological treatments (eg cetuximab: an epidermal growth factor receptor inhibitor). Furthermore newer techniques are being used to treat liver metastases (eg hepatic artery chemoembolisation).

❶ Patients are followed up with regular CT scans and carcinoembryonic antigen (CEA) monitoring.

Eighteen months later Doris is admitted to the surgical assessment unit with a history of colicky lower abdominal pain and increasing constipation for five days.

Q 4. **List two causes of *mechanical* large-bowel obstruction.** 2 marks

A **1 mark each for any of the following.**
Intestinal obstruction is either functional (ie lumen is not blocked but reduced

bowel motility, eg following surgery, peritonitis) or mechanical (ie blocked lumen):

- **Colorectal cancer: either at presentation or recurrence following treatment**
- **Volvulus (twisting of loop of bowel): may be relieved by insertion of a large-bore flatus tube**
- **Diverticulitis**
- **Faeces**

LEARNING POINT

ⓘ Causes of small-bowel obstruction include adhesions (eg following previous surgery), hernias, and strictures (eg Crohn's disease).

Q 5. **What signs would you look for in acute *mechanical* intestinal obstruction?** 3 marks

A **1 mark each for any of the following:**

- **Abdominal distension**
- **Abdominal tenderness (in strangulated bowel, eg volvulus, you may get peritonism)**
- **Visible peristalsis**
- **Hernias: check both inguinal and femoral sites**
- **Rectal mass on per rectal (PR) examination**
- **Increased (tinkling) bowel sounds (absent in paralytic ileus)**

LEARNING POINTS

ⓘ The four cardinal symptoms of obstruction are: pain (usually colicky but may be constant if strangulated), constipation, vomiting (with relief) and distension.

ⓘ Initial management involves nil by mouth (NBM), intravenous fluid resuscitation and correction of electrolyte imbalance, insertion of a nasogastric tube, analgaesia and anti-emetics (prokinetics, eg metoclopramide, are contraindicated in mechanical bowel obstruction).

Q 6. **Is this a small- or a large-bowel obstruction (please refer to Figure 13.4)? Explain your answer.** 2 marks

A **1 mark each for the following:**

- **Small-bowel obstruction**
- **Circular folds cross the full width of the lumen of the distended loops, indicating that this is small bowel**

SURGICAL

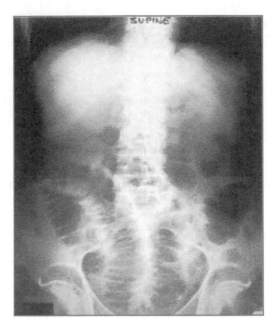

Figure 13.4: Abdominal X-ray is a patient admitted with acute intestinal obstruction.

LEARNING POINTS

ℹ Abdominal X-ray is primarily used to investigate the acute abdomen (also erect chest X-ray to exclude air under the diaphragm). Small bowel is recognised by circular folds (plicae circulares) that cross the full width of the bowel lumen (also tend to be more central); in the large bowel the haustral folds only go part way across the lumen (and tend to be more peripheral). In obstruction look for abnormal gas patterns (when supine) and dilated bowel (abnormal if small bowel > 3cm and large bowel > 6cm).

ℹ Patients presenting with acute large-bowel obstruction due to colorectal cancer may initially be treated with insertion of a colonic stent; Hartmann's procedure is used to treat malignant obstruction, which involves resection of the tumour with the proximal bowel diverted with a stoma.

Total: **15 marks**

SURGICAL CASE 4

Michael, a smoker of 40 cigarettes a day, attends his GP with a history of muscular cramp-like pain, mainly in one calf, on walking a short distance that is rapidly relieved by rest.

Q 1. **What non-invasive test confirms the diagnosis of peripheral vascular disease?**
1 mark

A **Ankle–brachial systolic pressure index (ABSPI).**

LEARNING POINTS

❶ The ABSPI expresses systolic pressure at the ankle as a percentage of the brachial systolic pressure (measured by Doppler): 1 – normal; < 0.5 represents severe arterial compromise.

❶ Peripheral vascular disease typically causes a cramp-like pain on walking (claudication distance) that is rapidly relieved by rest (intermittent claudication), after which the patient can walk further. The claudication distance is constant (there are no good days when the patient can walk further), although if exercise is increased (eg walking up hill), the pain comes on sooner. While symptoms are typically unilateral, disease is usually bilateral and revascularisation often unmasks claudication in the asymptomatic leg.

❶ Most patients with intermittent claudication do not require angiography as it is essentially a presurgical investigation, although duplex ultrasound scan may be used to identify the site of the lesion, the degree of stenosis and length of the lesion.

Q 2. **What are the main *modifiable* risk factors for peripheral vascular disease?**
2 marks

A **½ mark for each of the following:**
- **Smoking**
- **Diabetes**
- **Hypertension: β-blockers are not contraindicated in peripheral vascular disease**
- **Hyperlipidaemia**

LEARNING POINTS

- The management of intermittent claudication involves the modification of peripheral vascular disease risk factors, as well as regular exercise and aspirin (or clopidogrel if contraindicated). Bypass surgery or angioplasty ± stenting (lower long-term patency) is typically reserved for patients with critical ischaemia (see below) or disabling intermittent claudication.

- Patients with intermittent claudication have an increased risk of cardiovascular disease and are prescribed aspirin to reduce the risk of cardiovascular events (secondary prevention).

- Naftidrofuryl oxide (Praxilene) is a vasodilator and may be used to treat intermittent claudication.

Q 3. **What advice would you give Michael?**   2 marks

A **1 mark each for the following:**
- **Stop smoking**
- **Regular exercise**

LEARNING POINTS

- Stopping smoking improves circulation in both the short and long term (by slowing down the progression of atherosclerosis). The short-term effects of smoking on circulation include increased platelet aggregation, vasoconstriction and hypoxia (due to carbon monoxide binding to and reducing the oxygen-carrying capacity of haemoglobin).

- Patients should be encouraged to walk to near-maximum pain tolerance as this improves symptoms and prevents progression to critical ischaemia by stimulating the development of collateral circulation (although if they get chest pain, they should stop immediately).

Twelve months later Michael is urgently referred to the vascular surgeons describing a history of deteriorating claudication in the same leg, which has recently progressed to nocturnal rest pain. On examination, the affected foot shows signs of critical ischaemia.

Q 4. **What are the signs of a critically ischaemic foot?**   4 marks

A ½ mark each for any of the following:
- **Cold**

- **Skin discoloration: often purple–blue cyanosed appearance**
- **Hair loss**
- **Absent foot pulses**
- **Prolonged capillary refill time**
- **Necrosis (gangrene): usually confined to a toe. If infected, it is termed 'wet gangrene'**
- **Ulceration: arterial ulcers typically affect the pressure points of the heel, malleoli and toes, and are described as painful, punched-out lesions**
- **Venous guttering: collapsed veins looking like pale blue gutters (veins are normally full)**
- **Positive Beurger's test: elevation of the leg causes the foot to go white, as peripheral arterial pressure cannot overcome gravity**

LEARNING POINTS

❶ Critical ischaemia refers to arterial insufficiency severe enough to threaten the viability of the foot or leg, requiring surgical or radiological intervention.

❶ Angioplasty (with or without stenting) is typically first-line treatment (reduced mortality and morbidity compared with bypass) especially for stenoses or short occlusions of the iliac or superficial femoral artery, although it has lower long-term patency. Bypass surgery is used to treat diffuse disease or treatment failures, using either synthetic or long saphenous venous grafts.

Q 5. **Why is pain typically worse at night?** 3 marks

A **1 mark each for the following.**

Critical ischaemia is characterised by rest pain, which is worse at night due to:

- **Sleep-associated fall in systolic blood pressure**
- **Increased warmth of blankets causes peripheral vasodilatation, causing a further fall in blood pressure**
- **Loss of gravity-dependent circulation**

LEARNING POINT

❶ Patients with night pain often relieve their symptoms by sleeping in a chair or with their foot hanging out of the bed.

Michael undergoes an MR angiogram (shown in Figure 13.5) and his occluded left superficial femoral artery is treated by percutaneous transluminal angioplasty.

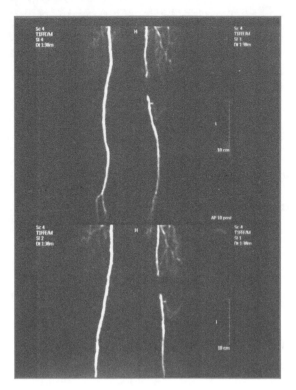

Figure 13.5: Michael's MR angiogram.

Two years later Michael presents to the Emergency Department with features of acute limb ischaemia.

Q 6. **List four causes of *embolic* acute lower limb ischaemia.** 2 marks

A **½ mark each for any of the following:**
- **Atrial fibrillation: account for approximately 80% of embolic causes**
- **Myocardial infarction causing a mural wall thrombus**
- **Aortic or mitral valve disease**
- **Prosthetic heart valves**
- **Abdominal aortic aneurysm (AAA)**
- **Subacute bacterial endocarditis (SBE)**
- **Patent foramen ovale (paradoxical embolus)**

LEARNING POINTS

ⓘ Acute ischaemia is caused by either emboli (30%) or thrombosis in situ (rupture of an atherosclerotic plaque). Emboli typically lodge at the common femoral bifurcation; if ischaemia is bilateral, it suggests occlusion of the aortic bifurcation. The history (eg recent myocardial infarction, underlying peripheral vascular disease) and examination (eg heart murmur, state of contralateral pulses: if good, more likely due to embolic cause) can help identify the underlying cause, which influences treatment (see below).

ⓘ It is highly likely that with Michael's past history of peripheral vascular disease his acute limb ischaemia is due to thrombosis in situ rather than an embolic cause.

Q 7. **Give six features of acute limb ischaemia.**   3 marks

A **½ mark each for any of the following:**

The six Ps:

1. **Pain**
2. **Pallor**
3. **Pulseless**
4. **Perishing cold**
5. **Paraesthesia: supersedes pain**
6. **Paralysis: unable to wiggle toes**

LEARNING POINTS

ⓘ **Incomplete** ischaemia (ie features 1–4) can usually be treated medically in the first instance (eg anticoagulation with intravenous heparin to prevent propagation of the thrombus and protect the collateral circulation while awaiting angiography).

ⓘ If embolectomy is performed, its adequacy should be confirmed by on-table angiography and thrombolysis performed, if inadequate. If acute ischaemia is due to thrombosis in situ, the treatment options are intra-arterial thrombolysis (catheter is advanced into the thrombus and thrombolytic therapy infused, eg tissue plasminogen activator), angioplasty or bypass.

ⓘ Paraesthesia and paralysis are key to diagnosing **complete** acute ischaemia, which requires emergency surgical revascularisation within 6 hours so as to salvage the limb. These patients need to go straight to theatre for surgical revascularisation, ie embolectomy or bypass; thrombolysis is not an option as it takes several hours to achieve clot lysis.

SURGICAL

Examination is suggestive of complete acute ischaemia. He is given intravenous heparin and taken straight to theatre for revascularisation of his leg.

Q 8. **Name three complications of reperfusion.** 3 marks

A **1 mark each for any of the following:**

- **Reperfusion injury (see below)**
- **Cardiac arrhythmias: due to metabolic acidosis and hyperkalaemia**
- **Acute renal failure: rhabdomyolysis causes release of myoglobin, which can cause acute tubular necrosis**
- **Acute respiratory distress syndrome (ARDS)**
- **Compartment syndrome: increased capillary permeability and oedema on reperfusion causes muscles to swell within their rigid osteofascial compartments, causing muscle necrosis. Treatment involves fasciotomy**

LEARNING POINTS

- The reintroduction of oxygenated blood following ischaemia causes more damage than ischaemia alone, termed 'reperfusion injury', due to production of highly reactive free radicals which activate neutrophils, which migrate into the reperfused tissue, causing injury.

- Reperfusion washes out the by-products of anaerobic metabolism (eg lactic acid) and cell lysis (eg potassium, myoglobin), causing arrhythmias, ARDS and acute renal failure.

Total: 20 marks

SURGICAL

INDEX

This index covers the answer section only. Page numbers in **bold** indicate the main subject(s) of each case.

effective, but that does not mean they should be considered legitimate. From another perspective, the astrological "learning community" is one that is effective at producing and sharing information, and is built around particular media and linguistic conventions, despite having no scientific basis for its claims (Thompson 2008). Whatever radical IL is to become, it must be able to assess the values underlying communities like these, reveal and criticise them.

Revealing contradictions in a learning community is part of being *vigilant* over it. Blaug's discussion (1999a) casts democracy as a constantly-updating, dynamic environment that supports empowering, inclusive activities, not a system, an end-in-itself. A democratic environment would have to be constructed around the understanding that communicatively rational organisational forms, and discourses, constantly tend to decay. A supportive environment would slow this decay, by allowing for the continuous review and possible transformation of practice (Habermas 1993).

Blaug describes two reasons for this tendency towards decay. First, there are hegemonic pressures, which work to deny counterhegemonic, decolonising spaces the resources (financial, intellectual) from which they would benefit, and exploit those resources that do emerge from the space – matters already discussed above. Second, Blaug argues that to understand the pervasiveness of hierarchies, actors in social situations must understand the benefits they bring to decision-making.

Hierarchies are attractive for a reason. The limitations on the ideal of the ISS – the continuous exercising of double-loop learning – include time, cognitive biases, and the structures of language which result in differing interpretations (which is why some dissensus always has value: Lyotard 1984). Hierarchical decision making saves time and cognitive work, and as a result may even improve the prospects of truly democratic decision making. Abrahamsson (1993, 92–4) argues that hierarchy is useful for democracy, a rational installation as it allows decisions to not just be taken, but implemented. But the trade-offs involved show why we must be vigilant about hierarchies (Blaug 1999a), whether at state level, within organisations, or within communities.

The different epistemologies underlying each form of rationality use resources in different ways. In a communicatively-rational environment, knowledge is *formed* by keeping ideas foregrounded, and under scrutiny. Resources are needed to create the necessary supportive environment, including allowing practitioners time to undertake this work, and keeping debate and discussion flowing around the landscape. By its very

criteria. Anti-organisational forms are often driving the movement, and the whole process: "thrives on diversity, works best when embedded in its own locality and context and develops most creatively at the edges, the overlap points, the inbetween spaces – those spaces where different cultures meet..." (anonymous author in *Do or Die* #8, 3).

For Habermas, social movements are one example of "counterinstitutions" that develop "within the lifeworld in order to set limits to the inner dynamics of the economic and political- administrative action systems". They aim "to de-differentiate some parts of the formally organised domains of action, remove them from the clutches of the steering media, and return these 'liberated areas' to the action-coordinating method of reaching understanding" (Habermas 1987, 396). Politically active communities would therefore seem to be a key agent of decolonisation.

Yet at this point Habermas failed to explore – indeed, almost pulled back from – the implications of his theories. He is notably weak on descriptions of how, in real-life political situations, these counterpublics could give rise to genuine change, by transforming practice. Can so abstract a theory be applicable to the real world, shot through with distortions, inequities and power? As Blaug (1999, 54) says:

> (A) quite extraordinary number of books and articles on Habermasian theory end with a somewhat nebulous benediction to its empirical promise. Often, an increase in popular deliberation in the making of political decisions is called for, and general praise is inevitably heaped on the public sphere as the appropriate space for such deliberation.... No one feels able to bring him or herself to actually address the empirical problem of how the normative insights might be translated into institutional shape.

This problem is reflected in the title of Blaug's book (1999a): the difficulty in moving from *ideal* to *real*, recognising the possible contradiction in the idea of "design for democracy". The contradiction is manifested if democratic institutions or processes are foisted on a community without the agreement of that community. Yet if democracy *emerges* from the community, the contradiction is effaced, and Blaug says (1999a, xv) that such learning processes should at least expect *guidance* from critical democratic theory. For critical theory to be a "living force" it must be developed in association with contemporary issues and problems (Forester 1985).

Blaug points out that hierarchism, like other aspects of hegemony, usually works not by direct coercion and the oppression of alternatives. Practitioners advocating the spread of new values, organisational forms, and ways of thinking may be detained as subversives, or subject to disciplinary action or dismissal, but more frequently the operations of hegemony are less direct, with actors denied the methodological or conceptual tools to evaluate and learn about alternative ways of thinking and working. Nevertheless, learning *can* take place regardless of the controls placed on it, and: "In such a learning process, it may well be that Habermas's regulative ideal can help us 'train our eyes'..." (Blaug 1999a, 100).

Yet, like any other abstract and generic theory of human behaviour, only in a *context*, at the *moment of application* (*ibid*, 13), can the validity of the theory – thus, *the validity claim of the theorist* – be opened to scrutiny. Theoretical speculation "can never be a substitute for direct experience, for making mistakes, for seeing others do it well" (*ibid*, 100). This is, ultimately, the problem with Habermas: his lack of attention to actual, embodied human experience, and the *methods* by which new insights emerge and are validated. He pays insufficient attention to everyday communication and activity to give guidance and, where he tries, it is to a limited audience. The social movement is certainly an arena in which new, democratic possibilities are actively explored and one that, in early phases at least (*ibid, 135ff*), is characterised by great energy. But democratic moments, "laboratories of experience", arise whenever existing practices, habits, or routines are called into question, including between friends, parents and children, colleagues at work, doctors and patients, etc.

This perspective on democracy – the possibility of a distributed authority that is consented to, not hegemonically, but in an active and consensual way – is a necessary counterpoint to Foucault's view of power (1980) as embedded in everyday social interactions. The claim that democracy not only can be, but must be, a lived, embodied experience, invested in everyday practice, reclaims the notion from hierarchism. Hierarchism, the idea that authority should be concentrated rather than distributed, has promoted a political system that reduces the powerful notion of democracy to a remnant – the vote, and only for certain groups[3]. This system of political representation is called 'democracy', but it is quite a different beast from the lived and embodied experience. It is testament to the power of the word that it is retained for the impersonal and instrumental voting system, or as a synonym for 'Parliament' or 'Law'.

The role of "counterpublics", whether in their full form as social movements or simply as a space within a landscape in which practice is questioned, has been undermined in Habermas's work since *The Theory of Communicative Action*. "[A]s Habermas himself has admitted, by 1981 he had given up on the hope that the economy and the state could be 'transformed democratically from within'" (Hirschkop 2004, 52, via Habermas 1992, 444). By *Between Facts and Norms* (Habermas 1996), the public sphere and its component counterpublics became, for Habermas, not the source of political change but more a "sounding board for problems that must be processed by the political system" (Habermas 1996, 359; cited in Hirschkop 2004, 52; also Gardiner 2004, 29).

Yet though this may seem an "admission of defeat", "what the public sphere loses in terms of decision-making power it more than compensates for in terms of its ability to track the problems of capitalism down to their private lair" (Hirschkop 2004, 58). What Hirschkop means here (cf. Habermas 1996, 365) is that in the *personal spaces* of individuals and communities the impact of "systemic deficiencies" – exploitation, impoverishment, surveillance etc. – in late capitalist society are most clearly revealed. It is the lifeworld that "is uniquely suited to the demystifying of these problems in liberal capitalist societies" (Hirschkop 2004, 58), precisely because the lifeworld is defined by intersubjective exchanges that allow it to remain adaptable and responsive, rather than structured around instrumental solutions to problems that become reified ends-in-themselves. Thus, counterpublics and communities are better suited to double-loop learning. Without allowing for the questioning of the premises which underlie ways of thinking, and the systems based on them, transformation cannot occur (Hirschkop 2004, 60): "Through the crevices in discourse which allow one to 'open up' the discussion of life experiences, citizens are able to connect problems experienced in individual life histories to wider social structures."

Counterpublics, then, are the spaces in which the notion of *expertise* is reclaimed, and community members can discover they have something *valid* to say on issues that affect them, directly and indirectly. Counterpublics help assert the worth of forms of knowledge-making and self-expression that have been devalued by colonisation generally, and/or specifically repressed in particular contexts.

There is a risk of relativism once again. To say that political activism is legitimate simply because it exists and is structured in communicative ways would accommodate, say, the unstructured networks that are gang culture and Al-Qaeda. Both networks, in their own way, may have been nature, this results in a more ephemeral and dynamic environment. In an instrumentally-rational environment, knowledge is *embedded* by devoting resources to the development of systems (hierarchies, procedures, technologies, etc.), which fix the results of decisions in place. This allows decisions to be implemented, but simultaneously leaves them less open to review and scrutiny.

Vigilance, therefore, is the process by which a community reveals these trade-offs, reviews them, and where necessary transforms them. Ideally, it does so in ways that do not retard the community's future ability to learn and transform its landscape. In other words, the information landscape is maintained in a sustainable way, by the members of the community themselves, but drawing on a supportive infrastructure. Habermas shows that it is a category mistake to expect this support from the state (the instrumental organisation *par excellence*), but there nevertheless need to be elements of this supportive infrastructure that go beyond simply encouraging discussion and consensus, which drains resources if not accompanied by more instrumental elements of support that allow decisions and transformations to be implemented. Hirschkop (2004, 62) points out that this instrumental activity, and the texts that must support it, are "unlikely to emerge from the interaction of well-intentioned citizens alone: it would require a specialised and organised practice consciously aimed at the emancipation of the existential language in circulation, which is itself in large part a product of the culture industry." What, then, are these "specialised and organised" practices to which Hirschkop refers? I answer that question simply: *radical information literacy*.

Therefore, if IL is the set of practices oriented towards the maintenance of information landscapes of any kind, radical IL is the subset of these practices oriented towards the maintenance of information landscapes within which communicative rationality is more likely to inhere, and therefore in which authority is more widely distributed.

***

IL, including radical IL, needs to be based on a range of learning outcomes that, as the phenomenographic school of IL has shown, encompasses generic skills and competencies, metacognitive skills, an ability to evaluate one's own context, and a facility with dialogue. Formal learning providers such as universities, schools, libraries, museums, and other training providers can potentially help in all these areas, thus contributing to radical IL. But there remains the danger of reifying this expertise. Like other delegations of cognitive work – to a hierarchy, a computer, a routine or habit – it can lead to decisions about the relevance of information not being kept under full scrutiny. Thus, the role of any formal learning or training provider, which, by definition, does not situate itself within the context in which such knowledge must be applied, must also be subject to the scrutiny of the community which seeks its guidance.

The creation of a *radical IL infrastructure* (cf. Landry et al 1985) is therefore a matter of developing communicative spaces in which a more democratic, distributed authority is apparent, and to provide the guidance that keeps the spaces sustainable (what Wenger, White and Smith (2009) call *stewarding*). These spaces may exist within particular communities, or may cross communities; both types are required. Guidance may be manifested in various forms of text, including technology. This guidance shapes practice by saving cognitive work: hence it needs to be periodically reviewed by the community members subject to it. The ultimate goal of a radical IL is the distribution of stewarding capacity throughout a community. This is not an end-in-itself, but a constant process. Hence, the goal of a radical IL practitioner is not to make themselves redundant, but to be constantly monitoring the environment for learning opportunities, keeping pace with the constant trade-offs required to stay vigilant over hierarchy, technology, routine, habit, and other trade-offs involved when cognitive work is saved.

Benhabib (1990; see also Nielsen 2002, 33) has critiqued Habermas's theory of discourse ethics for not being sufficiently context-sensitive. The model of radical IL sketched in the last few pages is an attempt to build on Habermas's generic philosophies and, from them, develop a more context-sensitive approach. Supporting a general case for a unitary, *critical* theory of IL entails showing (Ray 1993, 176–7):

> (F)irst, that existing forms of domination do not exhaust more varied potentials within modern structures; secondly, that an alternative, suppressed modernity continues to inform new protest potentials; and thirdly, that these have some realistic expectation of decolonising the lifeworld.

Habermas lacks the basis in *text* and *context* for this work to be fully founded on his theories, though they have provided considerable support. To go further into these matters requires an investigation of Bakhtin.

Notes

1. Habermas has been criticised for an overly idealistic view of 18th and 19th century public spheres, which writers such as Fraser (1992) point out were not as egalitarian as he claims (Habermas 1989); thus, the distribution of authority over text has never reached to the great mass of the population. The critique is valid, but should not affect his assessment of present trends.
2. See also Foucault's idea (1986, 24) of the *heterotopia* – not a place in which Utopia is made real, but one in which its claims are investigated, critiqued and contested – that is, *scrutinised.*
3. Suffrage is not universal anywhere; all countries deny it to children, even when matters affect them, and many still exclude prisoners, immigrants and other groups from voting.

6

Mikhail Bakhtin and IL

Abstract: This chapter explores the key concepts in Bakhtin's theories of communication and outlines their relevance for the study of IL.. These concepts, particularly the ideas of genre, chronotope, unfinalisability, and polyphony, or multi-voicedness, help show why information practices and information literacy cannot be a generic pursuit, but instead are context-dependent. The chapter also explores the difference between the human sciences and the natural sciences, and returns to the notion of strong objectivity to clarify why scrutiny of all validity claims is an essential aspect of IL.

Key Words: Bakhtin, genre, chronotope, unfinalisability, polyphony, strong objectivity, authority.

The role of this chapter is to root radical IL firmly in communication and democracy as experienced in everyday social settings and lived experiences, rather than as abstract ideals. To successfully build on chapter 5, the theories incorporated into radical IL must be attuned to the nature of trade-offs between different forms of thinking, which for Habermas were instantiated in instrumental and communicative rationality. Radical IL must incorporate the reality of colonisation and hegemony, yet simultaneously allow for the possibility of change in these social structures and, thus, how they govern the exchange of information and the making of judgments. All these conditions are met in the work of Mikhail Bakhtin.

Bakhtin wrote in the Soviet Union from the 1920s until his death in 1970. His work was popularised in the English-speaking world in the 1980s by commentators such as Holquist (2002; 2009) and Morson and Emerson (1990), and through two significant collected translations of his work (Bakhtin 1981; 1986). Linell (2009) cites him as the paramount theorist of dialogism. This chapter will review his key ideas, particularly the difference between dialogue and monologue, and the importance of *polyphony* or multi-voicedness in knowledge formation. For Bakhtin, literacy is applicable to every utterance, written or spoken, and not limited only to specialised texts (e.g. expert pronouncements, academic texts). He recognises the reality of authority over text, but also that, because of the nature of language, no 'final state' is possible in a communicative situation. Thus, there can be no *absolute* authority. Everything contains the possibility of change and transformation within itself at multiple levels, from the single utterance up to the structures of language and communication, and how meaning is created within them.

Bakhtin has been only infrequently invoked in the IL debate, and this chapter is the first full treatment of his work vis-à-vis IL. Nor are his ideas often connected to Habermas's. An exception is a paper by Nielsen (2002), who discusses how Habermas and Bakhtin both try to deal with "one of the most perplexing problems to face contemporary theories of creativity and action – diversity and the dilemma of reconstructing a transcultural (universal) ethics" (*ibid*, 24). Thus, both are concerned with how we retain diversity and polyphony while not collapsing into relativism, retaining normative criteria (in Habermas's case, communicative rationality) as a means of judging outcomes. Nielsen goes on to say (*ibid*, 27): "Neither thinker gives in to pluralism or a detached intellectual relativism yet each, in different ways, recognizes that modern societies develop 'polyphonically' (in multiple voices, perspectives, and simultaneous points of view)..."

Hirschkop (2004), Garvey (2000), and Gardiner (2004) also explore the similarities and differences in the work of Bakhtin and Habermas. According to Garvey (2000, 371), there are four issues on which they share common ground:

> First, they agree that before equality can be established in the social realm, it must be modeled by establishing egalitarian communicative relationships. Second, both strive to understand communication, not by analyzing language, but by analyzing how selfhood and intersubjective relationships are structured and mediated by communicative action. They both analyze communication as a social institution not unlike a political system or a religious tradition. Third, both assert the special importance of dialogic realms wherein relationships of power are partly neutralized by being brought into the foreground. Fourth and finally, each understands his analysis of communicative relationships as a mode of social criticism that can help to define a more ethical world by demystifying some of the ways in which domination is embedded in acts of speech and communication.

All are, in turn, true of a radical IL.

Also significant are the differences between the two authors. These show how Bakhtin's ideas can be used to overcome the problems which arise when applying Habermas to IL. This point of Gardiner's is pertinent because it revisits an idea which appeared in chapter 5: that (colonising) power involves shifting knowledge-formation structures out of the subjective and intersubjective domains, and into the objective (Gardiner 2004, 30):

> Whereas Habermas seeks to delineate sharply between particular realms of social activity and forms of discourse—between, for instance, public and private, state and public sphere, reason and non-reason, ethics and aesthetics—Bakhtin problematizes such demarcations, sees them as fluid, permeable and always contested, and alerts us to the power relations that are involved in any such exercise of boundary-maintenance.

Thus, for Bakhtin, power and authority are manifested in the very assertion that there can be 'objective' knowledge in the realm of human affairs. Instead, Bakhtin sees all such knowledge as essentially intersubjective. Authority is the means by which specific elements of understanding are assigned to one realm rather than another. Whether this authority can be considered legitimate or illegitimate depends on the context, but that does not mean the question is relativist and has no meaning. As with Habermas, Bakhtin develops clear normative criteria by which we can judge the legitimacy of authority: thus, *be literate in a given context*. These criteria – polyphony, dialogue, and an openness to transformation – can be shown to be true of 'objective' *scientific* knowledge, which has processes for claiming authority that open this claim up for scrutiny, but not of those forms of 'objectivity' which are claimed through the exercise of power, and close up channels of scrutiny. This is an essential move in defining radical IL.

Gardiner sees Habmermas's account of intersubjectivity as "overly abstract and formalistic" (Gardiner 2004, 30), and states that Bakhtin is far more sensitive to the plurality of "embodied, situational and dialogical elements of everyday human life" (*ibid*). He believes Bakhtin can fill lacunae in Habermas's conception of "dialogical democracy" by suggesting methods for judging the legitimacy of authority *in practice*: Habermas develops these methods in theory only.

Bakhtin helps reveal that these gaps arise from problems with Habermas's notion of consensus. Lyotard (1984) asserts the value of *dissensus* and conflicting opinions, and sees consensus, in Habermasian terms, as a dangerous imposition. This criticism can partly be countered by remembering that the ISS is specifically an *ideal*, which Habermas recognises is unattainable in practical situations. Nevertheless a 'perfect' consensus (the telos of communicative rationality) would, in principle, efface diversity just as effectively as would a 'perfect' system (the telos of instrumental rationality). Bakhtin would call both the perfect consensus and the perfect system *monologic* ways of thinking and working: that is, they allow only one voice to be heard. His counter-ideal, that of *dialogue*, is therefore quite different from Habermas's notion of consensus (Nielsen 2002, 25).

Dialogue is the key driving force of change in Bakhtin's epistemology. Its opposite tendency, the monologue, leads to the death of creativity and psychic stagnation. The "monologic way of perceiving of cognition and truth" (Bakhtin 1984, 81) is manifested in the *system*. As with Habermas's "system" – the consequence of instrumentally rational ways of viewing the world and engaging in activity – this notion describes *the product of a way of thinking*. A system can be driven by one voice and manifest only that one voice's values. Other voices or utterances must conform to the system, perhaps having to change words or position in order to be processed through it. The only cognitive relations one can have to a perfect system are conformity or error. In principle, a system can be "comprehended and fully contained by a *single* consciousness – in principle, by any consciousness with sufficient intellectual power" (Morson and Emerson 1990, 236). This invokes Zurkowski's vision of "information banks". From an instrumental *knowledge management* perspective, a 'perfect' information bank is one that contains all relevant information and answers, immediately and always accurately, any query put to it (Saracevic 1975, 326). The ideal system is convergent around a single voice and, to use the system effectively, the request must be shaped accordingly.

However, Bakhtin's work is "a highly rational attempt to imagine the world as incommensurate with systems" (Morson and Emerson 1990, 6). A monologic system can process inputs and outputs efficiently but, by definition, cannot grow and change, as anomalous, creative inputs would be rejected as errors. *In practice,* alternative perspectives (queries, criteria, meanings) always arise, evidence of *multiple* consciousnesses, interacting through dialogue. Because of the nature of language, and its essentially contextual nature, these interactions are innately *creative*, giving rise to new possibilities and practices (this claim will be explored further below in the discussion on 'unfinalisability'). Dialogue is thus essential to change, which by definition cannot arise from a monologue. Indeed, every monologue holds within it a basic contradiction: that it must, by *imposing authority*, acknowledge the reality of alternative voices, if only as things – potential hidden transcripts – which need to be repressed. What this means is that not only does instrumentality/monologism not prevent new possibilities emerging, it *cannot* do so.

Here Bakhtin is in agreement with Habermas, but we can now see how their notions of 'systems' differ. Bakhtin's system is rooted not in abstract forms of thinking but in *everyday language*. Language is not a direct way into people's brains. Because of the complexities and ambiguities of language, Bakhtin would not see it as possible to directly *transfer meaning* from a sender to a recipient (Linell 2009, 37). Meanings cannot be transferred, only signs. Language is a construction, but we think *through dialogue*. Hence, it is how dialogue, and the various elements of the information landscape in which it is embodied, are understood and used in diverse ways that reveals structure and agency (transformation) in Bakhtin's theories. This is why his work is wholly relevant to the development of IL generally, and radical IL particularly. Habermas's idea of colonisation is also useful, but too singular. It emanates in the same way from across the system and is experienced in the same way even across a variety of publics and counterpublics. Habermas was insufficiently interested in everyday lived experience to establish the variety of possible reactions – indeed, the variety of possible systems (monologic sources of authority) – and thus help with a study of how diverse information landscapes can be learned about and transformed. What is needed are theories that better explain the diversity of context, and how *both* this diversity *and* also the monologic nature of authority, are rooted in everyday communication and information. Bakhtin offers such insights.

Having considered so far how his ideas of dialogue and monologue help distinguish his work from Habermas's, this chapter will continue first with Bakhtin's concepts of *genre* and *chronotope*, which explain how an information landscape can shape communication; then, the notions of *utterances* and *unfinalisability*, which show how there are always unfulfilled potentials in any discourse; and finally, explore in detail the notion of *authority* in Bakhtin, with particular attention to how objectivity and intersubjectivity are, ideally, connected, but how authority rests in keeping claims to objectivity insulated from dialogic scrutiny.

* * *

For Bakhtin, it is in communication that the human world is created and, from this creation, future possibilities shaped, but not predetermined. This is not an abstract and idealised communicative event, as for Habermas. Rather, it is a "*practical* rationality, rooted in the actualities of the everyday and not detachable from specific conditions" (Gardiner 2004, 33). Thus, it is *prosaic*. For Morson and Emerson the concept of prosaics is:

> (A) form of thinking that presumes the importance of the everyday, the ordinary, the 'prosaic'... (1990, 15)

> (T)he everyday is a sphere of constant activity, the source of all social change and individual creativity... prosaic creativity generally proceeds slowly, begins in narrow spheres, and is hardly noticeable. For that reason we do not see it, and think that innovation must come from somewhere else. (*ibid*, 23)

Thus, focusing on the prosaic can help researchers and practitioners train their eyes, to see what often goes unnoticed, down to the significance of single moments of information exchange. As already noted, raising awareness of things often taken for granted is a key *learning process*; part (although not all: Morson and Emerson 1990, 36) of what it means to become literate.

Bakhtin shows that the meaning of any utterance is not given by the author, but nor is it wholly created by the recipient. Instead, there is a *dialogic* relationship between author and recipient in which there is inherent uncertainty, as the context of the author and recipient inevitably differ, though the degree of difference will vary from slight to extreme. All dialogue, then, can potentially destabilise existing practices and ways of thinking. Therefore, while prosaic communication can "display routinized, static and unreflexive characteristics, it is also capable of a surprising dynamism and moments of penetrating insight and boundless creativity" (Gardiner 2004, 41).

Learning about these areas of human communication depends also on establishing why there exist structural biases against prosaics. A focus on everyday life contexts and prosaic communication is atypical of formal education. Prosaic communication is usually not perceived as the 'domain' of the expert, the 'right' (that is, authoritative) location for knowledge[1]. An interest in prosaic communication, at least potentially, contests notions of authority which exist in those domains, seeking to question and possibly redistribute authority through widening access to these spaces and the forms of knowledge and information within them. This kind of challenge may be diverted in various ways. Access to a text, and the forms of authority invested in that text, may be directly restricted: one may be unable to physically access information without the requisite status (possibly invested in a technological device such as a password). However, access to the meanings invested in a particular dialogue can also be more indirectly concealed. Not all speakers will be *literate* in each context and their ability to become so may be limited.

These insights are explored by Bakhtin via developing the notion of *genre*. The popular notion of genre tends to be applied to literature and entertainment: the horror genre, the soap opera, etc. In each exist certain conventions. If a book called *Home on the Range* has a cover picture of an idyllic Midwestern US farm, a reader would be surprised if it was a horror novel. However, Bakhtinian genres "govern our daily speech, both 'outer' and 'inner'" (Morson and Emerson 1990, 275). Breure (2001, no pagination) says:

> For Bakhtin genres are not simply sets of rules and conventions, but ways of conceptualizing reality, forms of seeing and interpreting particular aspects of the world. They are connected with expectations about length and compositional structure. They are the fundamental molds in which we cast communication.

The concept includes (Bakhtin 1986, 60):

> (S)hort rejoinders of daily dialogue (and these are extremely varied depending on the subject matter, situation, and participants), everyday narration, writing (in all its various forms), the brief standard military command, the elaborate and detailed order, the fairly variegated repertoire of business documents (for the most part standard), and the diverse world of commentary (in the broad sense of the word: social, political).

In the 21st century Bakhtin may well have added the Facebook status update, the blog post, the comment on an online newspaper story, TV quiz shows, and more, as forms of speech genre.

As Andersen (2008, 349) says:

> To recognize a particular text type is to recognize a particular communicative situation and activity in which that type of text (genre) is used to accomplish a given task. In our everyday interaction with texts, whether as producers or recipients, genres are a means of orientation... and thus connected to literacy: The more we know about the communicative activities in which we are involved, the more we know how to understand and use the texts produced by these activities.

Genres are not just technical devices, therefore, but contribute to the stratification of society into distinct informational landscapes with specific characteristics. Professional groups develop not just specialised vocabularies, but also associated practices, boundaries, and ways of thinking that function to help form community identities, but also to exclude others (Bakhtin 1981, 289):

> (T)he language of the lawyer, the doctor, the businessman, the politician, the public education teacher and so forth... these languages differ from each other not only in their vocabularies; they involve specific forms for manifesting intentions, forms for making conceptualization and evaluation concrete... these possibilities are realized in specific directions, filled with specific content, they are made concrete, particular, and are permeated with concrete value judgments; they knit together with specific objects and with the belief systems of certain genres of expression and points of view peculiar to particular professions.

The genre is therefore a "human construction" that helps "determine how much selection and search power a searcher is in possession of" (Andersen 2006, 221–2). To be literate in a particular genre, however that is defined, is to have freer access to the resources of that genre, and wield them as an instrument. This is why information seeking is a sociopolitical activity, as its practices constitute aspects of the power structures in society (*ibid*, 222).

Genres are "ways of seeing" (Morson and Emerson 1990, 275): tools for analysis of practical communication, applicable to the study of particular landscapes. Genres and information landscapes, however, constructions which shape communication, are similar, but not the same thing. Genres are abstract, sets of "typified rhetorical actions based in recurrent situations" (Miller 1984, 159 cited in Andersen 2008, 350).

Like other abstract ways of organising and making judgements about information, genres require *situated interpretation* across diverse contexts, so becoming manifested within different information landscapes, in which the definitions and boundaries of genres are tested. The idea of, say, 'the legal genre' is a way of recognising texts, but does not fully elucidate the diversity of discourses which take place in legalistic contexts. Just as the UK Lake District and Australia's Great Dividing Range are both 'mountain regions', but recognisably different in specific form, so one law firm is a different landscape from another, even if both should be literate in the same genres. Therefore, the existence of genres does not invalidate the study of context. Genres are themes common to many landscapes, and each landscape may contain different genres.

The definition of genres is further enriched by Bakhtin's notion of the *chronotope*. This term links the Greek words for 'time' and 'place' and, again, has layers of meaning. It can refer to the particular sense of time and space that is characteristic of a genre. This is akin to Hall's studies of physical space, and how different cultures arranged their use of space, studies that informed his notion of "proxemics" (Hall 1968, 84): "...the way in which both time and space were handled [in a given situation] constituted a form of communication..." Saying that understandings of time and space vary between people is, emphatically, not suggesting that these concepts, as a physicist understands them, are relative. This position is castigated by Thompson in his discussion of counterknowledge (2008, 121–2), but in this case the argument is a straw man. Bakhtin is specifically making points not about the natural world, but about the human reaction to it. Particular spatial and temporal relationships between people do differ across landscapes. To pick two extreme, but nevertheless illustrative examples, time is thought of quite differently by a geologist than by a stock market trader. An 'urgent' communication may be perceived differently in a government department compared to an intensive care unit.

Chronotopes are not just an output of communication, however. They are a fundamental basis for activity in any landscape (Bakhtin 1981, 250). It is not just understandings of time and place, but the *physical and temporal location* of a speaker or text, that can define "parameters of value" (Morson and Emerson 1990, 369), and thus shape events. Bakhtin draws here also on Goethe, who saw (Bakhtin 1986, 42): "no events, plots or temporal motifs that are not related in an essential way to the particular spatial place of their occurrence... Everything in this world is a *time-space*, a true *chronotope*." Information or forms of expression that are "taken for granted in one culture [chronotope] may not even exist in another" (Hall 1968, 94). And individuals each have their chronotope, a specific place and time they occupy, uniquely, at every moment. Holquist (2009, 9–10) calls the chronotope "omnipresent": it is "the clock and the map we employ to orient our identity in the flux of existence", and thus, the basis of subjectivity. Just as the pronoun *I* has no intrinsic meaning but is filled with meaning when, and only when, employed by a specific person, so do the terms *now* and *here*, and cognates such as *then* and *elsewhere* (Holquist 2009, 16–17). At this individual level, the chronotope is the horizon of the speaker, the landscape in which they are present (cf. Steinerová 2010), the specific coincidence of time and place which forms the grounds for the structure of awareness of that person at that moment.

The diversity of genres and the effectively infinite variety of chronotopes give landscapes their heterogeneous and fractal characteristics. We may have single chronotopes but we are members of multiple communities, fluent in genres in varying ways, and we each bring our own level of 'outsideness' to any discourse. So, although the collective is a real basis for activity and ethics, these givens can be *transcended* by individuals. This is central to action. We each individually act at the nexus of many landscapes: "individual stylization" comes about as we try to act in ways that "satisfy conflicting obligations in a polyphonic milieu" (Cresswell and Baerveldt 2011, 274). Because we all live in multiple communities, "there is never a situation where one speaks from a single speech genre in isolation" (Cresswell and Teucher 2011, 115). The world is therefore a *polyphony* of voices – and it is through dialogue that we *experience variation* in the voices we encounter, learn from, and can engage with.

We therefore encounter many genres as we communicate, but do not use each equally well. Crossing the boundaries can cause difficulties. A text or utterance considered credible in one context may be questioned or dismissed as valueless elsewhere. A speaker may be literate in one genre of communication (e.g. academia, therapy) but less so in another (e.g. legal discourse, music). This is "not a matter of an impoverished vocabulary or style" (Bakhtin 1986, 80): in other words, a speaker's or text's 'illiteracy' in a classic sense. Rather, it relates to the unfamiliarity of that speaker, or lack of fit of the text, with context-specific features of the landscape: meanings, ways of using words, procedures, technologies, and so on, which constitute that landscape at that particular chronotope. Certain landscapes have come over time to be structured in ways that make them sympathetic to some genres over others, and if knowledge is not formulated and presented in ways that fit this structure, it will be rejected.

For example, the results of learning may be embodied in texts in diverse ways, not just in academic papers, official reports, or other such formal texts, but in the creation of technology, in oral narratives, in changed practices, on a blog, in conversations around a coffee machine (cf. Harris 2008, 253; Cresswell and Baervelt 2011, 267). The *authority* typically assigned to each of these media varies, yet this does not necessarily conform to the *value* that each may have in certain contexts. For example, the knowledge about how to safely fight a fire is clearly significant for humanity, but remains largely unwritten. Even where texts discuss technicalities (e.g. the design of effective fire extinguishers), practitioners in this landscape, as Lloyd showed (2007), still looked first to practice-based, embodied sources of information, such as the physical movements of colleagues, in which were encoded concrete experiences of previous fires (that is, relevant chronotopes). Tacit, rather than explicit, nevertheless that knowledge exists, is stored, is accessible, and is valuable. It shapes practice without wholly determining outcomes, nor closing off new possible insights. Yet because of the form it takes – harder to capture in an information system – it is less valued, and not addressed by competency-based approaches to IL.

Landscapes and genres are never the product of *design*, but products of evolution, which means they are always "imperfectly suited to their present use – and for that very reason are relatively adaptable to future uses, to which they will also be acceptably but not optimally suited" (Morson and Emerson 1990, 292). To retain relevance, genres – and by extension, particular information landscapes – must continue to evolve: but they can also fade away. They can "stubbornly" persist even when they no longer generate new insights (Bakhtin 1981, 85). Forms of authority within a genre may become more and more concealed, and as a result genres can become mythologised or symbolic, or degenerate into stereotypes or prejudice ('all people from X are Y...'). Structures of thinking in the individual mind can persist in the same way: this links to the earlier discussion of personal constructs and will be returned to below in the discussion of the 'authoritative voice'.

On the other hand, genres may also be subject to review following encounters with fresh inputs that may bring these collective assumptions into question. Again, this can happen at broad, macro-levels: for example, mobile technologies, and Skype, changed forever certain aspects of the genre that was the (landline) 'telephone call'. Or, it may take place at a more context-specific and local level.

It is possible to move between genres comfortably, bringing many different types of communication into one's own chronotope and becoming literate in a broader sense, able to "command a repertoire of genres of social conversation" (Bakhtin 1981, 85), which "enriches one's capacity to conceptualize and participate in varying aspects of social life" (Morson and Emerson 1990, 275). Orlikowski and Yates (1996, 542; cited in Andersen 2008, 354) note that this broad *genre repertoire* can be possessed both by individuals and by communities. If we see genres as "knowledge organizing categories" (Andersen 2008, 355) it can be seen how a wide repertoire of them gives an individual or a community a more flexible range of strategies to choose from – that is, it makes them more information literate (Andersen 2006, 225–6).

Facility may be acquired with surface elements of a genre: a sort of lay knowledge. I find astrophysics papers largely impenetrable. Yet, as a Humanities academic, I recognise in them features that are characteristic of the broader genre of the academic paper, such as its general intention, techniques such as the presentation of a methodology, a bibliography, and so on. I understand *why* these things are there, knowing that they give the text *authority.* I cannot, however, penetrate, and thus scrutinize, the authority of the paper using its more specific genres (e.g. the validity of its complex mathematics), though I can seek understanding from other media: for example, read about the research in the *New Scientist,* attend a public lecture, or engage in informal conversations with physicist friends. This may seem little more than the sign of a 'good education', but it is also information literacy in the broadest sense.

Bakhtin's work shows why crossing genre boundaries like this is essential. Linell (2009, 82–5) calls this 'outsideness' *alterity*, and recognises it as an essential element of dialogue. Each genre is a "combination of specific blindnesses and insights... adapted to conceptualizing some aspects of reality better than others. That, indeed, is why people and cultures need continually to learn new genres as the compass of their experience expands." (Morson and Emerson 1990, 276, citing Medvedev 1985, 131). The ongoing health of any landscape depends on its boundaries remaining permeable by fresh inputs, which by definition come from outside, as the validity claims present in one landscape are questioned at the point it comes into contact with another (Bakhtin 1986, 7):

> ...outsideness is a most powerful factor in understanding....
> A meaning only reveals its depths once it has encountered and
> come into contact with another, foreign meaning: they engage

in a kind of dialogue, which surmounts the closedness and one-sidedness of these particular meanings, these cultures.... Such a dialogic encounter of two cultures does not result in merging or mixing. Each retains its own unity and *open* totality, but they are mutually enriched.

Yet it is precisely at the boundary points between landscapes that authority is most clearly asserted. Boundaries are where communication crosses into a different landscape, and the systems and cognitive authorities within that landscape may struggle to accommodate the new perspective, particularly if they are monologic. Being literate in the genres that shape practice on both sides of this 'border' allows for the transformation of key elements of a text, or its re-presentation, to imbue it with authority in the other landscapes it must encounter. Literacy therefore helps bridge boundaries between cultures and thereby enrich them. This makes it essential for learning, and also gives it its political character.

Revealing the characteristics of genre and chronotope, and helping learners become literate in particular genres, is already a common learning method in IL. Competency-based IL does it implicitly, training learners to recognise features of authority, with a bias towards expert genres (academia, official publications, and pronouncements). The personal relevance and learning to learn frames of IL aim to help learners recognise their own chronotopes and the way each can best develop knowledge within them. Social impact views of IL would consider politically powerful genres such as the news media and engage in a critical investigation of the characteristics of that genre, whereas a relational approach would consider variation and difference between genres, and possibly aim to help learners acquire facility with multiple modes of communication, as called for by writers about transliteracy (Ipri 2010).

The critical eye can also be turned on the chronotopes and genres of IL itself, a task undertaken above, in chapter 4. The ACRL standards can be seen as a chronotope: see O'Connor (2009) who "uncovered the American political mythologies and assumptions inherent in the conception of information literacy, as reflected in the ACRL standards" (Julien and Williamson 2011, no pagination).

What Bakhtin can help with is to link these conceptions of IL as learning and IL as practice. To continue with this project it is necessary to more closely examine how prosaic communication is at the root of the processes by which genres, chronotopes and landscapes are transformed.

***

To say that 'outsideness' or alterity is essential for understanding genres, chronotopes, and landscapes may seem to invite the conclusion that these informational phenomena can be studied abstractly, like laboratory specimens, by observers who do not interact with the setting. Abstractions of the communicative process may be useful in generic linguistic and semiotic analysis, but they need to be recognised as abstractions (Bakhtin 1986, 69–70). Actual *transformation* of the landscape takes place not through treating it as a laboratory specimen, using methodologies oriented towards the *external* design of solutions to problems (such as an information system), but as a *laboratory of experience* (Melucci 1989), in which solutions to problems emerge from learning processes undertaken therein. The methods and studies may be explicit and formal, but these processes are also constantly occurring at the informal level. Just as Cervero and Wilson (1994) see organisational learning as a constant series of "micro-moments" in which practices are tested and validated, so Bakhtin sees every *utterance* as, at least potentially, a moment of learning. It is this constant process of checking and validating which invests all communication, potentially, with the capacity to transformation information practices and landscapes.

Bakhtin sees communication as a series of utterances with no start or end. Utterances can be as short as a word – even a gesture – or as long as a novel. Each is a move in communication. Single utterances hold within them, theoretically, the totality of previous communication: every utterance "must be regarded primarily as a *response* to preceding utterances of the given sphere..." (Bakhtin 1986, 91). Or as Morson and Emerson put it (1990, 137):

> Every time we speak, we respond to something spoken before and we take a stand in relation to earlier utterances about the topic. The way we sense those earlier utterances – as hostile or sympathetic, authoritative or feeble, socially and temporally close or distant – shapes the content and style of what we say. We sense these alien utterances in the object itself. It is as if the object were coated with a sort of glue preserving earlier characterizations of it.

And every utterance can be potentially replied to, even if that reply does not follow immediately (Bakhtin 1986, 68–9):

> An actively responsive understanding of what is heard (a command, for example) can be directly realized in action

(the execution of an order or command that has been understood and accepted for execution), or it can remain, for the time being, a salient responsive understanding... but this is, so to speak, responsive understanding with a delayed reaction. Sooner or later what is heard and actively understood will find its response in the subsequent speech or behaviour of the listener.

Utterances are shaped by genres, and so the genre will influence utterances' 'finalisability' as well as other features. The military command can almost be exhausted by a single utterance and response. Once one has heard a command and responded to it, there is nowhere else to take the dialogue, except to await another command. In creative spheres, there is almost no finalisation possible, except a "certain minimum of finalization making it possible to occupy a responsive position", that is, to make the next move in the creative conversation (Bakthin 1986, 77). Great texts, such as Shakespeare or Greek myths, retain 'genre potentials' more or less permanently: that is, they can continually be reworked as new communities use them for guidance on contemporary issues (and also, in many cases, see commercial potential, particularly with Shakespeare). For example, Purdue refers (2003, 658) to Walter Benjamin and the *transformative* power of great stories: like seeds preserved for centuries, stories "retain a germinative power" and "are begging to be retold".

These examples suggest that certain speech genres are more conducive to debate and creativity than others. Not all are equally able to develop new potentials. Orwell's essay *Politics and the English Language* (1950), and his invention of "Newspeak" in *Nineteen-Eighty Four* (1948) – a stripped-down language designed to eradicate subversive or non-dogmatic thought – specifically invoke this point.

In all, any attempt to understand meaning generically, independent of a listener's context, can at best derive some sense of the *potential* of an utterance, "but only when that potential is exploited for a particular purpose on a particular occasion is there real meaning" (Morson and Emerson 1990, 127). Indeed, it is genre and landscape that *carry* these potentials from the resources of the past into the present and future (Bakhtin 1986, 4). These structures support cognitive work, preventing speakers from having to engage in the long process of definition before making an utterance, e.g. indicating values, exploring the context, suggesting a sense of time and space (*ibid*, 60). Thus, they can also be conduits for the concealing of meaning, hiding assumptions from scrutiny, beneath awareness – thus, conduits for institutionalisation. It is in genres that *collective memory* can best be seen to reside (Wertsch 2009, cf. points made in chapter 1 above).

The genre framework can *explain* continuity from past to future, but genres do not define the future deterministically, as if the present and future can be understood merely from examining the past (Morson and Emerson 1990, 89):

> (I)n understanding genre we have not understood everything that is important about... acts or literary works. Genre provides the 'given', but the work or act provides the 'created', something new... each act of speech and each literary work uses the resources of the genre in a specific way in response to a specific individual situation. The genre – similar to the uttered word – is thus changed slightly by each usage...

Hence, landscapes are not made of the same ingredients, constantly recycled. Any landscape retains within it the possibility that entirely new perspectives and activities may emerge. Up to the scale of an entire culture, or down to the individual's chronotopic, personal landscape, all have within them potentials that cannot be completely specified (Bakhtin 1981, 37). That is, they are *unfinalisable*. The author remains a "captive of his [*sic*] epoch, of his own present", but can be "liberated" from captivity, and it is the scholar or critic – that is, the reader, the interpreter of the text – who "is called upon to assist in this liberation" (Bakhtin 1986, 5).

It is unfinalisability that both permits creativity, and means there is no possibility of designing a 'perfect' information system that can subsequently substitute for all necessary cognitive work in a particular situation. It could only do so if all possibilities were predefined, and could thus be coded into a series of algorithms. Such a system would become the aforementioned "single consciousness", yet could never create new possibilities or accommodate any anomalous inputs at all. No change would be possible in this perfect system.

Thus, for Bakhtin, *ethics* and *creativity* remain essentially intersubjective, only definable through constant attention to them via active cognitive work, undertaken through dialogue, and the constant scrutiny of utterances which that dialogue represents. A Bakhtinian ethics cannot rest on generic rules and principles. If there is a rule to apply to a situation, it always works, and the rule is known, then any *work* involved in that (ethical or other) decision disappears. At the other extreme, the ethical position that is total relativism – anything goes – also removes that work. The reality lies somewhere between these two positions, hence actors in social situations are always having to make *judgements* about ethics (Morson and Emerson 1990, 26) – ultimately, about information – and: "That work of judging necessarily involves a risk, a special attention to the particulars of the situation and a special involvement with unique other people at a given moment of their lives." This dialogic encounter opens any claim up to scrutiny when it encounters genres and other validity claims on which alternative perspectives rest. Thus, the act of co-constructing an ethical framework should be a mutual learning process for all concerned.

Ultimately the same is true of other creative acts. If all life were reducible to laws, and explicable by them – even if the laws are not yet known – "creation becomes mere discovery" (Morson and Emerson 1990, 38). Yet nor can creativity exist in a realm of completely random phenomena (*ibid,* 39). Creativity involves finding genuinely new and unexpected possibilities within existing structures and forms. These structures are the "congealed" products of former discourses (Bakhtin 1986, p. 165), but are unfinalised, so remain open to further transformation. Their heritage is stable, but only relatively so: nevertheless, it is this "relatively stable heritage" (Morson and Emerson 1990, 229) which permits true creativity.

***

Unfinalisability means that information and communication must be seen as *experienced and lived* phenomena, and cannot be fully understood abstractly. This epistemology, and the prosaic, polyphonic methodologies which grow from it, places Bakhtin's work in contrast to any theory of communication which is (Morson and Emerson 1990, 129) "concerned with how readers interpret texts *after* they are made". Bakhtin's epistemology instead "represents readers as shaping the utterance *as* it is being made" (*ibid*).

This calls into doubt any form of IL that is concerned only with the retrieval and consumption of texts that have been produced by others. IL must also incorporate attention to the *usage* and *production* of texts. Both usage, and subsequent production (or re-production) of text – which could include texts that are written, spoken, performed, photographed, etc. – open any text up to intersubjective checking of the values and assumptions which are encoded within it, and which underlie the landscapes with which it interacts. Usage and production are responses to the utterances of others, and how the *potentials* of a landscape are explored. The producer (or 'produser': Bruns 2009) can test their own assumptions about a genre or utterance, by opening it up to further responses, through publication. At a high level, this process of publication, review, and response could be considered a wisdom-based approach to information literacy (Bruce 1997), creating new possibilities that may ultimately transform ethical and social structures (see Morson and Emerson 1990, 288).

Yet institutionalisation empirically indicates that landscapes can not only be constructed around monologues but be *experienced* as monologues, denying the possibility that other voices or discourses could be more effective at addressing particular problems. "Extreme versions of official discourse are similar to autism in so far as they are totalitarian and do not recognize otherness; they abhor difference and aim for a single collective self " (Holquist, 2002, 52). That is, they are monologic.

As noted in the previous chapter, with regard to instrumental (monologic) and communicative (dialogic) rationality, it is not that monologism is undesirable in all situations. Both types are important. The assertion of a particular position is, at times, essential, in order to embed the results of dialogue into a landscape, the results of this process being *authority* and *information systems* of some kind. But the question is, how can these assertions – these authorities, instruments, systems – be scrutinised? How can we enter into a dialogue with them (cf. Johansson 2012)?

Authority is manifested in both the production and the consumption of utterances. An utterance will – and must – draw on forms of expression, characteristics of particular genres, that will either invite scrutiny of the claims inherent within it, or retard this scrutiny. Thus, there are two kinds of authority: the first dialogic, the second monologic.

A monologic 'authoritative' utterance would come from approved sources or be created to meet pre-ordained criteria, defined by an authority that could range from a Pope to a tenure committee. Because the subjective and intersubjective realms are intertwined, even a consumer's internal deliberations regarding a text will be subject to authority (Linell 2009, 133): "The 'authoritarian' voice is often akin to 'commonsense' or cultural assumptions that the individual does not question, and when the individual internalises the discourse, i.e. the ideas of this voice, it is often a kind of self-discipline in Foucaultian terms. These are the canonical, normally unquestioned views that become incorporated into the individual's self identity." Individuals also make secondary considerations (Wilson 1983), calculations of cost and benefit (like whether reading the book will secure a higher grade), or they may simply never question the authority that (they are told) is invested in the text.

Wilson (1983, 135–6) cites Becker (1967, 241) to show the strong links between monologic authority, information systems and hierarchy: "In any system of ranked groups, participants take it as given that members of the highest group have the right to define the way things really are... those at the top have a more complete picture of what is going on than anyone else. Members of lower groups will have incomplete information, and their views of reality will be partial, and distorted in consequence." But this is a *perception*. Wilson shows later (*ibid*, 154) that the manager, the overseer, still has a perspective that is therefore distorting the reality of what goes on at smaller scales (cf. Blaug 2007). The key organising factor here – how authority is imposed – is, therefore, not through any one individual's cognition, but the *system;* this is how the cognition of those at the top of the hierarchy comes to substitute for those of others in the organisation (Blaug 2007; 2010). While the relationship between the speaker and addressee of an utterance is an innately reciprocal one (Bakhtin 1986, 121–2), in situations where authority is asserted this reciprocity, this dialogue, may be skewed, denied, concealed, or simply ignored. Non-reciprocity is inherent to hierarchical systems of exchange (Graeber 2012), and in a non-reciprocal information exchange, one side can scrutinise the claims of the other, but not vice versa.

Yet the perceptions which support this imbalance always retain a potential to be challenged, by prosaic, everyday practice, whenever one enters into some kind of dialogue with a cognitive authority. In dialogue, the act of asserting something immediately invites critical, intersubjective attention to that assertion. A monologic assertion, conversely, "will probably be cited in a type of reported speech allowing for little opportunity to express agreement, disagreement, or other personal opinions. There may also be a tendency to 'depersonalize' and 'disembody' the authoritative figure's speech, so that it is not perceived as merely one person's opinion..." (Morson and Emerson 1990, 164; via Voloshinov 1973). Thus, when one encounters an information system, one tends to become a 'client' or an 'employee' (cf. Habermas 1987), an ID number, rather than a person, a unique identity. Nor will the system's processes be identified with the individuals who have coded it, and/or whose assumptions and values have influenced the design. As with the military command, there is little that can be done directly to respond to these kinds of system-generated utterances, except to withdraw from use of the system – which may not always be straightforward, or possible to do without incurring sanction.

Once again, however, it must be remembered that dialogue, the ideal communicatively rational form of speech, and monologue, the ideal instrumentally rational form, are complementary. Just as Klein and Truex (1996: see chapter 4 above) saw that instrumental action was needed *after* communicative actions in order to implement rational decisions, so monologic and abstracting statements about the human world may be both the product of enquiries and essential starting points for further enquiry (Gardiner 2004, 34). Problems of validity come not with monologic utterances *per se*, then, but arise when the claims inherent in these statements fall away from dialogic scrutiny, lose their provisionality, and become reified (Morson and Emerson 1990, 59).

For Bakhtin, dialogue is "centrifugal"; through dialogue, possibilities inherent in utterances are "pushed out" to individual speakers interacting within networks and communities, exploring ideas and forming knowledge polyphonically (cf. Hall 1968, 91 who used the term "sociofugal"). Yet each utterance can also be "centripetal" (Bakhtin, 1981, 272), meaning a force that pulls towards the centre. Specific genres and forms of speech can attract "words and forms into their orbit by means of their own characteristic intentions and accents, and in so doing to a certain extent alienating these words and forms from other tendencies, parties, artistic works and persons" (*ibid*, 290). As Linell (2009, 213) puts it, this contrast, between centripetal and centrifugal forces, is also a way of conceiving "the tension between, on the one hand, responding to and perhaps conforming with what the other has just said and, on the other, injecting new and perhaps divergent ideas, associations and initiatives to new communicative projects". All discourse can therefore be considered "a contradiction-ridden, tension-filled unity of two embattled tendencies in the life of language" (Bakhtin 1981, 272). Centripetal forces pull towards a unified language, devaluing idiosyncratic usages, dialects, and experimentations with form. This applies both in linguistic terms (e.g. academic papers are expected to be written in the 'high' form of any language and – increasingly – the English language), but also in terms of genre. It is hard to get any academic paper published that does not conform to, at least, the expectations of a given journal or editor, and there is no guarantee that one's institution will accept an unconventional publication when making judgements about promotion or tenure. Other professions will have their equivalents. Thus, a concept of 'literariness' is embedded into the landscape. It is how 'authoritative' people speak, it gives one credibility in a particular genre. Such discourses serve to "preserve local interests at the national level... or to defend the interests of cultural-political centralization..." (*ibid*, 382).

There is also variation within genres around how the speaker conceives of the addressee. Who are they? How should they be addressed, and what response do we expect from them (Bakhtin 1986, 96–8)? These also help define authority. One can make generalisations about particular genres here, but though this, like other abstractions, may provide useful general insights, these issues still need working out at the level of communicative practice, at the point in space and time (the chronotope) that specific utterances are made. Authority is therefore worked out at a continuum of levels, from the most abstract considerations (is the utterance phrased in ways that assert some kind of authority?) to very concrete and personal ones (does it accord with the reader's prior experience, will they face sanctions of any kind if they refuse to accept the authority of the utterance?). Factors such as emotion and personal trust also come into play.

Bakhtin still has to face the problem of relativism. Is all authority simply a matter of agreeing that something is true? Thompson (2008) would rightly call this counterknowledge. Is it morally right to refuse to accept authority of some kind, simply because one has chosen to do so, inside a specific chronotope? While justifiable in certain cases, this is by no means always true, and taken to its extreme would constitute a nihilistic rejection of any authority external to the self: the person would be a sociopath. How can these extremes be avoided within dialogism?

Bakhtin's solution is to posit that there *is* an ultimate, non-relativistic authority, but it is unreachable, so only ever approached or invoked in principle. Nevertheless, like the speed of light, which cannot be reached in reality but still governs physical reality, this authority is inherently present in all communication. The 'superaddressee' is an essential *psychological* element of effective communication, akin to an idealised listener, dispassionate, unbiased, and open to being swayed by the force of the better argument (cf. Habermas 1984). It is the ideal respondent against whom the real addressee's responses can be judged: "a constitutive aspect of the whole utterance, who, under deeper analysis, can be revealed in it. This follows from the nature of the word, which always wants to be *heard*, always seeks responsive understanding, and does not stop at *immediate* understanding but presses on further and further (indefinitely)." (Bakhtin 1986, 126–7). Thus, the superaddressee plays a role in Bakhtin's theory analogous to Habermas's ISS. Remove it, and the *possibility of progression towards ever-greater understanding* disappears (Morson and Emerson 1990, 125–6; Bakhtin 1986, 126–8). This would cast all speakers into a relativist dungeon, where one's chance of being heard depends only on random contextual events. Thus, the superaddressee is necessary to retain the possibility of validity claims. It is this notion – admittedly underdeveloped in Bakhtin's theories[2] – that makes his politics more than just reactive, a "constant struggle to maintain freedom in a world characterized by discursive cunning and infinite subtle forms of rhetorical coercion" (Garvey 2000, 385). Instead, the superaddressee gives his theory normative force, a belief that the worth of different communications can be *judged* according to criteria that are not just pragmatic, imposed through force, or habit.

But though these criteria are innately dialogic, monologue emerges when the superaddressee stops being treated as an abstract, unreachable ideal, and starts being reified as a concrete point in discourse which could be reached if only there were ways to get enough people to agree on something. At best, a speaker would be using rhetoric at this point, perhaps appealing to notions such as 'common sense', 'natural justice', or 'truth'. Further still, this is one way that dominant groups and their discourses try to position themselves as a final arbiter of validity, removing their claims to objectivity from all scrutiny, and possibly enforcing a position on others. This starts with depersonalisation of both speaker and addressee. This may be a valid move to make in discourse: many utterances can be quite validly described as generic. But the removal of the addressee from *personal* consideration also challenges the right of any given addressee to respond to the utterance, except in a similarly depersonalised way. When a speaker places their role or position at the forefront of consideration and speaks, not as themselves, but as a representative of something else, they become an *interface* to a system, expressing the cognitive authority of that system (cf. Blaug 2010). Depersonalisation has occurred. The ability to respond to the claims of the speaker is being instrumentally taken out of the exchange: thus, a monologue is emerging. The extreme is invoked in the superaddressee's "mirror image", the Fascist or Orwellian state police, the torturer, the panoptic surveillance society forcing conformity and having totally removed the individual from consideration or empathy (Bakhtin 1986, 126: Garvey 2000, 386).

In that these counterposed tendencies – monologic and dialogic forms of authority – are inherent in *all* speech, the counterplay between them (Morson and Emerson 1990, 219):

> (P)lays a role in all social groups, down to 'each small world of the family, friends, acquaintances and comrades in which a human being grows and lives' (Bakhtin 1986, 88). Authoritative discourses set the tone for action in a given sphere of life; and they are assimilated into the psyche to set the tone for a particular sphere of thought.

This is a Foucauldian view of the link between discourse and power (Foucault 1980, 93):

> (R)elations of power cannot themselves be established, consolidated nor implemented without the production, accumulation, circulation and functioning of a discourse...

Persuasive, authoritative voices, texts, or discourses nevertheless vie within us internally, and also within our landscapes. As we all struggle with this debate individually, we may see previously persuasive voices lose their authority. This, in the end, is the basis of transformation. Once an authoritative voice *has been* challenged, the potential always remains for it to be challenged again (Bakhtin 1981, 332). To defend itself, the claims of authority may be expressed in ever more monologic ways, closing off avenues of response. Yet (Morson and Emerson 1990, 355):

> Despite its pose of immobility, ennobled discourse undergoes constant change, in both literature and extraliterary life. Given the fact that the pose of immobility is just that – a pose, polemically ignoring vulgar life – such change is implicit in the very nature of the discourse. It carries the traces of whatever it is at the moment straining not to see. As new kinds of vulgarity and heteroglossia accumulate, new kinds of literariness arise to 'ignore' them.

* * *

One not only *can* enter into a dialogue with information systems (authoritative voices); one *must* do so (Morson and Emerson 1990, 222):

> (A)greement... is a truly dialogic relation, and to agree with a discourse is already to have tested it, deprived it of unconditional allegiance, and integrated it into one's own framework. One has told it in one's own words, and whether those words seem acceptable or unacceptable, they are still partially one's own. Conversely, mere hostility to authoritative discourse may leave its status as absolutely authoritative unchallenged... To take on responsibility with respect to a discourse, or to any kind of authority, it is necessary not to dislike it, but to enter into dialogue with it – that is, to *test*, *assimilate* and *reaccentuate* it.

This is the ideal of strong objectivity (Harding 1993, cf. chapter 1 above). Dialogue assesses the validity of a discourse while simultaneously allowing for the possibility of its falsification. Asserting the value of knowledge produced in context can therefore have a *positive* effect on the content of science (Harding 1993, 51) where the validity claims of the investigation were previously concealed. This ultimately produces "stronger standards for 'good method', ones that can guide competent efforts to maximise objectivity" (*ibid*, 52). In other words, it turns the authority from monologic to dialogic, strengthening it as a result.

Invoking these issues, of the validation of science, it is important here to revisit and restate the difference between human and natural science. The latter deals with non-human 'voiceless things', and monologic forms of knowledge are appropriate in this realm: knowledge developed through positivistic methods and systematic, rigorous, scientific enquiry. To assert otherwise would invoke the ire of writers such as Thompson (2008), who would attack those who, either through ignorance or in the name of such intellectual arguments as postmodernism, claimed that certain fundamental constants are in fact relativistic, or even depend on context. Such a view would recall the hoax wherein a physics Professor, Alain Sokal, fabricated a nonsense paper called "The Positive Hermeneutics of Quantum Gravity" and had it accepted by a journal, *Social Text* (Thompson 2008, 121–2). Yet the natural sciences are still dialogic at the level of *analysis* – and can and should have their claims to objectivity opened up to critical, and dialogic, scrutiny. Calling for a greater involvement in critical attention to the claims of science is no different from calling for greater public engagement with science, awareness of methods, and a willingness to engage in valid and reliable research *as a practice*, and this would be a political, liberatory process (cf Levine 2007).

It must also be stressed once more that the study of the non-human realm is fundamentally different from that of the human realm. Wilson (1983, 88*ff*) recognises this, going so far as to say that social science has nowhere near the same level of cognitive authority as natural science – partly because of the fundamentally ill-structured and unpredictable nature of the former, and partly because (1983, 89) "the business of the social sciences is everybody's business and not left by default to academic social scientists to investigate". In other words, it deals in large part with everyday, prosaic situations with which we are all at least intuitively familiar – not with natural processes that require specialised instrumentation to detect and analyse. Bakhtin was quite clear that the non-human realm requires a different epistemology from the human realm. The latter is transmitted by language, which introduces uncertainty and unfinalisability into the ontology, and requires an epistemology that is not positivist and empiricist (an approach which is quite appropriate in the natural sciences).

All in all, then, one can call into question the presentation and validity claims of particular utterances in the scientific realm without any need to claim that scientific constants are somehow relative: a nonsense perspective and one that would shatter any argument based on it. Gravity is a constant – it exists – it is not some rule written into a governing algorithm that we can eventually, with enough cognitive work, reveal, scrutinize, and transform, allowing us to fly through the air by will alone[3]. But the *utterance* 'Gravity is a constant' is one that is set into a context and which, by being stated, opens its validity claims up to scrutiny. If this were not the case then Sokal could not have written his hoax paper and *Social Text*, whatever its peer review practices, could never have accepted it. Indeed, by calling into question the specific *uses of language* in this case, and making a political point about peer reviewing practices in this journal, and postmodernity more generally, Sokal's paper was not nonsense at all. It was a very effective utterance, one made specifically in the *human* realm of knowledge-formation.

Thus, the non-human realm exists but has a different epistemology from the human, and scientific discourse remains in the latter (Bakhtin 1981, 351):

> In scientific activity one must, of course, deal with another's discourse – the words of predecessors, the judgments of critics, majority opinion and so forth... but all this remains a mere operational necessity and does not affect the subject matter itself of the science, into whose composition the speaker and his discourse do not, of course, enter. The entire methodological apparatus of the mathematical and natural sciences is directed toward mastery over *mute objects, brute things*, that do not reveal themselves in words, that do not *comment on themselves....* In the humanities... there arises the specific task of establishing, transmitting and interpreting the words of others...

The promotion of positivist methods in the humanities is not just inappropriate, therefore, it is actively exclusionary (cf. Harding 2003), as it seeks to create abstract forms of knowledge. At its extreme, this kind of abstract understanding "is completely separated from the living, ideological power of the word to mean – from its truth or falsity, its significance or insignificance, beauty or ugliness. Such a reified word-thing cannot be understood by attempts to penetrate its meaning dialogically: there can be no conversing with such a word." *(ibid, 352)*. However, as Bakhtin noted in *Towards a Methodology in the Human Sciences*, a study in the humanities must always deal with two or more subjects, each with their own voice and thus capable of dialogue. To treat these subjects as 'voiceless things' is a choice, which on occasion can be beneficial for certain tasks, but this choice should be made in the full knowledge that this does not (and can never) lead to full *creative understanding* and will always provide a limited view of the world (Morson and Emerson 1990, 98). More specific versions of this critique have been made in various fields, including Burrell (1997), who critiques the use of positivist and abstracting methods in organisational studies and Carr and Kemmis (1986) in education: chapter 4 above has already done much the same for IL.

Yet the fact that such work in the humanities continues nonetheless is a sign of two things: first, that there needs to be some level of monologism and temporary finalisation if any dialogue is to contribute to knowledge-formation – and second, a long-standing institutionalisation of the ensuing practices. Institutionalisation is centripetal, pulling things into a monologic interpretation of a field and constructing utterances in ways that limit possibilities for response, and Wilson (1983, 51) notes how various professions (not just academia) assert cognitive authority: "Professions generally aim to get and keep a monopoly on the right to criticize their own work by claiming that outsiders are incompetent to judge the merits and defects of their work". Institutionalisation of this sort does not occur because a particular view – originating from a specific moment in space and time, or a specific chronotope – is somehow 'more valid' than others. Bakthin's epistemology shows that such a view is impossible in a humanistic field of study: validity comes about through scrutiny. Thus, there is a need to study the fact of institutionalisation and how this in itself is representative of a particular landscape. As Douglas (1986) noted, the authority of monologic views needs to be asserted through some kind of structure through which the force can be channeled; some kind of control over the formation of knowledge, that exists in lived situations, not the abstract forms of langauge itself.

Technology and procedure – designed according to the dictates of instrumental rationality rather than communicative – play a significant role here. Technology becomes a conduit for centripetal force – the centralisation of knowledge-forming capacity – when the assumptions that have gone into its programming are concealed. A good example of this comes from Van Dijck (2010), who suggests that search engines like Google Scholar should be seen as being co-producers of knowledge. In Bakhtin's terms, the tool is shaping the utterance. However, its validity claims, indeed its very role in this process, are concealed, largely for reasons of commercial confidentiality. For example, at the time van Dijck wrote, Google Scholar had no connection to Elsevier's database, itself a significant shaper of academic text (van Dijck 2010, 577). Yet this challenge to its authority is not a clear part of the Google Scholar interfaces (input or output), hence it goes unscrutinised by those who use this tool to judge credibility and therefore validity of any texts that it helps find (in essence, Google Scholar is acting as a *locator*, level 2 of Kuhlthau's (1993) categories of mediation, introduced in chapter 3 above). All in all (*ibid*, 580): "In a network society, search engines like Google Scholar constitute a nodal point of power, while the mechanism of knowledge production is effectively hidden in the coded mechanisms of the engine, as well as in the unarticulated conventions of scholarly use, such as quality assessment and source presentation."

Intellectual property regimes are another example of how access to information can be defined in ways that are opposed to the polyphonic, evolving nature of text (Luyt and Azura 2010). Instead, in an instrumental way, they assert the rights, not even of the author necessarily, but the (corporate) publisher. "Commons-based" landscapes thus become enclosed and privatised (cf. Hess and Ostrom 2007). Luyt and Azura implicate institutionalised IL in this process: "In today's digital version of the enclosure movement, information literacy is implicated. Many of the information literacy standards explicitly acknowledge without criticism the tightening copyright regime" (Luyt and Azura 2010, no pagination).

This kind of authority can be asserted in more intersubjective ways, which nevertheless remain exclusionary. Mark (2011a, 5) investigates peer review, and generally notes the exclusivity of academic discourses: "In the culture of the academy, faculty are the experts and the process of naming is the purview of faculty. Faculty have a stake culturally, politically, and economically in expertise and hence a stake in naming and controlling dialogue." The authoritative voice here is systemic, not invested in an individual – but it remains exclusionary and unifying. The whole process of formal academic study can be considered as a way of acquiring the genre repertoire and, hence, legitimacy in this landscape (Mark 2011a, 6): "The purpose of papers and research assignments often is to train students out of the colloquial voice, to have students adopt the language and conventions of academia." She also asks (2011b, 25): "What if educators constructed a theory of information literacy where students' opinions about information were as valid as professors'?" Chapters 7 and 8 address this task in part, but note straight away that this question poses an explicit challenge to the notion of the authoritative voice, and an admission that within HE students and faculty – and the library – occupy different contexts. Mark also says that (2011b, 25): "Freire wrote that the teacher confuses the authority of knowledge with his or her own professional authority, which she or he sets in opposition to the freedom of the students". The point is about how the student should ascertain *for themselves* the authority of the knowledge, and not simply accept it because the professor (or librarian) has said it is authoritative.

Historically, this has always been the professed aim of higher education, particularly in its later stages: indeed, PhDs oblige such challenge to occur, with a requirement that the thesis is a report on original research. This kind of work is based around practices that fuel the creation of new knowledge *within the discipline*: all good science, though (cf. Goldacre 2008), is presented using genre conventions that hold its claims up to intersubjective scrutiny through certain conduits, principally the conference and journal, but with increasing contributions from new media. Nevertheless, the university and academia as institutions also serve to exclude large proportions of the population from contributing to dialogues which originate within them, even when matters affect them directly or indirectly – as do all institutions. This has important consequences for how libraries and universities can contribute to radical IL, but that is a subject which should be left for another chapter.

Bakhtin has offered much to the study of IL, and to radical forms of it. His work shows how authority can be embedded in landscapes in different ways, and how this is a *communicative act*. Yet it is precisely because it is communicative, and hence informational and dialogic, that it can be challenged, for no ultimate and final *cognitive* authority can possibly exist, even if it can be invoked via the 'superaddressee'. Extant structures of information processing, being the congealed products of former discourses, shape utterances in various ways, but they cannot, for all time, determine the content of these utterances, nor dictate how people will respond to them. Thus, while there is clearly structure, there is also agency in a Bakhtinian world. Dialogue is that form of knowledge-formation which opens validity claims up to scrutiny. It is an *innate* challenge to the authority of more monologic forms and it is only through such challenge that the validity of monologic statements can be truly determined.

Thus, while Bakhtin does not share Habermas's views on the desirability of consensus, and would problematise the distinctions Habermas draws between spheres of human action, he nevertheless supports the position that *communicative competence* of some kind is essential if *transformation of cognitive authority* is to have a chance of occurring through dialogue. It is this competence which constitutes information literacy in a broad sense (Whitworth 2007), and this is a competence which can only be exhibited in prosaic, everyday communicative practice, a lived experience. Bakhtin's work shows definitively that information and communication, and the sociolinguistic structures which have evolved over time to shape them, are fundamental to human activity: hence, so is IL. IL is educational – or at least, learning-based – in large part, and libraries and universities are among the professional groups in society well placed to help nurture IL in certain populations. But to declare that IL is *solely* educational, *solely* oriented to texts that can be found in a library, higher education institution, or search engine, *solely* rooted in one or other frame; these are all examples of monologic thinking. They neglect the empirical diversity and polyphony of human responses to information, the role of uncertainty and unreason, and the role authority plays in each particular context. The remaining chapters of this book will explore the consequences of this statement.

Notes

1. Ethnomethodological and other studies may focus on prosaic communication (Linell 2009 has several examples) but even here, the study is typically driven from within specialised context of the academy, and not by the prosaic concerns of the research participants.
2. The superaddressee concept does not emerge into Bakhtin's writing until just before his death.
3. Compare this with the ontology expressed in the fictional, computer-generated world of *The Matrix* (1999, dir. the Wachowski brothers), where all this is the case, and gravity can be ignored by those who have achieved a high enough level of awareness of the rules by which that world functions.

Practising IL

Abstract: This chapter examines practice-based views of IL in more detail and links them with the phenomenographical view, via the idea of mapping the information landscape. Producing such maps is the outcome of a learning process, often engaged in unconsciously. Practice and transformation — thus, the experience of information literacy — can be controlled when these learning processes are not sufficiently relational to allow all experiences of variation to appear in a map (outcome space).

Key Words: Information practice, socialisation, reflective practice, mapping.

By this point it is assumed that the need for a practice-based approach has been justified. Limberg et al (2012) stated that sociocultural practice theory was one of the three key theories of IL, along with phenomenography and discourse analysis. But though Limberg et al discuss each theoretical field's implications for IL, their paper is not a synthesis of phenomenography, practice, and prosaics, in the way that this book is. That synthesis can now be completed, by returning to some ideas which have emerged from the IL-as-practice school and using them to explore that school's methodological connections with IL-as-learning. By doing so it can be shown how both views of IL can support radical IL, or IL as *transformation*. These connections arise through the notion that the information landscape is a space that can be mapped, that producing such maps is the outcome of a learning process, but also that practice and transformation can be controlled when these learning processes are not sufficiently relational to allow all experiences of variation to appear in a map (outcome space).

The previous three chapters, 4–6, have explored institutionalisation, colonisation, and authority, and justified the conclusion reached at the end of chapter 3, that the phenomenographical enquiry must be a *critical* one if it is to reveal (map) not just the variation within a landscape, but the unequal distribution of both cognitive authority itself and the resources needed to scrutinise that authority. Hence, a critical view of the learning-practice link will demonstrate why not all experiences of variation will be equally supported by the structures of authority and information exchange within a landscape. Unequal distributions of cognitive authority are a result of the need to periodically embed the results of discourse in information systems and texts. However, unequal distributions of the resources needed to scrutinise and, if necessary, challenge and transform authority are manifestations of hegemony. *Pace* Hamelink, Gramsci and Freire, then, radical IL seeks to address this latter problem of distribution, and it does so not through setting standards, focusing on technology or proposing alterations to any existing information system, but rather by influencing practice. In short, radical IL seeks directly to close the theory-practice gap.

* * *

Hultgren (2009, 45) defines *information practice* as a concept which: "can be used to identify and define sets of information related activities and procedures that are created collectively. They can be described as socially sanctioned and structured tools which social groups use to monitor their worlds". Practices include those for "scanning, actively seeking, and avoiding information, and for being identified as an information seeker. Such activities are socially and culturally embedded, they are learned through interactions with others and they are used not only to generate information relevant to the actor's situation but also as a means of orienting in the world, gaining control over one's life and to demonstrate one's position in the world" (*ibid*, 54).

Lloyd notes that (2010b, 249, via Schatzki 2006):

> Practices are constituted as open-ended, spatio-temporal manifolds of actions that are organised in three ways. First, an understanding of how to do things (practical understanding), e.g. explaining, questioning, and describing. Second, rules i.e. the formulations that prescribe, require or instruct. Third, teleoaffective features which structure emotions that are acceptable or prescribed for participants in practice.

Like cognition, practice is distributed across mind, body and world, having an "affective and embodied" dimension as well as a cognitive one (*ibid*). Analysis of practice cannot therefore just reduce the practice to the action of an individual, but must focus on "how the practice is constructed corporeally and socially and how these features are interwoven and mesh together within a social site" (*ibid*). Texts of various kinds do play a significant role in constructing practice, but practice-based investigations of IL highlight the blinkers which IL tends to wear, particularly as taught through the content and competency frames: namely, seeing IL as applicable only to certain types of texts, those which can be found through a library or a search engine. Even forms of IL which look beyond just written texts, and include video and imagery, retain an implied emphasis on what has been (or could be) subject to *publication*. What IL-as-practice impels is an acknowledgement that IL is relevant to *any* text, including sociotechnical information systems as a whole and also social relations. Practice is therefore an innately intersubjective concept (*ibid*, 250):

> All practices are social therefore they are not constituted as individual self-sufficient activity, but are located within and through group activities – formed, interwoven and sanctioned through a dialogic intra-group process. This suggests that there is an intersubjective dimension to the concept, its dimensions and arrangement, which facilitates the development of shared understanding and shared skills (Schatzki, 2001). In writing about practice as the property of groups, Kemmis (2006) suggests that they are 'shaped through histories and traditions that locate practices in such a way that they are "inherited" already formed, by contemporary practitioners, who in their turn, become the custodians and developers of practices' (p. 2.) Therefore practices are understood, organised and conducted through the discourses that characterise and shape a setting...

Drawing on all these observations, Lloyd comes to see information literacy as certainly more than an outcome of a learning process, and also more than just a tool to achieve certain ends. Instead, information literacy is fundamental: it is *the source of practice*. In general (Lloyd 2012, 773): "[i]nformation landscapes reflect the modalities of information (agreed upon sources) that people draw upon in the performance of their practices in working or everyday life, and therefore constitute the intersubjective agreement that informs our situated realities..." Therefore, focusing on how IL emerges in a setting is a way of investigating the information exchanges, genres, and artifacts that (*ibid*, 772): "reveal the nature of a setting, particularly in relation to what information and knowledge are sanctioned and legitimized". IL therefore does not exist *independently* of the landscape (*ibid*, 774):

> (P)articipating collectively in a social setting bring[s] practices such as information literacy into being, and shape[s] it in ways that are collectively agreed upon through negotiation, and in ways that reflect the practice traditions of the setting. In effect, people engage with a discourse that governs agreements about what is accepted as information and knowledge, and also what activities are acceptable in the performance of becoming information literate (Lloyd, 2006; Sundin, 2008).

These are significant conclusions, as they explain why IL cannot be a generic practice, *even when it draws on standards*. IL is an understanding of what "modalities of information... are considered credible and authoritative", but this enquiry varies, in both methods and results, from landscape to landscape (*ibid*, 777). The outcomes of such enquiries govern practice, because they establish conventions of information exchange, or "practice architectures" (*ibid*, 775, via Kemmis and Grootenboer 2008):

> (P)ractice architectures provide the enabling or constraining preconditions for practice by orchestrating the activities of individuals who are co-located and co-participating in a particular setting thus enabling individuals to become drawn into its collective practices...

Thus, there is a strongly social and intersubjective aspect in how we become drawn into collective practices, and thus enter a practice community (*ibid*):

> When we are stirred into a practice (by mediators such as teachers, other workers, or people in our communities, or by the material objects that inhabit our contexts), we are drawn into the information landscapes that compose a setting. We are also introduced to the ways of knowing that connect us to the arrangements that enable us to become aligned to socio-cultural, material-economic and historical traditions of the setting. We learn how to take on professional or occupational identity and learn to identify and affiliate with

others in the same field, through the practices and performance of our occupation; we learn to become members of a community in the same way.

This process of socialisation is, again, not solely cognitive, but distributed across mind, body, and world (technologies, information systems, social relations, and ways of using words). In the first place, from the very earliest stages of becoming a practitioner, "it is through language that the object and its background are differentiated for the novice" (Gherardi, Nicolini and Odella 1998, 282). However, non-linguistic communicative elements: that is, embodied acts such as pointing, doing things in a certain order, movement through a physical space, or operation of a technological interface, also play a part. The structures which socialise novice practitioners are also constrained by information systems designed around assumptions and values that may or may not be explicit. "Accordingly, one of the most important skills that a novice must learn is 'how to see'" (*ibid,* 282); that is, reveal and learn the practices that comprise the landscape. At first, novices tend to apply context-independent rules, or practices from other landscapes and communities they are familiar with. As competence increases, and they become more embedded in the landscape, they may seek guidance from formalised educational resources, e.g. textbooks, web pages: here the content and competency frames of IL can certainly play a part in their becoming proficient. But one also learns to recognise non-textual elements of practice, and "situational elements which depend on the context" (*ibid,* 276). Through processes like these, novices *learn* to become more practiced within a given landscape – they become more literate in its genres and acquire an authority that may also be recognised in similar settings (such as a different organisation in the same sector). This cannot be done simply by reading about practice, but engaging in it, becoming part of a community of practice (Wenger 1998, Wenger et al 2009), and acquiring ways and habits of engaging with that community's information landscape that remain unique to the individual, but which are also intersubjectively conditioned by the community.

So far, this section has provided a general definition of practice and described *ideal* ways in which actors in a social setting learn to become practitioners – that is, comfortable with the genres and systems that exist within their landscape, and invested with a certain amount of cognitive authority therein and, consequently, able to change their practice and that of others. However, this ideal is not always reachable in practice. Practice may be developed in ways that retain for an individual the awareness and opportunity to keep his/her practice under review, leaving the assumptions beneath practice open to scrutiny, but communities of practice can be closed and parochial, even dysfunctional. They may also be disempowered, deliberately or not, by practice architectures that reflect more dominant interests in the community, such as those further up an organisational hierarchy. Different landscapes and practice architectures will be differently configured, depending on the intersubjective understanding of questions like: what information is appropriate to share or not share within a context? What information is shared in a communistic way and what hierarchical? What genres marshal and guide these exchanges? What forms of knowledge and practice are considered valid? Whose inquiries construct practice, and embed it into information systems? What support can be drawn from the landscape generally: is it set up in ways that privilege certain viewpoints, or is it a landscape that allows a multitude of voices (Bakhtin's "polyphony") to establish their own authority over information? If the latter, is this a cacophonous and formless diversity, what Keen (2007) would see as "the cult of the amateur"? Or are there structures which offer conduits for these intersubjective agreements to become instrumental action: that is, ways to channel dialogue into the transformation of practice? And once such transformation has occurred, can it be kept under review, and made the subject of further enquiries, or have more monologic forms of cognitive authority come into play, producing an information system that is closed to subsequent scrutiny? Do actors have access to all available cognitive tools and the full experience of variation within the landscape, or are aspects of it closed off behind non-reciprocal forms of information exchange, possibly the abstract construct of "confidentiality"[1]?

These various questions can potentially be answered by philosophical speculation, or by scientific, abstracting research, conducted from a position external to the community. But the results of such inquiries cannot change a landscape until they are *put into practice*. Carr and Kemmis (1986, *passim*) see this as the fundamental characteristic of professional activity in education. They mean not that practice should be performed automatically, being merely a response to stimuli developed externally, such as standard operating procedures, guides to 'best practice', standards, and so on. These *resources* can assist a practitioner, for certain, but it is incumbent on the good practitioner to always *reflect* on their applicability in a particular chronotope: that is, *make a judgement as to their relevance in a particular setting*. In that this is the core driver of IL, it can be seen how being information literate is essential to becoming a practitioner.

Reflective practice is called for by many other authors in the Education field (e.g. Schön 1983; Brookfield 1995; Reason and Bradbury 2001; Loughran 2002; for IL educators see Whitworth 2012). All see it as a way of raising awareness of how knowledge formation can become constrained by the constructs and categories of description that have shaped an individual's upbringing and training. The existence of such 'constraints' is not a negative: we must limit our informational intake somehow, in order to save cognitive work. And, to some extent, information seeking itself is an activity "focused on discovering, or becoming aware of, the context in which the individual is embedded and how the system of categories that describes it works" (Hultgren 2009, 76). But reflective practice is more active and critical: it involves the scrutiny of the act, and the assumptions which underlie the act – double-loop learning, in other words (Argyris and Schön 1999). Reflective practice is how practitioners can enhance their awareness of their professional status and validity claims regarding their activity, and promote these at the expense of generic claims and the consequent engineering of their landscapes by 'experts' (in academic research establishments, in governments, wherever).

Reflective practice does not 'just happen', however: as with other aspects of radical IL, there needs to be a supportive infrastructure, and also some level of individual motivation (Hultgren 2009, 85):

> Reflection on the motives for, and meaning of our activities occurs only if the actor sees pragmatic reasons for doing so; otherwise our activities tend to be a 'matter of course' and a part of the 'natural attitude' – things we do without paying much attention to the actual 'doing' and of which information seeking is a case in point. Reflection is a choice one makes, a kind of stepping aside for a moment in order to articulate knowledge of the social context of our activities, even if it is only to oneself.

Nevertheless, this kind of constant evaluation of practice – reviewing the assumptions underlying acts, as well as one's progress towards the act – is what constitutes double-loop learning: thus, the scrutiny of validity claims and cognitive authorities within a landscape that must periodically take place. The theory of radical IL therefore suggests that reflective practice is not just something which should be adopted by professional educators, but which is *fundamental to learning throughout society,* including informal learning. Through such cognitive work, all validity claims are scrutinised and their applicability in particular contexts is tested in practice. That is, the community would be continually validating its practices through double-loop learning.

It is this kind of *governance* – now expressed not in a monarchic, or oligarchical, but a *collective* authority – that is the essence of a democracy considered as a practical, lived experience. It is also, if linked to valid methodologies for researching the world, how one avoids counterknowledge and secures "strong objectivity" (Harding 1993).

A few paragraphs ago, a range of questions were posed, the various answers to which would reveal some of the diversity within real information landscapes. Not all practice architectures will be constructed in ways that are as conducive to transformation as others. In these characteristics of landscapes reside the power relations which can put a brake on transformation and the redistribution of cognitive authority within a landscape. The IL-as-practice approach fully acknowledges that communication, and hence information, has an embodied aspect: "... embodied persons are not simply constructs, but are *productive bodies* capable of activities that change the nature of their lives... their natural habitats and... their social scenarios" (Burkitt 1999, 2). Systems of information processing acknowledge this, as within them, relations of power "constitute attempts to restrain and curtail bodily powers through regulations around the formation and exercise of capacities and agency" (Burkitt 1999, 3). In other words, restrictions are often placed on the ability of social actors not just to state that practice should be transformed, but to then transform it. These restrictions can be direct, with undesirable practices subject to sanction; they may also be indirect, with practitioners denied the financial, intellectual, or linguistic resources they need to either develop practice, or to properly scrutinise and evaluate it.

At times there are valid reasons to restrict practice and the ability to transform it. This is recognised most clearly in the conventions of democratic practice, such as checks placed on the ability of a monarch or oligarch to wield the political system as an instrument in their own interest. The ability to transform a practice may be limited because of valid and – importantly – open and scrutinised agreements from members of the landscape. This may be for entirely pragmatic reasons, such as to avoid open conflict or danger (seeking to transform the practice that one should not operate heavy machinery while drunk will likely be rejected or sanctioned, for obvious reasons), but it may also be because of shared values that can be regularly reviewed. However, cognitive authority also comes into play. Socialisation is not a passive thing, a mere acquisition: the newcomer is not a 'social dope', but straight away an actor, a product and producer of the landscape (Gherardi et al 1998, 283). Yet novices also tend to have limited *authority* within the landscape, and again this can be linguistic and communicative, rather than formally bounded by organisational constraints such as rules and sanctions. Gherardi et al observed authoritarian styles of language in use by more established practitioners, "where no effort was made to help the novices learn from what they did" (*ibid* 289): thus, not orienting their practice toward any kind of distribution of their authority. In part this was also because expert practitioners did not necessarily include the genre of *teaching* in their repertoire (*ibid*, 292–3): some experts are brilliant teachers, others less so, as every former student knows. But senior members of groups also exhibited "jealous custodianship of their expertise" and the influence that comes with it (*ibid*, 290). Wilson (1983, 63) noted that: "An innovation made by one with no particular authority will not become fashionable unless taken up by those who do have authority, who legitimize the innovation, making acceptable for others to try and exerting an influence that may lead others to try." Thus, one's position in a social network, as well as within an organisational hierarchy, and the cognitive authority or capital which one has acquired within a landscape, will be factors in how easily one can shape one's own practice, and that of others.

* * *

Studies that use a practice perspective have highlighted issues with information processing in organisations that other views of IL may have missed. This perspective shows how macro-level organisational factors and micro-level practices combine to form information landscapes. For example, Urquhart & Rowley (2007) examined student information behaviour and concluded that it was affected by macro factors such as the ICT infrastructure, policies, funding, and organisational leadership, which comprised the practice architecture in this case. Huvila (2010) described how in corporate finance firms in Finland, decisions about information were made not primarily on the basis of relevance, but on how individuals thought the information would affect their chances of success at work. This in turn was defined differently by different people, some in terms of the organisation's profits (short-term, longer-term), others with reference to salary, promotion, prestige, or work-life balance. Huvila points out that understanding these effects makes it possible, within a particular context, to predict what sort of sources will be preferred, and thus design appropriate assistive strategies. In this regard his objectives are similar to the "Aggregate-then-Curate" project of Whitworth, Garnett and Pearson (2012): see chapter 8.

Workplace studies show how IL can be relevant to organisational operations and practices that are not always present in formal education. Chou, Chen and Pu (2005; 2008) conducted a study of Taiwanese civil servants' propensity to engage in collective action, measured with reference to their level of IL. The context for this study was the introduction of e-government in Taiwan, and the authors postulated that low levels of IL were retarding the move in this direction. They concluded individuals with higher levels of IL were more likely to seek to transform practices in response to the move.

Zhang, Majid and Foo (2010) examined IL vis-à-vis "environmental scanning": that is, an organisation seeking information about its wider environment as a way of perceiving and responding to risk (see also Nara 2007). This is an interesting idea as, while it is conceptually indistinguishable from developing a general awareness of the environment, which we all do at a subconscious level – Bates (2002, 128, cited in Tavares et al 2011, 127) claims that 80% of information is absorbed this way, and Blaug (2007) notes that this always forms the first stage in cognition – it describes the need to foreground this process of scanning, periodically bringing it into conscious awareness. But Zhang et al (2010, 722) specifically say that their review ends at the point at which the scanning process results in information, with everything after that – *viz*, decision-taking – being a "strategic management issue". This limits the criticality of their idea, as it is describing only single-loop learning. Against what criteria is the scanning taking place? Are these open to scrutiny and review? They say (*ibid*, 726) that wider informational distribution improves decision-making and helps produce consensus – but that also, in practice, many organisations restrict access to information for reasons of confidentiality, which as noted above is an essentially abstract, depersonalising feature of a practice architecture. No attention is paid to the impact of this on actual practices, nor to how such an assertion could be challenged, *as part of the same environmental scanning process* – that is, the process of learning about and mapping the information landscape (see below).

More generally, Tuominen et al see studies of practice as an essential foundation for the effective teaching of IL (2005, 341). The approach (*ibid*, 342): "calls for empirical research efforts to analyze how specific communities use various conceptual, cultural, and technical tools to access printed and digital documents and to evaluate and create knowledge." This is absolutely correct. But radical IL demands attention to the question of what *kind* of research can not only illuminate practice, but subsequently offer practical guidance to participants wanting to transform practice. Clearly, one can learn to do things better; the "cult of the amateur" (Keen 2007), in this case interpreted as poor quality information processing, is by no means an inevitability. One can be taught better practice, and one can be open to learning it. This does not just apply in a workplace: indeed, to assume that it does is another way of imposing and institutionalising a limited perspective. One can, for example, learn how to do things like political campaigning better: research into social movements reveals that once certain individuals have engaged in activism the first time, they become more *practiced* at it, and more inclined to engage in this kind of practice at a later date (Wall 1999, 96).

Limberg et al (2012, 107) write that:

> Within a sociocultural perspective people's activities should be studied in relation to the tools through which the activities take place and based in the social practices where the activities are carried out. Hence, a sociocultural perspective often favours ethnographically oriented research, in which rich qualitative descriptions of people's activities in their 'natural' settings form the basis of analysis.

Such study would also need to be *critical*. Fay (1975) criticises interpretive paradigms of social research for neglecting issues of power, focusing only on subjective issues and ignoring the role of linguistic, cognitive, and technological artifacts in shaping the views of participants in interpretive research. For transformation to take place, it is important not just to know what people think, but to know why they think it. This is what offers studies a critical dimension (Fay 1975): it also requires some kind of dialogue, as Bakhtin identified. This does not prevent some kind of formal study, external to the landscape, taking place – as noted earlier, such alterity is essential for dialogue to occur. 'Scientific' studies of a particular landscape can take place, as can training or professional development schemes. Yet, whenever an analysis is undertaken from outside any landscape, to be relevant within the landscape the results of the analysis must be interpreted with relevance to situated understandings of practice. Through both this investigation and application, and their own learning, conducted within the community, people learn about information needs and how best to respond to them. This response may involve retrieving information to help meet goals that have already been set (single-loop learning), but it may also involve reflecting on practice and reviewing goals in light of the information found (double-loop learning).

* * *

Chapter 8, below, explores practical strategies which exist for developing reflective practice and double-loop learning within individuals and communities, ideally enabling them to undertake these kinds of evaluations from within their own landscape. Before moving on to that discussion, however, it is necessary to complete the theoretical synthesis of IL-as-practice with IL-as-learning. The first step in this is to recognise the implications of extending IL beyond just the evaluation of texts, and into an understanding of all potential information sources within a landscape, particularly including other people.

If knowledge is seen as developing through an interaction of practice and information, then any other person becomes a potential information source. The idea that only those in particular *roles* have cognitive authority in a context is characteristic of bureaucratic information systems (Weber 1947), and Wilson (1983) shows how, empirically, we assign cognitive authority in many more varied ways than just by role. Badke (2010; 2012) criticises the institutionalised approaches to IL within HE that have been focused principally on published texts and the idea that IL teaching is role-based, taking place formally, usually in a library. Yet they have not been successful at improving student research skills, a valuable characteristic of "graduateness" and useful outside the academy in organisations and communities (cf. Levine 2007, Whitworth 2009 ch. 13). He notes that these institutionalised views of IL do not encourage students to appreciate how their own status as practitioners in this area can help novitiate colleagues. This potential, but underused, arena for the sharing of practice could compensate for cognitive differences and tensions between how students perceive their information needs, and how faculty do (Badke 2010, 134):

> Leckie (1996) discussed an 'expert researcher' model inhabited by faculty members. Professional academics work within narrow fields where they have a strong understanding of their literature. For many of them, keeping up with a few journals and staying in contact with colleagues is more useful than doing the kinds of research performed by their students, who know little about the field they are studying and, thus, must cast a wider net to find relevant material for research projects. Leckie concluded, 'The expert researcher simply cannot imagine (or refuses to think about) the continuum of problems that undergraduates have in using even a moderately-sized academic library' (p. 206).

Such circumstances are ripe for the formation of communities of practice between the learners, which operate 'under the radar' of their teachers and institutions (Wenger 1998). In these communities, information is exchanged regarding shared learning needs and how these can be fulfilled. The key concept to note here is not the question of whether or not students *should* teach other students the practices they need to adopt in order to be seen as information literate within this particular landscape. Badke suggests that they *are* doing it regardless: indeed, that this is a natural part of what it means to become socialised into academic practice. Learners generate their own context, drawing on a range of informational resources to do so, including but not limited to technology (Luckin 2010; Luckin et al 2010). It is precisely because communities like these share practices that are *not* those sanctioned by the 'host' institution (in this case, the university, its teachers, and librarians), that they tend to be 'under the radar': the evaluation strategies and rubrics which help the institution fulfil its informational needs, being systematised and usually not open to scrutiny by the students, are harder to apply to these practices. Hence, they tend to go unseen.

Generally, what is happening in this example – and similar processes can be viewed in other types of organisation (see the example of the insurance claim processors with which Wenger opens his book (1998)) – is that, first, initiates into this practice are making judgements about the various resources available in this landscape, and concluding that other students are more relevant and contextually-useful information sources in this case than the IL training being offered by the library. But because the *categories of description* developed in the university-as-institution do not encompass this particular practice, or experience of variation – in this case, how students can and do learn IL skills from each other – the activity is hard to see. The *outcome spaces* around which the university has built its information systems do not accommodate it, just as the outcome spaces of the insurance company in Wenger's example did not accommodate the practices which claims processors actually engaged in on the shop floor, including the exploiting of social networks in order to learn how to do the job more easily, networks through which they would learn shortcuts to 'official' procedure.

What is being described here, then, are examples of where the outcome space, the map of an information landscape, has omitted key elements of the practices which actually occur in this landscape. Thus, they are not seen by those who drew the original maps, even when these practices are clearly relevant and significant to the members of the community of practice.

Some may consider this argument as stretching the definition of phenomenographic enquiry and outcome spaces too far, even if it is remembered that what is being discussed here is a typical, but hypothetical, situation. It may be that the university has reviewed its IL provision via a process of phenomenographic enquiry, but more likely is that other, more positivistic, methods and quantitative data were used (e.g. library use, student grades, occurrence of plagiarism in submitted work, etc.). The product of these enquiries will be texts such as reports, academic papers, and elements of information systems such as rubrics, self-assessment questionnaires, tutorials, and the like. Yet even if these texts would not normally be considered an outcome *space*, they remain *outcomes of enquiry*. Epistemologically, they are a map of the information landscape, but one which reflects only the limited experience of variation that has emerged from the institution.

To see outcome spaces in this way requires the idea to be extended from meaning only some kind of written or drawn text. Maps are not simply pieces of paper: they are cognitive depictions of reality (Wandersee 1990). One can have a personal, inner 'mental map' of something – both Kelly's and Bakhtin's theories make this clear – and a map can also be encoded in collective memory, which is why we can usually direct a stranger to some location in the vicinity without consulting a paper map. Landmarks within a landscape may also exist, or signposts can be built, which either make a map less necessary or complement one. The erecting of a signpost is a way of making knowledge of a map more explicit. Due either to innate or to built-in characteristics, some landscapes are easier to map (and/or navigate) than others. Either way, understanding any map depends on familiarity with certain conventions of a genre. What goes on to a map, and what is left off it, are *choices* that are made partly depending on the audience for the map, but also on the message that the mapmaker – or whomever is driving the creation of the map – wants to promote. Certain features of the landscape will be centralised within the structure of awareness depicted on the map, others marginalised or omitted altogether. This can take place for many reasons, often quite subtle ones. For example, the present author has been to all the continents except South America, and on each has seen world maps that depict his current location in the centre. One could interpret this as an innate patriotism or even jingoism, and indeed, many maps are guilty of this, more-or-less overtly. But this positioning could also be seen as sensible design, a gentle piece of cognitive assistance. Presenting the *most context-specific* information in the centre of a 'map' gives the reader a known starting point and allows them, for example, to make the greatest number of observations of distance relative to the current position. Therefore, making a map context-specific is also a way to make a map more engaging and useful for particular audiences.

Either way, a map – an outcome space – will become a useful guide to a landscape if it offers *relevant information* to its users. Phenomenography is oriented to producing "lean, thin" descriptions of landscapes rather than the sort of "rich, thick" understandings of it that are acquired through immersion in a landscape over a period of time (Christine Bruce, personal communication), but that is exactly why the analogy of a 'map' is a useful one. All maps are, obviously, simplifications and representations of reality. In phenomenography, the outcome space is viewed as a tool for exploring and revealing variation (Andretta 2007b, 156), not a definition of a phenomenon, which is inevitably much richer and thicker than can be accommodated by the technique of mapping. Nevertheless, the formally conducted phenomenographic enquiry, which produces a written-up, tabular, or diagrammatic outcome space (map of the landscape) that is intended to be purposefully used, cannot be conceptually separated from other types of communicable outcome, based on other forms of enquiry that may be positivistic or interpretive, formal or informal, analytical or intuitive, but which all produce *informational resources within the landscape*. The images produced by Steinerová (2010) and Whitworth et al (2014), or the textual maps of Tavares et al (2011), are equivalent to other resources in an information landscape: like any map or text, they have informative potential, but will acquire actual meaning and relevance only when applied by practitioners in a given landscape.

The key critical question therefore becomes not just what is on the map, but who has drawn it, how, and why. Whose perspectives influence the experience of variation, and thus the map of the information landscape? What methods have been used?

Practice is the *lived-in embodied experience of variation within a landscape*. That "experience of variation" can be elicited in various ways, but, crucially, many methods for doing so are not *relational* (Bruce et al 2006): that is, they aim to elicit only a limited view of the landscape. The outcomes of such enquiries will tend more toward monologic forms of knowledge than dialogic or polyphonic. Content and competency-based approaches to information literacy focus on assessing learner conformity to extant mental models of a landscape, manifested in the information systems and texts which have been allocated authoritative status by dominant actors within that landscape. These approaches will see certain types of practice, those which accord to standards and rubrics, and which take place in certain physical and informational locations (the classroom, the library), but neglect others. The mapping of the landscape in these cases has been engaged in by external interests, evaluating the landscape according to their own criteria, rather than being embedded in those practices, within the landscape, around which practitioners gather (in this case, students). Results of such enquiries will be less relevant to the research subjects *but may be foisted on them anyway*, even if *their* full variation of experience will not have been explored, and the research results will therefore be more likely to be depersonalised, objective, and generic. Systems designed around this outcome space will be less likely to meet the needs of participants. A system may be created that delivers information according to generic assessments of 'need', but not context-specific ones. Or, if IL teaching focuses only on the learning to learn and/or personal relevance frames, the emphasis will be on subjective mental models of a landscape. Important as these enquiries are, they again will not allow for the full experience of variation because within these frames the learner/ practitioner is not exposed to the maps, and hence the understandings of others, whether within the same community or from outside it.

On the other hand, where the learning about the landscape is actively engaged in by the participants, where learning is socially situated, where it takes place in (relational) ways that encourage a wide exploration of the variation in practice, then the full[2] experience of variation of these participants will be more likely to become embedded in the outcome space: the texts, systems, and genre repertoires of the landscape. The resources produced through this active learning will be more relevant to members of that community and, if sufficient variation exists within the map, possibly relevant to other communities as well. This permits the distribution of stewarding capacity (cf Wenger et al 2009), providing useful resources to those seeking to nurture the information landscape through developing a broader genre repertoire, as well as more technical skills (which include the various frames of IL). Through this practice, potentials are worked out and the 'genre memory' drawn on, but also slowly transformed.

This process can become reified, when a practice becomes embedded into technologies or routines and is no longer being scrutinised. The *epistemological mistake* that Carr and Kemmis (1986) discuss becomes manifested when the outcome space *does* get treated as a "definition of the phenomenon", rather than merely a tool which, through practice, can have its relevance judged by those who are actually engaged with the phenomenon. The phenomenon would become defined in *monologic* ways. Problems may then arise within a landscape around the lack of relevance of the information systems to learner needs, because their experience, the mental models they use to orient themselves in this landscape, will not be reflected in the system.

Yet when problems like these arise, they do not have to cause alienation, information obesity, and other such pathologies – though they may well do so. Despite the pressures weighed against it, people and communities *can and do* raise such tensions back up into awareness and, through dialogue, learn about and attempt to address them. Raising awareness in this way is an essential *teaching* role in any given landscape, and the outcome of teaching is an outcome space: resources for subsequent learning, thinking, and practice. The better the maps – meaning, the more the teaching captures the full experience of variation – the more effective a guide they become to the subsequent nurturing of the information landscape. These maps can draw on technical, scientific enquiries, but can never be *fully* technical, as Bakhtin showed (and as Carr and Kemmis show). Thus, the creation of these outcome spaces must also be a dialogic and participatory process. And an approach that was not just relational, but also critical, would, as noted earlier in chapter 3, raise awareness within practitioners and community members of the structural causes of inequality within the landscape, and permit the scrutiny of the validity claims that support cognitive authority therein. The facilitation of this process – the *teaching of IL* – does not inhere only in formal education, but in all practice.

Wilson (1983, 123) describes how in a society that was "unanimous... in matters of cognitive authority", "everyone would know who the leaders are... who the teachers are...". Yet (*ibid*), such unanimity is "unlikely without strong and deliberate control over the formation and expression of opinion." One reason IL has lost its political heart, epitomised by Hamelink's vision of it as an emancipatory, community-led learning process, is that because it is an essentially educational activity, perceptions of it have suffered from the same institutionalised blindness as affects many studies of 'education': that it is largely the activities of professional teachers which are considered significant in the outcome spaces of relevant enquiries. Yet the work and methods of both the practice and phenomenographical schools of IL demand the conclusion that it is precisely by such *role-based* definitions of cognitive authority that the full experience of variation in any given landscape can easily be limited, by limiting who is *entitled to research and draw maps of an information landscape.* As such, research and mapping should be seen as a fundamental, relational teaching and learning activity, thus, these conclusions suggest the fully universalist character of IL. IL is for all, *and all can teach it.*

Notes

1. 'Confidentiality' cannot be defined except with reference to an abstract boundary drawn between communities, one of which is defined as having a legitimate right to access to the information and the other of which is not. To assert that something is innately confidential (e.g. 'National Security') is a prime example of how language is used by the powerful to prevent scrutiny of validity claims. When the term is invoked, it is hard to translate 'confidentiality' as substituting for anything other than 'We know this information, but without even telling you what it is, we have decided that you cannot be trusted with it.' Confidentiality is the antithesis of dialogue.
2. Or at least, fuller; one should see the idea of capturing the 'full' experience of variation as akin to the ISS: an ideal, worth striving for even if one acknowledges that it can never actually be reached due to inherent constraints such as time and uncertainty.

Reclaiming IL

Abstract: This chapter explores empirical examples of a radical approach to the teaching of IL, investigating the usefulness of narrative-based approaches to teaching: action research; Bakhtinian pedagogies, and more. It investigates what might be done inside the library, but also beyond it, in classrooms and workplaces, communities and families. Radical IL happens whenever the assumptions around which we base our learning and practice are called into question and scrutinised in democratic, participatory ways. Methods presented here help practitioners 'train their eyes' and see when others are doing it well, so these experiences can be evaluated and applied in a different context, as appropriate.

Key Words: Teaching, decolonisation, creative understanding, action research, collaboration, transformation.

The synthesis of IL-as-learning and IL-as-practice is now complete. IL, or more precisely, information literate behaviour, can be defined as *practices that sustain learning and the potential for transformation within communities and their landscapes.* Radical IL is the subset of these practices which lift those potentials up into practice, transforming information landscapes through scrutiny and review of the cognitive authorities that penetrate them. As Hamelink noted, these practices are diametrically opposed to the 'pushing' of information *onto* communities: something that can now be defined, more precisely, as the design of information systems which do not accommodate the experiences and categories of user groups. Hamelink's critique was directed mainly toward the broadcast media, but the synthesis of learning and practice within radical IL shows how these hegemonic and colonising practices also work through many other arenas for information exchange, the structuring of information systems, and the use of centripetal forces in language.

Radical IL seeks to counter these tendencies, wherever they may be found, and thus reclaim the political heart of IL. It attends to how authority over texts can be redistributed in a landscape. Methods for exploring this, in and via practice, lie with critical phenomenographical approaches that attend to the experience of variation within the landscape but also recognise that not all of these experiences are granted equal potential to transform practice, and are able to reveal the reasons why they are not. Empirical examples of this approach will be explored in this chapter. Like Linell (2009, 387–8), however, I do not want to use the theoretical distinctions I have presented to assign all existing literature and/or practical work to one 'side' of the debate or the other: in his case monologism versus dialogism; in mine, institutionalised versus radical IL. Nor do I claim that all IL practitioners must now adopt radical practices, at least, if they want to attain certain political ends. What the framework should be used for is *learning to see*: as a way of noticing, assessing, and evaluating trends and examples of work, and casting judgment over whether such work is oriented to the scrutiny of cognitive authority (double-loop learning) or to its acceptance (single-loop).

What this final chapter must now do is to explore what this theory means for practice, offering guidance where it can (cf Blaug 1999a; 1999b). Radical IL is not presented as a new 'standard' or rubric, nor as a form of assessment or, generally, some new approach which all IL teaching must hurry to adopt. Radical IL is already happening, and has been for millennia. It happens whenever the assumptions around which we base our learning and practice are called into question and scrutinised in democratic, participatory ways. The theoretical discussion presented here, and the critical phenomenographical methods that emerge from it, help practitioners 'train their eyes' and see when others are doing it well, so these experiences can be evaluated and applied in a different context, as appropriate.

Radical IL is also a theory that suggests why change is difficult. Institutionalisation, authority in texts, and the presence of unscrutinised assumptions and values in many landscapes helps to explain why collaboration, whether between librarians and faculty or between communities and formalised educational institutions, has proven so elusive. It shows that any institution, by its very nature, restricts choice and thus becomes an information filter. At the same time, radical IL fully embraces the *possibility* of transformation in any social setting, and the information landscapes, genres, and personal constructs that drive these settings. It is not about designing practice, but learning to see the practices that exist, and understanding their consequences, experiencing their variations, and facilitating transformation. It is not relativist: certain practices can be viewed as information illiterate, if they contribute to a reduction in learning capacity by closing off the exploration of alternatives (double-loop learning), or if they exclude certain communities from participation in information-processing activities and decisions which affect them. Critical theory must be premised on these kinds of practices, ones that diminish the negative effects and cognitive costs of authority (such as coercion, alienation, surveillance) in workplaces and communities. Ultimately, radical IL is a guide to remaining vigilant over direct democracy and small-scale decision-making, and assists the creation of decolonising forms of organisation and community-building, with a particular focus on the importance of the information landscape to these endeavours. It counters colonisation's tendency to separate capital (of all kinds, including financial, human and social capital, as well as capital in the Bourdeuian sense (Bourdieu 1990)) from the communities which have generated it.

Radical IL is political: but so is IL, and all social science in fact (Carr & Kemmis p. 144):

> Inevitably... social science is political: what is done depends on the way social processes of knowing and doing in particular situations are controlled. Critical social science thus requires a political theory about social life and, equally importantly, about its own processes and their effects on social life. The political theory of critical social science is democratic and rests on Habermas's theory of communicative competence and, in particular, on the idea of rational communication in which decision-making is guided, not by considerations of power, but by the rationality of arguments for different courses of action.

Communicative competence, in this sense[1] (see also Whitworth 2007) is fed by the effective distribution of IL throughout a community – that is, distributing the ability to make reasonable and methodologically-valid judgments that sustain that community's information landscape into the future. As the foundation of practice, radical IL thus drives the "organisation of enlightenment [which] is the organisation of the learning processes of the group" (Carr and Kemmis 1986, 146). The development of context-specific, defensible, and rational forms of knowledge is absolutely essential to this. Social change demands that (Harding 1993, p. 50):

> (I)t is not only desirable but also possible to have that
> apparent contradiction in terms – socially situated knowledge.
> In conventional accounts, socially situated beliefs only get to
> count as opinions. In order to achieve the status of knowledge,
> beliefs are supposed to break free of – to transcend – their
> original ties to local, historical interests, values and agendas.

This 'breaking free' can take place when knowledge becomes expressed
generically and monologically. And there are times when this must take
place, or society would be mired in endless discussion. However, this
process also contributes to colonisation, whereby the values, assumptions,
and forms of thinking that shape generic knowledge become concealed
within information systems. As a result, double-loop learning – scrutiny
of not just the effectiveness of a decision, but the premises underlying
that decision – becomes more difficult. Thus, information systems
become less flexible: enquiries must be shaped according to the needs of
the system, rather than the other way around. The system thereby denies
resources to alternative perspectives, and a fuller experience of variation
is more difficult. Monologism, single-loop learning, systems, and
standards are all thus interconnected.

The colonisation of knowledge formation in this way can be – and
often is – *decolonised,* based on epistemologies and methodologies that
are dialogic, and methods that are practice- and practitioner-based.
These enquiries redistribute authority over knowledge products. They
also test and validate texts and systems (written, technological, cognitive)
that are based on this knowledge. "Strong objectivity" (Harding 1993)
therefore becomes not just a philosophical position, but a practical one,
and critical phenomenography offers methods that permit such scrutiny.
Such a view is questioning and critical, and emphatically not anti-
scientific: instead, it strengthens and spreads valid scientific practice,
while still permitting (indeed, impelling) critiques of the colonisation of
science by the steering media of money and power. These kinds of
critiques are essential for democracy (Angus 2001, 10): "When understood
radically, democracy is about the processes of public decision-making to
which economic, social and cultural institutions must be subjected in
order to be legitimate and binding upon citizens. Such a radical concept
of democracy is concerned to *judge* social, economic and political
institutions, not presuppose their legitimacy." And (*ibid*, 48): "To
confuse democracy with institutional arrangements is not only to put the
cart before the horse, it is to miss the essence of the process altogether
– which is movement and creativity, the desire for change, for inclusion."

Strong objectivity is not monologic, an attempt to *impose* a consensus; it is dialogic, polyphonic, dynamic, and challenging (*ibid*, 55). Access to good quality information is one capacity needed to sustain the democratic quality of a group's interactions and, thus, the distribution of authority throughout the landscape, but also needed are (Blaug 1999a, 145): opportunities for deliberation, that is, problems to address; fora of some kind in which the community can undertake the process of learning about itself, which may now include digital fora (see also Wenger et al 2009) but which are not limited to them; motivation, and good morale. These all help provide the necessary energy. Being information literate requires having access to good information, but it also requires these other resources. Money and formalised teaching and training can also be valuable resources, but as these are also conduits of colonisation, to accept them a group has to remain vigilant over the trade-offs which arise when they are used.

This kind of active, self-aware, democratic involvement in a broad range of communities and landscapes has been called "*deep*" citizenship: "the activity of the citizen self acting in a variety of places and spaces" (Clarke 1996, 3). Deep citizenship has no fixed beginning and end, no single conception of the 'good life', but a number of possible ones, dynamic potentials that can be manifested in a range of different locations and contexts (*ibid*, 18–20).

The remainder of this chapter investigates pedagogical approaches and locations which are already undertaking relevant work in this area. It discusses the importance of action research as a way of bridging the theory-practice gap, and examines the political pressures that will inevitably be brought to bear on a radical IL, discussing how these must become learning opportunities whenever possible. Because the book has been, in part, a critique of the institutionalisation of IL within the library, but has also acknowledged the depth of IL expertise that exists there, there are passages below which discuss the library in particular, but the general concerns of the chapter are broader. There is a need not only to discuss the potential contributions made by both formal and informal learning, but also the links between the two types, and how each can strengthen the other by helping with the scrutiny of each other's validity claims.

* * *

Landscapes can be understood at a variety of ways. They can be examined according to generalisable principles. For example, in many valleys of northern England, it is not hard, once one knows what to look for, to see evidence that proves glaciers covered the landscape relatively recently, but have now disappeared. Such evidence is not visible in, say, Queensland. One needs to know very few details about either context to draw this conclusion. Rather, one needs to be able to apply more generic rules, such as looking for U- rather than V-shaped valleys and items such as erratics (boulders left behind by retreating ice). This kind of knowledge, an active, but generalisable, awareness of one's surroundings, would in this case be based on a basic understanding of the 'objective' scientific discipline that is geology, but would still be developed in personal and subjective ways (see Bakhtin's (1986, 32) anecdote about Goethe).

However, to gain a more holistic, dynamic, and intimate appreciation of the landscape – to understand what it is like to actually *live* in the landscape – one cannot rely on summary data and generic enquiries. One must develop a deeper understanding of the specific context, a "chronotopic visualizing of locality and landscape" (Bakhtin 1986, 36). Both types of inquiry involve learning, but the second, situated type forces the inquirer to enter into dialogues with the sources and forms of knowledge existing within the landscape. It also requires more time and active involvement. Both types of inquiry would be facilitated by a teacher, but in the first case that role would probably be satisfied by a single person or textbook, whereas in the second case, the role of 'teacher' would spread throughout the community within the landscape, and into the landscape itself, in both its informational and natural forms.

We undertake both types of learning at different points in our lives. The latter type is slower, more diffuse and, for that reason, far less visible than the first, but it is also more fundamental. Knowing what constitutes cognitive authority in the first type of learning environment is important, but that knowledge must, in turn, be based on the sort of deeper understandings of the many information landscapes we encounter. It is at this deep level of understanding that radical IL works. As a result, it specifically effaces the difference between formal and informal education, between the office of 'the teacher' and the practice of 'teaching'. Hence the statement which ended chapter 7, also captured in the epigraph that appeared at the beginning of part 2, from the movie *Ratatouille* – "Anyone can cook".

That statement does need qualifying, however, in order to avoid relativism. While the statement that 'all can teach IL' is an inexorable consequence of the argument thus far, there remains a difference between teaching that is IL-oriented (and information literate in its own right), and teaching that is not. That is, there remain normative standards against which practice can be judged. The statement "Anyone can cook" is explored in *Ratatouille* by the character of food critic Anton Ego. He originally disparages it, as he believes it trivialises the art of cooking: popularising the notion, in this context, of the "cult of the amateur" (Keen 2007). But by the end of the movie, stunned by the great meal he was served by the (rodent) protagonist, Ego is moved to say: "Not everyone can be a great cook, but a great cook can come from anywhere".

So it is with IL teaching. Anyone can do it, but it takes care, attention, and practice to do it well. It involves guiding and facilitating the exploration of an information landscape, so can involve both of the forms of knowledge formation discussed just above. The formal educational provider clearly has a role to play, but so must informal learning, and good or bad teaching can be found in both sectors. And the normative standards which govern good teaching are not to be found in the simple assignation of the role of 'teacher' in a particular context. Carr and Kemmis (1986, 89) write that: "... to describe somebody as 'teaching' is to implicitly appeal to a background of rules operative in a particular society which specify what is to count as teaching. Indeed they constitute the very possibility of teaching at all." These rules may be drawn in exclusionary ways, around the possession of certain qualifications, the membership of a certain subset of an organisation's employees (those whose job description specifies a teaching role), or generic, objective statements in the academic literature about what makes for effective teaching. Carr and Kemmis counter these generic rules by examining in detail how rules can also be *practice-based*. Good teaching practice means, in any setting, that teachers must also become researchers, reflecting on their practice rather than separating theory and practice from each other, depersonalising both (1986, 127) so research is done 'on' practice. Instead, research becomes integrated into practice.

As with teaching, the notion that 'research' is something esoteric, for initiates only, is ultimately part of the boundaries drawn in society around knowledge-formation; it is an expression of authority and may even be subconsciously perpetuated by the academic community (as discussed at the end of chapter 6, e.g. via Mark (2011)). In any case, it is this kind of continuous self-reflection and application of generic principles within one's own context that Carr and Kemmis hold up as the normative standards for good teaching practice. This is not to dismiss the usefulness of more quantitative and generic measurements of learning outcomes – such as grades – but emphasising practice rather than outcomes makes the point that desirable outcomes cannot arise without good practice underlying them.

Effective IL teaching takes place when the process of reflection and experience of variation is facilitated *within the learning environment.* The roles of 'teacher' and 'learner' within such an environment may at times be fixed and clear but they can also be dynamic and fluid: either way, the basis of the teaching is dialogue. The environment may exist within formal educational institutions, but it has the potential to arise in any social setting.

There exist many documented examples of teaching and educational practice that encourage students to explore variation in information, and/ or draw on investigations of these methods to argue for transformation in practice, whether in higher education specifically (e.g. Whitworth, Fishwick & McIndoe 2011; Bruce et al 2007, 51–55; Hepworth and Walton 2009; Andretta 2012), or outside the academy (Sayyad Abdi et al 2013, Yates et al 2009). Studies of the *impact* of these practices are harder to find. Herein lies an issue with the genre that is the academic paper. These texts' conclusions cannot *evolve*: they should be judged as utterances to which practitioners can respond, but it is harder to judge the responses unless follow-up studies may take place. Indeed, where such follow-ups have been done, the response to such teaching may even be negative, as it has been with Andretta's project (2012). This invokes the more difficult questions, of how institutionalised biases against democratic and critical forms of knowledge-formation work to deny resources to alternative approaches like these, but that will be returned to below.

Technology skills are a factor, as many papers have discussed (Brandt 2001, Reffell and Whitworth 2002, Scoble 2011), but the retheorisation of IL conducted here has shown that digital literacy is included in IL: it is one aspect of it, just as are scientific literacy, media literacy, and so on. Technologies are texts, so can be read, critiqued, scrutinised. As a subset of IL, digital literacy needs to be developed in dynamic and holistic ways, not just skills-based, moving "from following steps to applying concepts" (Brandt 2001, 81), but that is beyond the scope of this book (see Whitworth 2009, however). Views of digital literacy development which are more in tune with radical IL have been propounded by Luckin and colleagues (2010), and Garnett and Ecclesfield's Emergent Learning Model (2012) applies similar ideas to the organisation of learning resources more generally: this model was adopted in the MOSI-ALONG project (see below).

A pedagogical approach to consider is one inspired by Bakhtin's notion of "creative understanding". A truly creative understanding of a text goes beyond understanding a text as the author intended. Indeed, it is the act of understanding by other readers that really gives a text its potential, by imbuing it with multiple meanings: "creative understanding continues creativity, and multiplies the artistic wealth of humanity" (Bakhtin 1986, 142). While one can still recognise the authority invested in the author's creation of a text (hence the etymological similarity between the words 'author' and 'authority', just as there is a common root to 'community' and 'communication'), it is only by critiquing an author's intentions, and transcending them to some extent, that the full creative potential of communication is realised (Morson and Emerson 1990, 55):

> Outsideness creates the possibility of dialogue... for any culture contains meanings that it itself does not know, that it itself has not realized; they are there, but as a *potential*... Only dialogue reveals potentials. It does so by addressing them, by provoking a specific answer that actualizes the potential, albeit in a particular and incomplete way. At the same time, the questioner necessarily undergoes the same process, which helps him comprehend unsuspected potentials in his own culture. The process, then, is multiply enriching: it educates each side about itself and about the other, and it not only discovers but activates potentials. Indeed, the process of dialogue may itself create new potentials, realizable only through future activity and dialogue.

In this dialogic epistemology, neither side simply turns themselves into the image of the other – accepting authority unquestioningly – but both engage in dialogue. This is why the roles of 'teacher' and 'learner' become fluid and less clear. "As Bakhtin would say, intelligence is a matter not of the given but of the created" (Morson and Emerson 1990, 214); this creation is a *joint* project (Matusov 2011, 115[2]):

> The goal of education is not to make students have the same understanding as the teacher, but rather to engage them in historically valuable discourses, to become familiar with historically, culturally, and socially important voices, to learn how to address these voices, and to develop responsible replies to them without an expectation of an agreement or an emerging consensus.

Generally, appropriate pedagogical techniques will facilitate the experience of variation, guide the creation of an outcome space that will subsequently be relevant and useful to the community, and sustain their ability to learn into the future. Good teaching practice would then be manifested in the ongoing scrutiny and review of these techniques, to make sure they remain appropriate and relevant.

It is not the place of this book to discuss radical IL pedagogy in detail. Many guides already exist to IL teaching (e.g. Mackey and Jacobson 2011, Hepworth and Walton 2009, Andretta 2005, Bruce 2008), and to reflective, constructivist, and critical pedagogy more generally (Loughran 2002; Shor 1996; Mezirow 1990). 'Bakhtinian' pedagogies have also been presented: see below, and also White (2009). Geijer & Olstedt (2009) invoke Bakhtin, and also Mezirow (1990), a writer with a critical perspective on staff development, in their discussion about the importance of dialogue in vocational education, aimed at helping learners develop professional identities and resist erosion of their status and autonomy. Generally, all will share a pedagogy that encourages dialogue and the experience of variation (polyphony).

One, more specific, suggestion will be made here, however. Various authors have examined *narratives* as a valuable means of raising consciousness and becoming aware of other experiences of variation. Linell (2009, 243) observes that the narrative is an intuitively useful way of organising information, giving experiences shape, form and order by embedding them within a "plot" and using the narrative to forge links between "the exceptional and the ordinary". In his definitive study of conspiracy theories, Knight (2000) observes that one reason these forms of counterknowledge are attractive is that they exploit the narrative form, as well as features of certain fictional genres, to construct a theory of how the world works into which evidence can be easily slotted, even when it may seem to challenge the conspiracy theory. Narratives (Linell 2009, 243–4):

> (D)eal with the unexpected, create a viable account or a good story by showing the deviance in relief to the normal order of things. A good story presupposes some 'normal' background setting, introduces certain complications, and then accounts for the resolution of the problems and the restoration of normality (it accounts for why the deviation from the norm occurred)... narratives are not just retrospective accounts of past events... they involve active attempts to shape the present and the future.

Within narratives, one can see signs of the information landscapes that have shaped them. For example, Wertsch (2002, cited in Linell 2009, 244) shows that both Russians and Americans presented narratives about their countries' history in characteristic ways, emphasising emotion and the fight for freedom in the American case, the preservation of indigenous culture and the expulsion of foreign invaders in the Russian. At the very other end of the scale, personal construct psychology also encourages (amongst other things) the learner to explore and scrutinise personal narratives of change, and blockages to change: in their book on the subject, Fransella and Dalton also present case studies as narratives (e.g. 2000, 27–30). Purdue (2003) considers narrative a useful tool to use at the beginning of group professional development sessions, with participants offering stories and experiences, seeing parables as a kind of extant collective map of a landscape. Broidy (2007) did much the same to teach gender issues in information. Watkins and Russo (2005) took the technique outside the academy, undertaking work of this kind with communities in Queensland, Australia. Whitworth, Garnett and Pearson (2012; see also below) researched the links that could be built between informal learning communities and formal learning organisations in Manchester, UK. One technique used was when a city museum helped local communities present their narratives through helping them create 'Cabinets of Curiosities', video-based presentations of technological artifacts in which were encoded information that was relevant to communities or individuals, creating resources that were relevant to subsequent community learning. Popular culture offers narratives for analysis, and material to use in reflection: Ward (2006) suggests the use of images and music; Detmering (2010) uses films, specifically *Burn After Reading, Thank You For Smoking* and *W*. The present author adopts this approach in his teaching, using Morgan Spurlock's film *Supersize Me,* and the accompanying book (Spurlock 2005), as an illustration of various forms of information gathering and information concealment, with the film itself being an example of self-generated, justified research and conclusions[3] used to address a question of political and social interest (the effect of fast food on health) (Spurlock 2005). Herman (1998, cited in Luyt and Azura 2010) encourages students and teachers to use local and alternative media as resources for learning, as opposed to an increasingly concentrated corporate media, recognising that the stories, enquiries, and critiques present in these media will be more relevant within specific contexts.

Reflection can also be promoted by encouraging learners to develop their own narratives, either in an ad hoc way or systematically, perhaps through writing a journal or, more publicly, creating a blog. These are valuable tools in reflective practice (Loughran 2002) and also can become texts, through which narratives can be shared with colleagues and discussion ensue. They can also become data for analysis. Narayan (2012) asked twenty people to record their interactions with information each day, using the data to study information behaviour in prosaic settings. Her method sought to overcome limitations which affected Kuhlthau's and other information retrieval studies (Saracevic 2007b): namely that the act of assigning research subjects an information task immediately constrains their activity and risks making the behaviour artificial or, at least, applicable only within the context from which the task emerged. Her subjects were not engaged in specific tasks, however: she sought to have them record *every* engagement they had with information over the study period. Narayan expressed concern in her thesis that even then, the journal could not be a wholly objective source of data about her subjects' information behaviour, because the act of keeping the journal may have changed their behaviour (the so-called "Hawthorne Effect"). However, this is precisely the effect being encouraged here. Narratives like these can be useful for information counselling, helping reveal personal constructs (cf. Kuhlthau 1993; Fransella and Dalton 2002). Describing and reflecting on events allows values and assumptions to be foregrounded, one can trace trains of thought and sources after the fact, and so on: this is the original intention of the term *journalism*, so one might call it 'personal journalism'. With the blog, this self-presentation can be made more public. Narratives like these draw attention to how the image of the author is constructed, and thus, the image of authority present in the narrative. This, in turn, allows the claims of the author to be reviewed, and judged as more or less relevant within the reader's chronotope and landscapes.

The criticism that encouraging this kind of self-presentation contributes to 'information overload' and the 'cult of the amateur' can be effaced if the material is published in an *information literate* way, e.g. by attending to metadata, accessibility, use of language: in short, making the information of good quality. The sort of assistance that is needed here, for the effective (micro-)production, retrieval, and use of this kind of information, may be drawn from libraries, teachers, and other professionals; it may also be drawn at times from fellow members of one's community and social network.

Ultimately what radical IL pedagogy seeks is to develop "informed participation" (Wilson 1983, 144) in the decision-making structures of society. This is an ideal, and, as Wilson admits (*ibid*, 145), not often attained in our less-than-ideal democratic society. Yet this is precisely the point: it is this low level of informed participation that radical IL seeks to address.

* * *

Though LIS gave birth to IL, and libraries nurtured its early growth and development, radical IL must transcend the library. Yet the library, despite the challenges it has faced in the decades since Zurkowski first called for the spreading of IL, remains the most significant source of *technical* IL expertise. What radical IL work, then, can be done inside and across the boundaries of the library, under the restrictions posed on librarians' practices, whether due to colonisation or institutionalisation? What role should a library take in maintaining the spaces of a radical infrastructure – that is, information landscapes that are supportive of attempts to scrutinise and redistribute cognitive authority?

Simmons' paper (2005) is worth discussing first, and in some depth. The paper adopts some of the *elements* of radical IL, and is probably the best other example of academic work that links Bakhtin with IL. But it does not turn the critical investigation back on the library itself.

Simmons suggests that librarians should teach genre theory as part of their information literacy instruction. She proposes that this work could help embed students in different HE disciplinary cultures, supporting the argument that it is necessary to teach IL with reference to a particular context, and not generically. Simmons also invokes ideas of Bakhtin's, to support claims that librarians can and should aspire to become a *bridge* to academic landscapes rather than fully enter them, by claiming that librarians are in a particularly convenient place within the university to undertake this work (2005, 298): "Librarians are simultaneously insiders and outsiders of the classroom and of the academic disciplines in which they specialize, placing them in a unique position that allows mediation between the non-academic discourse of entering undergraduates and the specialized discourse of disciplinary faculty." She claims librarians have a particular ability to notice what is not visible to others embedded within these different academic cultures or genres (*ibid*, 299; here see also Becher and Trowler 1989). Simmons (2005, 298) describes how: "domain-specific rhetorical processes are seen by the faculty members who work within the domain as the 'normal' or 'natural' or 'correct' way of writing, reading or researching; and they expect their undergraduate students to be able to learn and adopt these ways of communicating without explicit instruction." However (*ibid*): "Because faculty members in a discipline are immersed in the discourse of one discipline, it can be difficult to see (and explain to students) how this discourse is different from other fields' discourses and how students can negotiate the language of their chosen discipline... [faculty members'] prodigious, focused knowledge can hinder the ability to make visible and explain to undergraduate students the rhetorical practices that have become inseparable from the faculty members' own ways of communicating."

Simmons wants librarians to adopt a genre-based approach to teaching as a way of moving beyond the ACRL standards, developing students as "participants in scholarly conversations" (299) – thus, informed participants (cf. Wilson 1983, 144). She invokes Freire on page 300, and critical information literacy (via Pawley (2003) amongst others) on pp. 300–301. Her methods are sound: she does not view any genre as fixed and authoritative, that is, another set of standards, but sees the notion as dialogic. There is a need to illustrate to students that there is a diversity of landscapes (or disciplinary discourses), each of which is constructed by various kinds of cognitive work undertaken in different locations. This will have academic benefits: (305):

> In order for undergraduate students to be able to locate, understand, evaluate and use information [ACRL standard], they need to recognize the disciplinary epistemological conventions that shape the knowledge... by learning that there are differences between discourse communities, students will be able to move from one discipline's research practices to another.

But Simmons also wants students to (302):

> (B)egin to see themselves as participants in a disciplinary conversation with the potential to effect change in the conventions instead of simply learning to conform to the established patterns within a particular 'community of practice' or academic discipline.

She makes the claim that if undergraduates learn that knowledge is dialogic, they will be better equipped to enter a particular community of practice. Thus, there is a claim that through this kind of instruction, students become better prepared to become, at least, novice practitioners in a discipline, through having gained a general view of "the landscape of scholarly work" (305).

These are all laudable ends. However, some problems emerge when these Bakhtinian lenses are turned back onto her claims. It is difficult to justify the notion that, even in relative terms and within the HE landscape, librarians can somehow be 'genre-neutral' or, at best, more familiar with the discourses of entering undergraduates than are academics. There is little support for this claim. On page 306 she brings in some assumptions about the qualifications of librarians; on pages 307–8 there is reference to work done in LIS bibliometrics: "the information science literature in bibliometrics attends to disciplinary characteristics in research practices of varying disciplines". This may be true but information science literature is not necessarily going to be part of the everyday context of librarians teaching IL, and nor is it only the landscape of different academic disciplines that Simmons is claiming librarians are best placed to deal with, but also the landscape of entering undergraduates. There is no evidence for that latter view.

Simmons' suggestions also remain firmly rooted in HE. They are no more likely to overcome institutional boundaries and biases than other pleas for collaboration. Leckie and Fullerton (1999, 7) agree that there is no evidence that "faculty will be eager to embrace a librarian-centred pedagogical discourse that is essentially foreign to their experiences and ways of thinking". Seeing the university as a realm in which students can be thought of as novice participants in constructing academic landscapes is a worthy aim, but it does not challenge the notion that the "landscape of scholarly work" is in fact a very limited view of the landscapes they will go on to enter, whether in the workplace or in private and community life.

Despite these issues, Simmons' approach is an interesting one and does recognise that becoming a practitioner in a given field involves more than simply absorbing content, but requires an understanding of conventions and other *practices* which have constructed a landscape over time.

Elmborg has written two papers which make brief reference to Bakhtin. In one (2006, 58), he refers to Bakhtin to support pedagogies in libraries and IL that embrace dialogue and polyphony, arguing against a "monologic" classroom "where one dominant voice and style of speaking is authorized while others are controlled". At its extreme this would "create an educational system that eradicates individuality and institutionalizes the status quo". In Elmborg's other reference (2002) he discusses the reference interview as a speech genre employed in libraries. He reveals the genre's assumptions and practices, with particular attention to the idea that the user can precisely outline their needs and the librarian precisely answer them: Elmborg uses Bakhtin to suggest this is not only an unjustified assumption, but it creates "library anxiety" (cf. Kuhlthau 1993). He makes explicit reference to Bakhtin's point that otherwise literate people can have difficulties making use of the conventions of a genre with which they are unfamiliar, and says (2002):

The problem delineated here runs deep in the culture of academic reference. The reference interview puts students in an untenable position. They are asked to participate in a strictly defined genre without being told the rules. When they sense that they are expected to play a role in the transaction, they become anxious and inarticulate... the reference interview and subject classifications can be seen as powerful agents for channelling students into categories of thinking that reflect authorized disciplinary constructs in the academy. 'Good questions' track automatically into such categories. 'Bad questions' do not.

Hence, the need for librarians to adopt more of a *mediator* role, as advised by Kuhlthau (1993); something which obliges dialogue and a creative understanding of the perspective of the user.

Work has been done at Høgskolen i Bergen, Norway, to create an online information literacy tutorial, *Søk og Skriv* (Search and Write), and written up by Skagen et al (2008) and Torras i Calvo (2012). These papers invoke Kuhlthau, and ideas of information anxiety and communities of practice, to discuss how the aim of the tutorial is to inculcate new students into the *practice* of academic study. Both mention Bakhtin briefly, but do not develop the theoretical links. However, the example is worth invoking because it does at least show how this perspective on education, building on Bakhtin and other authors (like Kuhlthau) already invoked in this book, can lead towards a practice-based approach to IL education.

The papers mentioned so far concentrate largely on the internal practices of the library, but others have examined practices at the boundaries, and how the library therefore relates to informal learning spaces and communities. In a radical IL, provision of boundary spaces is not intended to prescribe practice, but to cross the gap that is the "false narrative isolation of lifeworld problems from larger structures" (Hirschkop 2004, 64). In radical IL there certainly remains a role for the expert. Some professional groups do have a grounding in forms of knowledge that are suited to the promotion of IL, but one can be members of multiple communities, and in radical IL it is the role of 'experts' to promote dialogue and the experience of variation, not to instruct. Formal learning providers can be used as resources to challenge the break between the felt, lived experience of real people and the macro-level structures that, albeit not exclusively, cause and intensify problems. These spaces could be resources in a negative sense as well, operating in ways that give rise to critiques and hidden transcripts in their own right. Through such critiques, the relevance of the provider could be challenged, possibly leading to a positive response (the provider's practices change to accommodate the needs of the community), possibly negative (the relationship between provider and community breaks down).

Scoble calls for "Pro-am" [professional-amateur, as in golf] links, as a direct response to the criticism of Keen (2007): he recognises that collaborations like these (Scoble 2011, 241):

> (A)re obviously nothing new, but the ways in which the relationship is conducted and supported is radically new, and both parties can now take advantage of the following:
>
> - share the same data sources;
>
> - use similar tools that were once too expensive or difficult to use; and
>
> - communicate much more easily with each other through new media tools.

He is right about the added capabilities offered by Web 2.0 technologies, also noted by Spiranec and Zorica (2010), but the differences between the landscapes and cognitive authorities of the 'Pro' and the 'Am' still need to be accounted for.

Some librarians have managed to embed a more politically-oriented approach into IL curricula. See Broidy (2007) for instance, who created a course entitled "Gender and the Politics of Information", albeit building on past successes and emerging from a Women's Studies department, so not starting from scratch. The course was approved only because it was (*ibid*, 499):

> (P)erceived as a course that 'belonged' to an academic department and not to the library.... The incorporation of the skills portion became a covert activity. We needed to devise strategies for presenting information-seeking techniques within the context of the intellectual core of the course. In other words, we had to teach basic skills while maintaining the integrity of an upper division seminar.

But this quote also highlights the essential cognitive tension here. The library was perceived, *even by the librarian*, as concerned only with 'basic skills'. This amounts to a near-admission that the library is unqualified to go beyond this. One could argue that this is a collective construct that the library profession needs to overcome, but though this was much the same as argued for by Kempcke (2002), in the paper which was critiqued at the end of chapter 4, taking a belligerent approach to it is not a constructive approach. What is needed are *spaces for dialogue* with the other groups, not hectoring of them.

It is admitted that, here, the argument shares much common ground with the mainstream IL literature (e.g. Secker and Coonan 2013; Badke 2012; Kakkonen and Virrankoski 2010). McCrank said back in 1991: "If the aim is truly comprehensive information literacy, then libraries must cooperate with other information agencies more than ever. They will need alliances with nonlibrary admistrators, civic and religious leaders, educators, and academicians." Alliances like these are essential not just for strategic reasons, that is, to attract resources and support (though they are that), but because they help extend a community, jointly developing ways of thinking and thus building stewarding capacity from within. Instead of just consulting 'outside' experts, the expertise is brought into a shared community. But if these alliances are to emerge they are not going to do so around some shared interest in understandings of 'IL' which librarians can perceive but academics (or other groups) for some reason cannot. If alliances are needed, then active work needs to be put into building them, including negotiation and bargaining (Cervero and Wilson 1998) but also cognitive work. Cognitive work here means double-loop learning, with librarians reviewing and, if necessary, adapting their perspectives, learning about the contexts of the other stakeholder groups they wish to work with. 'IL' is too fundamental and abstract a notion to motivate activity, just as political alliances are unlikely to be motivated by a shared interest in 'politics' *per se*, but something more specific. What, then, are the hidden transcripts within an organisation (whether a university, or something else) around questions such as learning (the quality of the student experience), professional development and the erosion of professional autonomy, certain features of information systems, and the need for transformation in particular practices? Where information specialists and non-specialists find common ground in these terms, joint understandings of IL, *relevant to this shared context*, can then be negotiated.

'Operational proximity' can help form alliances: that is, the informal conjunctions that arise within information landscapes due to the literal sharing of a working (or other[4]) space, thus, a *context* (Tagliaventi and Matarrelli 2006). For example, Bridgland and Whitehead (2004, 56) mention the benefits of information specialists having offices inside academic departments for some time each week. Weiner (2012) offers useful advice to librarians about understanding the organisational dynamics of different contexts and tailoring IL advocacy accordingly. It is clearly going to be easier to work with sympathetic allies first, or 'academic champions', even though McGuinness (2007) questions whether this approach is useful. But alliance-building tactics can be proactive and creative, acknowledging the blocks to change which are endemic to HE institutions as currently structured. The institutionally limited perspective on IL that is typical (but understandable) within a library may mean that very good work in IL, even in radical IL, may just not have previously been noticed within academic settings.

However, a fresh look at research and teaching interests of faculty could take place, now using lenses that go beyond just 'IL' as explicitly named to also encompass interests in constructivist and critical pedagogy, professional development and reflective practice, community development, cognition, communication, human geography, and political theory – to name but a few. Professional development units within universities (and other organisations) could become another conduit (McGuinness 2007, 33) but, as noted here, these can also be conduits of colonisation and institutionalisation. However, there are other organisations which play valuable roles here, particularly trades unions. Alliances for radical IL could encompass student union activists as well, and reach off campus, via public engagement and "service learning" (see Warschauer 1999).

Libraries can also come to see themselves as a *space*, rather than a *service* (Elmborg 2011), re-working their information systems and practices to support dialogic knowledge-formation rather than more instrumental kinds, but this is a longer-term project. Nevertheless, it is an idea worth developing. In the first place, the information systems literature does offer guidance on how to design systems in more flexible and open ways, such as Checkland's "soft systems methodology" (see Checkland and Holwell 1998, for example): these are useful insights, but not covered in further detail here, firstly for reasons of space, but also because such a methodology would still rest on knowledge-formation practices of the type being discussed throughout this book. More usefully discussed here are insights into how the library can come to define its general role in dialogic knowledge formation.

Wilson discusses the distinction between the *didactic library* and the *liberal library* (1983, 188–91). Essentially, the difference is that in the liberal library, the librarian is not supposed to allow any of his/her own judgements regarding the cognitive authority of any text to affect the inclusion of that text in the library, whereas in the didactic library, texts are selected because they accord with learning outcomes that the library has been set up to promote. Thus, the didactic librarian is acting as cognitive authority for the users by, in turn, implicitly stating – via inclusion of the book in the library – that these texts also possess cognitive authority. As Wilson says (1983, 189): "Not only might there be such libraries, there are plenty of them." They arise wherever selections are made based on some principle of cognitive authority – whether works are suitable for children, whether they are of sufficient relevance for the user community that the library seeks, and so on.

That being the case, how could a librarian possibly be liberal, bearing in mind that the physical space in all libraries is limited somehow? Even the use of digital technologies to compensate is itself limited by funding and other constraints. Wilson argues that the driving force in the liberal library would in fact be *demand*. This may seem a plea for a pure 'free market' in books, and one that would lead to any liberal library becoming filled with bestsellers and celebrity biographies, but Wilson acknowledges that this kind of full libertarianism is an extreme that is rarely reached. The greater significance of the idea of the liberal library is that its basic founding principle is that the choice of text is made, not according to the librarian's notion of cognitive authority, but to (*ibid*, 191): "prefer one text over another to the extent that the first is more likely than the second to be found satisfactory by a user of the library". To put this principle into practice would require the liberal librarian to be engaged in a constant *dialogue with users*, and, through this, trying to develop a dynamic and creative understanding of their context – thus, co-creating an environment in which *the user community is more likely to find relevant texts*. What the librarian particularly brings to this co-creation is not, therefore, an uncaring laissez-faire attitude, but a professional skepticism (*ibid* 194): "The liberal librarian can be viewed as a professional skeptic about claims to knowledge or claims of the superiority of one opinion over another... Pyrrhonian skepticism [is] the attitude of one who neither asserted nor denied the possibility of knowledge but continued to enquire, though always unsatisfied that knowledge had yet been found." In other words, the effective librarian recognises that the library is *unfinalisable*.

Librarians may well ask what practical steps can be taken here and now – in one's chronotope, that is – to help bring about this long-term goal of an evolving space in which dialogue with users and this kind of professional skepticism can evolve? But specific actions depend on the context, so cannot be dictated here. Instead, what is required is to promote professional development activities, freer access to texts and/or guidance with organising and navigating open educational resources, evaluation of where operational proximity and other non-hierarchical forms of information exchange can be exploited, and other tactics suggested above, all of which help develop a supportive environment within the library for the transformation of practice, and also contribute to the radical information infrastructure of society: a Zurkowskian "information services environment" devoted to the centrifugal redistribution of cognitive authority, not its centripetal centralisation.

In the public library sector, radical IL work is taking place. Ferguson (2012) describes how public libraries develop social capital in communities, with the promotion of IL a key strategy. He notes that public libraries are most valuable resources within the information landscapes of voluntary associations and ethnic minority communities, and that because libraries remain physical spaces and not merely virtual ones, they are rooted in local contexts, particularly those of marginalised groups. In essence they have become more low-income oriented as Internet access has spread. Public libraries have played a critical role in helping individuals and communities through the post-2008 economic downturn (Rooney-Browne 2009, 348, cited in Ferguson 2012, 25). Radical IL certainly supports these views, but it also suggests why the funding cuts being faced by public libraries at the present time, most incisively in the UK, are a *consequence* of their context-specific, potentially decolonising role, not just a constraint on it. However, O'Beirne observes that there are contrasting perspectives on the reasons for the public library movement (see also Black 1996), including radicalism, but also including social control, the education of the population in technical skills required by industry. Nor has every country experienced a 'public library movement'.

The role of the library in IL has been explored with reference to Habermas by Elmborg (2011). He, via Buschman and Leckie (2007), invokes the idea of the public sphere as an image of what a library should aspire to as a *physical* space: an environment or architecture designed around democratic principles and supporting learning and transformation (Elmborg 2011, 341). Then, invoking Harvey (1989), he describes how the instrumental rationality of late capitalism depends on the increasing collapse of space and time, seeing them as inefficiencies, as obstacles to the production, movement, and consumption of goods, particularly informational goods (Elmborg 2011, 342):

The Enlightenment project of human emancipation has been increasingly ineffective as a means to resist the capitalist restructuring of culture (hence the transformation of the public sphere chronicled by Habermas). While we might see ourselves as autonomous and rational, the culture we live in undermines our autonomy and subverts our rationality.

Yet, within this reality, communities can still work to define spaces in particular ways (*ibid*). Within formal organisations, like the library, *boundary* spaces can exist in which two cultures – now interpretable as two *contrasting rationalities*, ways of thinking and communicating – can come together. Indeed, all learning providers can become boundary spaces (or landscapes) in this way, depending on the context: that is, the specific set of practices being constantly developed within the landscape. Elmborg (2011, 349) observes:

> We [libraries] can become bookstores in an effort to beat bookstores, or we can work to build libraries and librarianship around the concept of shared social space where real people engage in real struggle for meaning and purpose in a landscape of increasingly rapid human movement and social change.

Yet the landscape of institutionalised IL is still a dominant one, and we cannot simply ignore it, claiming that a radical IL is needed and should be self-evident to educators or, more pertinently still, those who provide the resources to them and develop the criteria by which their 'effectiveness' will be measured. Elmborg (2011, 345) observes that:

> Like cathedrals, temples, and other culturally symbolic spaces, libraries evolved to fill one sociocultural function, and they are so filled with the essence of their identities that they tend to resist appropriation or reinvention. Through the rhetoric of those who resist library change, we hear the fear that the library might become something other than the absolute institution it has always been.

* * *

Ultimately, the location for a radical IL lies outside the HE institution, even if work inside HE can, as it always has done, contribute to the radical infrastructure through becoming a space in which resources can be found to assist the relevant research and theorising[5] . It is how bridges are built, between informal and formal educational processes, that matters: the bridges must become conduits for two-way traffic, not just the imposition of cognitive authority from the formal realm of education onto the informal learning processes of society, thus ensuring dialogue between the two.

Radical IL work can focus directly on creating community-generated, alternative information banks in the sense described by Hamelink. The "cult of the amateur" (Keen 2007), a deterioration of the quality of the online information landscape *in toto*, is not an inevitability. Communities who wish to create online spaces or "digital habitats" (Wenger et al 2009), and use these to store and present elements of their information landscape, can be helped to learn the necessary technical skills, communicative competence, and reflective, dialogic practices needed to keep these spaces of good quality, dynamic and open to new inputs.

This objective drove the MOSI-ALONG project which took place in Manchester, UK in 2011 (Whitworth et al 2012)[6]. Essentially, MOSI-ALONG sought to enact the co-creation of museum collections that Simon (2010) terms "the participatory museum". It did so by brokering alliances between community groups – informal learning spaces which in this case included local historical societies, urban gardeners, and webmasters of community web sites – and formal and non-formal[7] educational providers in Manchester including museums, the university, social media experts, video production specialists and the BBC (British Broadcasting Corporation).

Evaluation of the project, mainly using observational and qualitative methods, led to the framework termed "Aggregate-then-Curate" (Whitworth et al 2012). This outlined the process of creating *good quality and sustainable* online content collections, identifying seven stages, from the initial, subjective impetus to produce a text and the validation of this by close collaborators (friends, colleagues), through the process of creation and, possibly, eventual accreditation which could take various forms such as funding, further commissions, course credits etc (for more detail, see Whitworth et al 2012). The quality and relevance of online content was, through this process, validated by both the formal learning providers and the informal learning processes within the community. The communities driving the creation of these particular information landscapes focused their validation of the process more on the content of the collection, whereas more formal learning processes focused on technical issues and how the content was presented and structured. Both were essential: relevant content will not be found if there is no use of tagging or other metadata, and other technical qualities (whether a video is in focus, for example) will also affect its reception.

Aggregate-then-Curate thereby constitutes a framework through which collaborators could jointly identify those areas in which the community most needed guidance, in order to nurture their information landscape (or as Wenger et al (2009) would put it, steward their digital habitat). Use of the framework to analyse various case studies arising from the project also permitted the conclusion that where one or more of the seven stages were omitted from the content creation process, the content would lose quality and relevance. An example of this was seen with a set of online resources intended to be used for ICT skills training in the community, but which had not been open to community participation in their creation. As a result, they were underused due to a perceived lack of relevance to the user community (*ibid*).

The process of online content creation can only be one element of IL, but MOSI-ALONG has wider relevance, as it highlighted some problems with sustaining formal/informal learning collaborations. Whitworth et al found that it was at the point of *curation* where the greatest tension existed between the community's interest in content, and the information professionals' interest in structure. Where community content was offered to the museum partner, curation – the restructuring of that content to offer learning pathways – was always done on the museum's terms, not the community's. In this respect, MOSI-ALONG's bridges remained one-way. However, more of a two-way dialogue was seen in another case study, the redevelopment of a community web site for a suburb of Manchester[8], as brokering contacts between the site's webmaster and social media specialists provoked the addition of a Twitter feed to the site that then substantially diffused the cognitive work required to keep the site up to date. Through this, the webmaster removed significant constraints on her time and the site became more relevant and useful to users: accreditation then came with direct use of the site by the city council (Whitworth et al 2012). These are limited case studies, and not generalisable, but nevertheless show that in this context, a productive dialogue could be facilitated between 'pros' and 'amateurs', and that social media greatly facilitated the nurturing of a useful and relevant information bank in this case. This bank was constructed more along Hamelink's lines than Zurkowski's, being essentially under the control of the community, and thus an actively stewarded part of their information landscape.

There have been other projects which have tried to broker such alliances, by developing the IL skills of marginalised communities. Bruce's work with the Puerto Rican community of Paseo Boricua in Chicago (Bruce and Bishop 2008) is a more involved, longer-term version of MOSI-ALONG. Kanyengo (2009) recounts work done by libraries on HIV/AIDS issues in Zambia (in an environment, incidentally, in which the library has not been able to afford any journal subscriptions since the 1980s, and relies entirely on donations). Dorner and Gorman (2011) have done work in Laos: they recognise the constraints imposed by a poor overall level of education, but claim that IL can be a starting point, and help development, because of its basic rooting in *literacy*. External advisors can help develop IL, even in these extremely marginalised areas of the world, but must understand the local context and cannot just apply the ACRL standards (Dorner and Gorman 2011). The authors also reported a lack of relevant information in local languages, and that even where donor agencies and foreign governments declare a lack of influence over what is taught, they establish *de facto* control over curricula due to supplying resources.

Ultimately, when considering IL in the community, what this means is not that 'community' should be seen as the *location* for pedagogical work, but it is also the *content* (Harris 2008, 252) and *outcome* of the work. This combination can be seen in the work of Tavares, Hepworth and Costa (2011), who conducted participatory action research (see below) with a community in Brazil. The participation (Tavares et al, 2011, 128) improved the success rate of this development project, and its longer-term sustainability, because it enhanced the ownership of the discourse among the community. The problems they faced (such as lack of access to services) could be presented as information problems and, thus, potentially addressable (*ibid*, 134). Evaluation was integrated into the process: not just evaluation of its impact on information searching, but on members' collaboration and participation in community life. Thus, community itself became an outcome of the research (*ibid,* 136): "through the course of intervention there was a growing awareness of rights and a sense of responsibility and a desire to participate in the democratic process".

The same impetus also drives the notion of 'service learning', whereby work done within a formal educational setting is made directly relevant to the communities around that setting through an activist outlook and the nurturing of informed community participation (Warschauer 1999; Riddle 2003). Rockquemore and Schaffer (2000) reported that students engaging in service learning did initially manifest alienation and despair at the magnitude of problems faced by communities, and the seeming inevitability of them but, as the course progressed, they overcame this anxiety (cf. Kuhlthau 1993) and were increasingly engaged: that is, embedded in the context.

Eubanks (2011; 2013) examines the question of social justice in the information age: her book contains a dozen examples of projects but her theories are drawn mainly from her work with the YWCA in Troy, NY, US. This work was collaborative, action research driven by the community; Eubanks was therefore helping her subjects develop their own laboratories of experience, rather than using them as laboratory specimens. Like Feenberg (2002), Eubanks is committed to "popular technology"[9]. Access to technology is perceived as a human right in the digital era, but Eubanks notes that many lower-income and marginalised populations are already firmly "plugged in" to information systems, as the consumers of digital content produced by the mass media, low-status workers in menial information industry jobs, the subjects of surveillance, and so on. Therefore, 'access' alone is not empowering: it may even be colonising and hegemonic. However, the popular control and ownership of technology must also be based on participation (in policy decisions, construction of networks), common ownership (of networks), and healthy communities, virtual and otherwise (see also Seale 2010, who presents a similar definition of "digital inclusion", and Whitworth et al 2012). In offering guidance to academics, librarians, and those within communities who wish to assert control over their information systems, Eubanks stresses the importance of one's personal experience of what it means to be a critical technological citizen: that we are all experts about what technology means in our own lives. But this subjective view must also be made intersubjective by having a social justice framework at the centre of one's IL work. Coalition-building needs prioritising, through meeting people in their own context.

A crucial role in Eubanks' Troy work was played by an "activist lab", a technological space for use by members of this community. When the computers were just provided alone, use was limited, but once the space included "lab hostesses" – people who lived in the YWCA, and who spent time in the lab as a human face – then use increased hugely: not because the lab then contained "experts" but almost the opposite; users responded positively to hostesses "who looked like them". In other words, there was a clear common context. There was no imposition of practice; no declaration of how the lab should be used (e.g. a fixed schedule of training sessions). Users were instead encouraged to reflect on their own activities first, and then once a focus for the use of the lab was so found (cf. Kuhlthau 1993), the hostess would help the user find out how the technology could help. An example of this (Eubanks 2013) is that a *potential* user might come in and simply want to play the guitar in the lab. After letting them do this (subject to them not disturbing other users), the hostess might have suggested the use of digital recording and editing software such as Audacity, as a way of opening a dialogue with the user about their potential requirements.

Eubanks' work shows that one can work on IL at a very local and contextual level, yet still reveal macro-level structures of constraint, both in theory and practice, and that stimulating a community to engage in its own research and reflection lies at the roots of transformation. Access to technology and expertise alone is not only inadequate to overcome colonisation, it is a conduit for it. Dialogue, self-reflection, and learning are the micro-level processes which drive any change.

* * *

The term "action research" (AR) has begun to appear within discussions of how to facilitate dialogue, and the experience of variation. Hughes, Bruce and Edwards (2007) draw on it specifically, relating reflection and AR directly with the seven frames of IL. Narrative and reflection were mentioned above as ways to scrutinise one's own practice, but AR makes this more systematic, and turns it into praxis (Reason and Bradbury 2011, 1–2):

> (A)ction research is a participatory, democratic process concerned with developing practical knowing in the pursuit of worthwhile human purposes, grounded in a participatory worldview... a practice for the systematic development of knowing and knowledge, but based in a rather different form from traditional academic research... action research is about working towards practical outcomes, and also about creating new forms of understanding, since action without reflection and understanding is blind, just as theory without action is meaningless.

AR has an essential role in combating limited views of professionalism, whether these views come from within the profession or from outside it. In Carr and Kemmis's view it is what allows educators to *justify their validity claims*. AR is built around a cycle, or rather a spiral[10], of practices: planning, acting, observing (or recording), and reflecting (Hughes et al 2007, 73–6). Three areas of improvement are intended: improvement of a practice; improvement of the understanding of a practice by its practitioners, and improvement of the situation in which the practice takes place (Carr and Kemmis 1986, 165). AR can be used to raise awareness of a context, at a macro level (e.g. within a whole profession: *ibid,* 8), the meso-level of the community, and the micro-level, personal context. It is oriented not to the development of theory, but nor only to practice: instead, theory and practice come together in *praxis,* a dialogue between theory and practice which is intended to "remake the conditions of informed action and the knowledge which informs it" (Carr and Kemmis 1986, 33). Thus, it remakes the *information landscape.*

AR is an epistemology that closes the separation between researchers/ policymakers on the one hand, and practitioners on the other (*ibid,* 216). The "epistemological mistake" that is the theory-practice gap has developed into a "cultural or political mistake" (Carr and Kemmis 1986, 218), creating professions with (*ibid,* 2) "limited views of [their] professionalism" (Carr and Kemmis write about education specifically, but it applies more widely than this). This passivity is conducive to conformity, with educational standards specifically mentioned by Carr and Kemmis as part of this process. AR, as a means of countering this view and promoting professional practice, is driven by democratic and participatory impulses, simultaneously seeking contributions to both social science and social change (*ibid,* 165; Reason and Bradbury 2001; Gustavsen 2001). Notions of standards and control are incompatible with unfinalisability (*ibid,* 26):

> (E)ducation is essentially a process or an activity. It takes place in social situations of great complexity.... While the technical view of education sees teaching and learning behaviours as elements in a system which can, in principle at least, be controlled as means to given end, the practical view asserts that the social world is simply too fluid and reflexive to allow such systematization. It regards social life as in principle fluid and open. Such control as is possible in the social process of education will only enter through the wise decision-making of practitioners – through their deliberation on practice.... But the events of school and classroom life will always have an open, undetermined character. The action of those in the situation will never completely control or determine the unfolding of classroom or school life.

Professional practice is thus fully context-specific, dependent on the educational 'micro-climate' in which the practice occurs, something which can change from day to day (*ibid*, 37). It is through AR that relativism is avoided, and the practices of educators (which, remember, can now be located in any setting) are scrutinised and given validity. This is all part of achieving "strong objectivity" (Harding 2003), the revealing of assumptions, opening them up to scrutiny. The purpose of this kind of research "is to ensure that the observations, interpretations and judgments of educational practitioners can become more coherent and rational and thereby acquire a greater degree of scientific objectivity" (Carr and Kemmis 1986, 124).

AR can be formal, engaged in through the same methods as in other research, such as surveys, questionnaires, observation. Methods vary from reflection via narrative and anecdote (Horton 2011), to more systematic techniques. Hughes et al (2007, 77) note its applicability to information literacy learning needs analysis, curriculum development, pedagogical strategies, and monitoring and evaluation of IL programmes.

At the individual level, personal constructs can block change. Personal construct psychology (PCP) is effectively a form of self-reflective AR, thus applicable to IL. The personal construct psychologist seeks to help the client raise awareness of constructs that can block learning, and works to transform them, both of which challenge the client's *inner* 'authoritative voice'. PCP as a practice has been best worked out by Fay Fransella (e.g. Fransella and Dalton 2000), and Kuhlthau's work remains the best treatment of the PCP-IL connection, with the caveat that her work remains library-oriented.

However, personal constructs cannot explain all reticence to change practice. Broader, meso- and macro-level structures also must be investigated by AR (Carr and Kemmis 1986, 189): "much teacher action is the product of custom, habit, coercion and ideology which constrain action in ways that the teachers themselves do not recognise..." AR here can become a way of developing informational products from processes that communities and community members engage in all the time, though not always effectively. Kemmis relates this directly to Habermas's notion of communicative action, noting that the first step in AR is not the research itself, but (Kemmis 2001, 100, emphasis in original): "*the formation of a communicative space* which is embodied in networks of actual persons... A communicative space is constituted as issues or problems are opened up for discussion, and when participants experience their interaction as fostering the democratic expression of divergent views".

AR can be a way of mapping the experience of variation that is evident in these "divergent views". This mapping process can be explicit, using techniques like group concept mapping, which promote reflection and develop outcome spaces (Johansson 2012, 6–7). Kuhlthau also suggests that concept mapping and other visualisations such as timelines and flowcharts can be useful for "charting information and... visualizing emerging ideas" (Kuhlthau 1993, 181). She sees the visual and nonlinear elements of the technique as significant here, allied to the importance of composition and production as a way of promoting thinking and (for her) helping with formulating a focus. Steinerová (2010) asked her subjects to create visualisations of their information horizon, an idea conceptually related to the outcome space. Johansson (2012, 2) sees visualisations as information media that, even more than text-based media, have the potential to be "*evocative* and *non-blackboxed* information resources that inspire new questions and enable repeated analyses from alternative perspectives rather than as enunciative tools providing true answers". Tippett's work on using concept mapping to promote reflection on small-group decision making has taken place in various communities from workplaces to marginal communities in Southern Africa (Tippett, Handley and Ravetz 2007). She does not invoke IL directly, but is clearly oriented to scrutiny of cognitive authority within information landscapes. Whitworth et al (2014) have applied the same techniques as Tippett et al to studies of two academic libraries in Norway, using concept mapping, other visualisation techniques, and social network analysis to map changes in the communities' information landscape over a period of organisational change. This work is in its early stages at the time of writing, but the desired outcome is to use these visualisations to reveal how these groups collectively make judgements about relevance, a question that has long been neglected by information science (Saracevic 2007b).

***

The techniques listed so far – narratives, concept mapping and other forms of visualisation, action research, dialogue, constructivist and critical pedagogies, small-group decision-making – are nothing new, but their importance to IL can now be justified theoretically. What they all have in common is their attention to the micro-scale, the psychology of the individual actor, their relationships to diverse communities, and the information horizons of each. In that radical IL is specifically community-oriented, communicatively-rational, and prosaic, it is correct that no mention has yet been made of how standards, national policies, specific curricula, and assessments could promote it. These are the tools of instrumental and institutionalised education. While radical IL can and must respond to these, and perhaps incorporate them in particular contexts if they are seen as appropriate there (selecting them from a range of alternatives, and keeping this decision under review), they should be seen as *potential* resources, and not essential elements of a radical IL.

What is more significant, and must be at least raised, as the end of the book approaches, are the institutional biases against these practices, the macro-scale, system-wide means by which transformational and democratic activity is denied financial and social capital, and thus cognitive support. This issue has been raised throughout, particularly when criticising mainstream IL literature in chapter 4, so it cannot be avoided here.

There are micro-level, personal reasons why AR does not take place more often in professional and community contexts. Lack of time is an obvious one. Nor does everyone wish to undertake this kind of work: "involvement in decisions is not attractive for everyone in all relevant choice situations, all the time. The capacity for beliefs, attitudes and concerns is larger than the capacity for action" (March & Olsen 1979, 14). Even if these are personal constructs, they cannot be simply wished away. There is no point simply demanding that teachers, or any other professional, engage in some new activity that they do not have the capacity to engage in. At the same time, these kinds of constructs can be exploited by hierarchism to justify the delegation of cognitive work away from communities ("this system will save you time"). Nor should the galvanising effect of hidden transcripts be underestimated: even the most apathetic community can at least potentially be roused by injustice, incompetence, or a simple incompatibility of perspective, a contradiction arising between what they are told and what they see or do for themselves. More significant are not that these sparks of rebellion never arise: rather, that when they do, their potential energy can be drained away by meso- and macro-level structures that then re-entrench themselves around whatever discourse provoked the critique.

Even if nonconformity and dissent "provides the gene pool for social innovation" (Korten 1990, 214), it is also at least potentially disruptive to an organisation: "there is no such a thing as learning without conflict, for any modification of the knowledge distribution is perceived as a way of subverting the established knowledge/power relations within a social context..." (Gherardi et al 1998, 276). Therefore, organisations tend to approach decisions as analytical problems, to be answered with the *appearance* of due process and objectivity, even when it is clear that to actually implement the content of a (rational, instrumental) decision, communicative actions – bargaining, negotiation, the reaching of a consensus – must then take place (March and Olsen 1979, 89–90; Cervero and Wilson 1998). Carr and Kemmis (1986, 197) note that:

> The organisation of enlightenment in action research thus gives rise to conditions under which the organisation of action can take place as an attempt to replace one distorted set of practices within another, undistorted set of practices. Such action is always political action; new practices always challenge established institutional interests. They express a realignment of tendencies towards empowerment and emancipation, on the one hand, as against tendencies towards the entrenchment of sectional self-interests, on the other. At every moment... any action research project will contain some balance of both of these tendencies.

Effective, transformational AR is as much about managing conflict and achieving a sense of community as it is about the results of the research itself (*ibid*):

> Since it is undertaken by a particular group with particular self-interests of its own, and under particular historical conditions of relative power or powerlessness, it is always subject to distortions by these self-interests. By aiming to involve others in its progress, however, it can expand the community of self-interests it represents...

Thus the importance of alliance-building in AR, just as in radical IL more widely. These drives are implicitly refuting the idea that the *authoritative voice* in a landscape can come from outside the community of participants in the practices that constitute that landscape (cf. Carr and Kemmis 1986, 211), yet expanding the community in this way also involves a risk: moving beyond what is known, into what is unknown, a step that might go wrong (Carr and Kemmis 1986, 185). Managing emotion is also important and cannot be avoided, as people tend to shy away from interpersonal conflict (Blaug 1999, 153–5).

One should not expect support for direct democratic processes, such as radical IL, to emerge from most state apparatuses. At a transnational level, there has been support from organisations like UNESCO, and Sturges and Gastinger (2010) invoke the UN Declaration of Human Rights, particularly the right to "seek, receive and impart information and ideas, through any media and regardless of frontiers" as the basis for IL. But, (*ibid*): "while Article Nineteen provides excellent inspiration, like any simple statement of a human right, it does not offer supporting arguments that might indicate the specific dimensions and potential structures of an information right." In any case, we live in an era where certain governments and media interests, particularly in the UK, regularly propose withdrawing from certain binding human rights agreements (e.g. that of the EU). The "responsibility on governments, professionals and civil society activists for the (active) creation of suitable conditions for the effective exercise of intellectual freedom" that Sturges and Gastinger mention is one adopted with varying enthusiasm by each group, but the basis of radical IL in theories such as Gramsci's and Habermas's suggests it is a category mistake to demand that a government do more to support the development of radical information infrastructures, although it is true that some states, such as Norway, do offer more protection than others (*ibid*). Clarke (1996, 62) observes that the state is not a necessary requirement for politics, and "there is a perfectly defensible view that the state inhibits politics and distorts citizenship."

Graeber (2012, 382–3) goes further still:

> (I)t could well be said that the last thirty years have seen the construction of a vast bureaucratic apparatus for the creation and maintenance of hopelessness, a giant machine designed, first and foremost, to destroy any sense of possible alternative futures. At its root is a veritable obsession on the part of the rulers of the world – in response to the upheavals of the 1960s and 1970s – with ensuring that social movements cannot be seen to grow, to flourish, or propose alternatives; that those who challenge existing power arrangements can never, under any circumstances, be perceived to win. To do so requires creating a vast apparatus of armies, prisons, police, various forms of private security firms and military intelligence apparatus, and propaganda engines of every conceivable variety, most of which do not attack alternatives directly so much as create a pervasive climate of fear, jingoistic conformity, and simple despair that renders any thought of changing the

world seem an idle fantasy. Maintaining this apparatus seems even more important to exponents of the 'free market', than maintaining any sort of viable market economy.... To begin to free ourselves, the first thing we need to do is see ourselves again as historical actors, as people who can make a difference in the course of world events. This is exactly what the militarization of history is trying to take away.

Because validity claims and cognitive authority can only be truly tested in contexts that are not those from which they originated, these other contexts are grounds from which hidden transcripts (Scott 1990) and, eventually, challenges to authority emerge. However, the rhetorical moves made by colonising forces are often based around the *denigration of contextually-relevant, situated knowledge* and also deterministic views of humanity that deny the possibility of internal and individual transformation and change (as an example, consider the arguments made in favour of mass surveillance and subsequent use of the data gathered for 'profiling' purposes). Asserting the value of this kind of knowledge in turn drives depersonalisation (Morson and Emerson 1990, 405) which, in turn, detaches the individual from their context, sometimes forcibly so (Graeber 2012, 437).

Yet even here, there must remain some grounds for hope *(ibid):* 'To begin to free ourselves, the first thing we need to do is see ourselves again as historical actors, as people who can make a difference in the course of world events. This is exactly what the militarization of history is trying to take away." This accords with Hamelink's words (1976, 123): "The process of becoming the object of one's history has to start with the awareness of the immediate context and the consciousness that this context is changeable..."

Is this a forlorn hope? Certainly, the path is a difficult one, and change will not be rapid. But empirically, the work is being done in places, now as it has been in the past, as writer/activists such as Eubanks (2013) prove, as well as many others already cited in this section. What these projects must concentrate on, more so than data gathering, is the active *evaluation* and *communication* of their results to other interested communities – whether these are presented in academic form (but outside the academic publishing establishment, and/or in open access journals) or using other genres such as narrative, awareness-raising workshops, and so on. In this way can both the theory and practice of radical IL continue to evolve. This book is not the end of the process – nor indeed, its starting point – it is merely a move in the ongoing dialogue around direct democratic practice, and how we can learn to be better citizens. The present author will continue his work in this area and others will also do so. The hope is that the theory and practice of radical IL will continue to evolve as we all learn about how we must challenge the cognitive authority currently invested in powerful and influential information systems, open the claims of the powerful up to active scrutiny, and realise we have the power to transform our local contexts through active dialogue and work.

* * *

In summary, radical IL picks up Hamelink's early, tantalising but underdeveloped views on IL, and returns to them with new theoretical lenses, developed by those authors which have previously analysed IL in dialogic terms – particularly those working in the phenomenographic and practice schools of IL. The ideas originating from these schools have been synthesised through the idea that through everyday, prosaic explorations of the various information landscapes we inhabit, we are, collectively, constantly drawing maps of these landscapes that help organise and visualise the resources available to us for learning and transformation. But only rarely do we become fully conscious of this process – usually doing so at times of rupture, when the validity claims we habitually accept are called into question by new information or anomalous experiences. These can cause anxiety and denial, but they can also provoke learning experiences, sometimes of great energy. Participation in such a project is a learning process in its own right, and if reflected on and assimilated into a worldview, one realises that one can, indeed, learn to become more political – a conclusion recognised by the social movement literature (e.g. Diani 1995; Wall 1999, 96). The question is whether organisations who may seek to facilitate this kind of process can withdraw from control of it at the appropriate point.

In 1990 Korten looked forward to the need in the 21st century for a 'fourth generation' of transformative political actors that stood outside the governmental sector – in other words, NGOs (non-governmental organisations, for instance the Red Cross, Greenpeace, or more local charities and voluntary groups). He saw the first generation of NGOs as those that organised immediate relief efforts in times of suffering (e.g., the Red Cross); a second generation that focused also on building communities without the necessary provocation of a disaster (e.g. Voluntary Service Overseas or VSO); and the third generation, which many NGOs have reached, as campaigning for change in government policy and against transnational organisations like the IMF (e.g. Greenpeace). Korten then defined the fourth generation as organisations that would aim at "energising decentralised action" (Korten 1990, 120), for example, Dr Y C J Yen's *literacy* movement in China in the 1920s–30s:

> Copies of the texts... appeared in provinces and towns throughout the country, and not even James Yen knew how many classes were in fact being taught or how many schools were operating. In a more conventional project... these conditions would have been a sign of poor management. In a true movement it is a sign of the vitality of an idea with a power to spread by its own momentum, wholly beyond any central control or monitoring.

A form of radical IL can be seen in Yen's example. It raised the ability of the mass of the population to engage with what had previously been elite dialogues, improved their ability to engage with information generally, and was decentred and community-focused. In modern parlance, Yen's texts 'went viral'. The example also suggests that to distribute stewarding and authority, to create the intersubjectively-validated elements of the radical infrastructure, more than just introspective reflection is required. It requires the production of texts. This is itself a 'risky' business, requiring reflection: we cannot be sure of our recipient, or even that we will be externalising our own 'inner speech' accurately (Morson and Emerson, 1990, 215). Nevertheless, only by producing such texts, narratives and maps of various kinds can ideas enter into dialogue with one another. It is in this *production* that radical IL can be 'measured', not by the creation of rubrics and standards. By the production of texts, and their validation *as utterances*, the responses made to them by others, can the impact of radical IL be seen, and it can come to be defined as more than just an abstract concept. But these are not the same criteria of success as will be expected by organisational hierarchies.

Subordinate members of a social and organisational structure – the 'lower classes' if one likes – are worked harder. This work is both physical and cognitive. These classes lack not technology as such. As Eubanks shows (2011), most are already plugged in to information systems. But rather than facilitating learning, these systems are essentially extractive. The huge information banks which Zurkowski anticipated are now manifested in sites like Google and Facebook, with the brute processing power required to make use of these data well beyond the reach of the ordinary citizen and, indeed, many corporate entities. But to call for such power to be redistributed to communities misses the point. What the disempowered need, and what transformation depends on, is not this kind of instrumental force, but a flexible genre repertoire, an ability to communicate effectively in a variety of landscapes, to learn from the resultant dialogue and, ultimately, to understand how to transform one's own world, and the cognitive authorities which constrain it.

Work and authority are diametrically opposed. Authority, as instantiated in a monologic information system, forces other people to do cognitive work to adjust to it. Just as radical IL redistributes authority, so it redistributes work. The sort of holistic, situated understanding it implies takes time and effort to achieve – there is no 'magic bullet' in this case – but the investment is worth making. Radical IL redistributes the benefits of work: that is, it more equably distributes capital of various kinds, and it redistributes the negative, colonising, unsustainable effects of work, effacing them with positive impacts on communities' ability to sustain their own information landscapes and continue to retain learning potentials into the future. Radical IL highlights not just the financial, but the cognitive debt that our increased reliance on instrumental rationality owes to the products of communicative rationality. For that reason it is opposed by the hegemonic institutions that are funded by these debts.

Notes

1. This is quite a different usage from the idea of competency as manifested in Bruce et al's (2007) competency frame of IL education.
2. Note the difference between Bakhtin and Habermas's views on 'consensus', epitomised by the last line of this quote.
3. The question of the 'validity' of Spurlock's research is a matter for critique, of course: but it cannot be denied that he at least attempted to root his conclusions in scientific analysis through the employment of three medical specialists to evaluate the results of his experiment (that is, the effects on his body). He also presents his methodology and justification for the study at the beginning of the film. In short he shows himself to be aware of the genre of academic study and though, like any academic study, his findings can be critiqued, they should be critiqued on the right terms. His book (2005) also plays a role here. In the teaching being referred to here, students follow the film by engaging in discussion of these matters.
4. I came to know one of the University of Manchester's librarians, Ian Fishwick, not because of some formal connection made on campus but because we live in the same town and often share a commute. This link became strong enough to produce a jointly-authored book chapter on IL pedagogy (Whitworth, Fishwick and McIndoe 2011).

5. This book is an example: for all that the ideas are mine, building on the work of other individual authors, the book could still not have come into existence without more institutional forms of support from at least three universities: The University of Manchester, Queensland University of Technology and, in a lesser but still significant way, Charles Sturt University. The same will have been true of almost all the other books cited here.

6. MOSI comes from the name of one of the project partners, the Museum Of Science and Industry. 'ALONG' is then a backronym. The project was funded by JISC (*www.jisc.ac.uk*).

7. Formal educational providers are those which offer accredited courses of some kind. A non-formal provider is an organisation with an educational mandate but which does not offer courses, such as museums, libraries and public service broadcasters. See Garnett and Ecclesfield (2012).

8. *www.whalleyrange.org* (last accessed 6th August 2013).

9. see *www.populartechnology.org* and also the Detroit Digital Justice Coalition (djc.org)

10. A cycle implies that one simply moves round and round the same points, whereas with a spiral there is a sense of progression.

Bibliography

Abrahamsson, B. (1993). *Why Organizations? How and Why People Organize.* London: Sage.

ACRL (Association of College and Research Libraries) (2000) *Information Literacy Competency Standards for Higher Education.*

Adamson, W. L. (1980). *Hegemony and Revolution: A Study of Antonio Gramsci's Political and Cultural Theory.* Berkeley: University of California Press.

Aharony, N. (2010). Information literacy in the professional literature: an exploratory analysis. *Aslib proceedings,* 62(3), p. 261.

Alexandria Proclamation (2006), ed. S. Garner: *Report of the High-Level Colloquium on Information Literacy and Lifelong Learning.* Alexandria: Egypt.

American Library Association (1989). *American Library Association Presidential Committee on Information Literacy: Final Report.* Chicago: ALA.

Andersen, J. (2006). The public sphere and discursive activities: information literacy as sociopolitical skills. *Journal of documentation* 62/2, p. 213.

Andersen, J. (2008). The concept of genre in information studies. *Annual review of information science and technology* 42/1, 339–367.

Andretta, S. (2005). *Information literacy: A practitioner's guide.* Oxford: Chandos.

Andretta, S. (2007a) Information literacy: the functional literacy for the 21st century. In S. Andretta, ed. *Change and Challenge: Information literacy for the 21st century.* Adelaide: Auslib (pp. 1–13).

Andretta, S. (2007b). Phenomenography: a conceptual framework for information literacy education. *Aslib proceedings* 59/2, 152–168.

Andretta, S. (2011). Information literacy: a term whose time has passed? *Journal of Information Literacy,* 5(1), 1–4.

Andretta, S. (2012). Facilitating information literacy education (FILE). *Handbook of library training practice and development* 3, 49–75.

Angus, I. (2001). *Emergent Politics: An essay on social movements and democracy*. Winnipeg: Arbeiter Ring.

Argyris, C. and Schön, D. (1999). *On Organizational Learning*. Oxford: Blackwell.

Babalhavaeji, F., Isfandyari-Moghaddam, A., Aqili, S. and Shakooii, A. (2009) Quality assessment of academic library performance: the case of an Iranian academic library. *Malaysian Journal of Library and Information Science* 14/2, 51–81.

Badke, W. B. (2008) A rationale for information literacy as a credit-bearing discipline. *Journal of Information Literacy* 2/1.

Badke, W. B. (2011). Why information literacy is invisible. *Communications in Information Literacy*, 4/2, 129–141.

Badke, W. B. (2012) *Teaching Research Processes: The faculty role in the development of skilled student researchers*. Oxford: Chandos.

Bailey, P., Hunsberger, M. and Hayden, K. A. (1998). The diverse faces of critical literacy: only knowledge or also social action? *Alberta Journal of Educational Research*, 44/2, 120.

Bakhtin, M. (1981). *The Dialogic Imagination: Four Essays by M. M. Bakhtin*. Ed. M. Holquist. Austin: University of Texas Press.

Bakhtin, M. (1984). *Problems of Dostoevsky's Poetics*. tr. C. Emerson. Minneapolis: University of Minnesota Press.

Bakhtin, M. (1986). *Speech Genres and Other Late Essays*. Ed. C. Emerson & M. Holquist. Austin: University of Texas Press.

Bartlett, F. (1932) *Remembering: A study in experimental and social psychology*. Cambridge: Cambridge University Press.

Basili, C. (2011). A framework for analyzing and comparing information literacy policies in European countries. *Library Trends* 60/2, 395–418.

Bates, M. (1986): Subject Access to Online Catalogs: A Design Model, *Journal of the American Society for Information Science* 37, 357–376.

Bawden, David (2001) Information and digital literacies: a review of concepts. *Journal of documentation*, 57/2, 218–259.

Becher, T., & Trowler, P. (1989). *Academic tribes and territories*. Buckingham, UK: SRHE/Open University Press.

Becker, H. (1967) Whose Side Are We On? *Social Problems* 14, 241.

Beetham, H., McGill, L. and Littlejohn, A. 2009. *Thriving in the 21st Century: Learning Literacies for the Digital Age*. Glasgow, UK: The Caledonian Academy.

Behrens, S. (1994). A conceptual analysis and historical overview of information literacy. *College and Research Libraries* 55/4, 309–322.

Black, A. (1996). *A new history of the English public library: social and intellectual contexts, 1850–1914.* Leicester: Leicester University Press.

Blaug, R. (1999a). *Democracy Real and Ideal: Discourse Ethics and Radical Politics.* Albany, NY: SUNY Press.

Blaug, R. (1999b). The Tyranny of the Visible: Problems in the Evaluation of Anti-Institutional Radicalism. *Organization* 6/1, 33–56.

Blaug, R. (2007) Cognition in a Hierarchy. *Contemporary Political Theory* 6/1, 24–44.

Blaug, R. (2010). *How Power Corrupts.* London: Palgrave Macmillan.

Blaug, R. and Schwarzmantel, J. (2001) *Democracy: A Reader.* Edinburgh: University of Edinburgh Press.

Bohman, J. (1989). System and Lifeworld: Habermas and the Problem of Holism. *Philosophy and Social Criticism* 15, 381–401.

Booth, S. (1997). On phenomenography, learning and teaching. *Higher Education Research and Development* 16/2, 135–158.

Bourdieu, P. (1977). *Outline of a Theory of Practice,* translated by R. Nice. Cambridge: Cambridge University Press.

Bourdieu, P. (1990). *Homo academicus.* Stanford, CA: Stanford University Press.

Brandt, D. S. (2001). Information Technology Literacy: Task Knowledge and Mental Models. *Library Trends* 50/1, 73–86.

Breivik, P. S. (1985). A vision in the making: putting libraries back in the information society. *American Libraries* 16/10, 723–723.

Breivik, P. S. (1986). Library based learning in an information society. *New Directions for Higher Education* 56, 47–55.

Breivik, P. S. (1991). Information literacy. *Bulletin of the Medical Library Association* 79/2, 226.

Breivik, P. S. and Gee, E. G. (1989) *Information Literacy: Revolution in the Library,* American Council on Education, Washington DC.

Breivik, P. S. and Gee, E. G. (2006) *Higher Education in the Internet Age: Libraries Creating a Strategic Edge.* Westport, CT: Praeger.

Breure, L. (2001) *Development of the Genre Concept.* Utrecht, NL: Department of Information Science, University of Utrecht.

Bridgland, A. and Whitehead, M. (2005). Perspectives On ... Information Literacy in the "E" Environment: An Approach for Sustainability. *The Journal of Academic Librarianship* 31/1, 54.

Broidy, E. (2007): Gender and the Politics of Information: Reflections on Bringing the Library into the Classroom. *Library Trends* 56/2, 494–508.

Brookfield, S. (1995). *Becoming a Critically Reflective Practitioner.* London: Sage.

Bruce, B. C., & Bishop, A. P. (2008). New literacies and community inquiry. *The handbook of research in new literacies*, 699–742.

Bruce, C. S. (1997): *The Seven Faces of Information Literacy*. Adelaide: Auslib.

Bruce, C. S. (2008): *Informed Learning*. Chicago: ACRL.

Bruce, C. S. (2013) Information literacy research and practice: an experiential perspective. In Kurbanoglu, S., Grassian, E., Mizrachi, D., Catts, R., Akça, S., & Spiranec, Sonja (Eds.) *Proceedings of the European Conference on Information Literacy (ECIL 2013)*, Hacettepe University Department of Information Management, Istanbul, Turkey, p. 6.

Bruce, C. S., Edwards, S. L. and Lupton, M. (2006) Six frames for information literacy education. *Italics 5/1*.

Bruner, J. S. (1973) *Beyond the Information Given: Studies in the Psychology of Knowing*. New York: Norton.

Bruner, J. S. (1986) *Actual Minds, Possible Worlds*. Cambridge, MA: Harvard University Press.

Bruns, A. (2009) From Prosumer to Produser: Understanding User-Led Content Creation. In *Transforming Audiences 2009*, 3–4 Sep, 2009, London.

Burchinal, L. G. (1976) The Communications Revolution: America's Third Century Challenge, in *The Future of Organizing Knowledge: Papers Presented at the Texas A & M University Library's Centennial Academic Assembly*, Sept. 24, 1976, Texas A & M University Library. (See also *http://personalpages.manchester.ac.uk/staff/drew.whitworth/burchinal.html*).

Burrell, G. (1997). *Pandemonium: Toward a Retro-Organisation Theory*. London: Sage.

Burkitt, I. (1999) *Bodies of Thought: Embodiment, Identity and Modernity*. London: Sage.

Bush, V. (1945) 'As We May Think', Atlantic Monthly, July: available at *http://www.theatlantic.com/doc/194507/bush* [last accessed 6th Dec 2013].

Calhoun, C., ed. (1992). *Habermas and the Public Sphere*. Cambridge, MA: MIT Press.

Carr, W. & Kemmis, S. (1986). *Becoming Critical: Knowing Through Action Research*. Geelong: Deakin University Press.

Cervero, R. and Wilson, A. (1998): *Working the Planning Table: The Political Practice of Adult Education*. San Francisco: Jossey-Bass.

Chang, C. and Liu, E. (2011). Exploring the Media Literacy of Taiwanese Elementary School Students. *The Asia Pacific Education Researcher* 20/3, 616–623.

Checkland, P. and Holwell, S. (1998) *Information systems and information systems: Making sense of the field,* Wiley.

Chen, K., Lin, P. and Chang, S. (2011) Integrating library instruction into a problem-based learning curriculum. *Aslib Proceedings 63/5.*

Chou, T., Chen, J. and Pu, C. (2005): Collective Actions: The Case of e-Government Development. *9th Pacific Asia Conference on Information Systems* (PACIS 2005).

Chou, T., Chen, J. and Pu, C. Exploring the collective actions of public servants in e-government development. *Decision Support Systems* 45/2, 251–265.

Clarke, P. B. (1996). *Deep Citizenship.* London: Pluto Press.

Conant, J. B. (1951) *Science and Common Sense.* New Haven, CT: Yale University Press.

Cover, T. and Thomas, J. (2012) *Elements of Information Theory.* London: Wiley.

Crawford, J. and Irving, C. (2011) Information literacy in the workplace and employability agenda. In A, Pope and G. Walton, (eds). *Information literacy: infiltrating the agenda, challenging minds.* Oxford: Chandos (pp. 45–70).

Cresswell, J., and Baerveldt, C. (2011). Bakhtin's realism and embodiment: Towards a revision of the dialogical self. *Culture & Psychology* 17/2, 263–277.

Cresswell, J., and Teucher, U. (2011). The body and language: MM Bakhtin on ontogenetic development. *New Ideas in Psychology* 29/2, 106–118.

Curl, S. R. (2001). Subramanyam revisited: Creating a new model for information literacy instruction. *College & Research Libraries* 62/5, 455–464.

De Boer, A. L., Bothma, T., and du Toit, P. (2011). Enhancing information literacy through the application of whole brain strategies. *Libri* 61(1), 67–75.

Demo, William (1986) *The Idea of "Information Literacy" in the Age of High-Tech,* Tompkins Cortland Community College, New York.

Dentler, R. A. (2002). *Practicing sociology: selected fields.* Greenwood Publishing Group.

Detmering, R. (2010). Exploring the Political Dimensions of Information Literacy through Popular Film. *Portal* 10/3, 265–282.

Dewey, J. (1909). *Moral principles in education*. Houghton Mifflin Company.

Diani, M. (1995). *Green Networks: A Structural Analysis of the Italian Environmental Movement*. Edinburgh: Edinburgh University Press.

DiMaggio, P. and Powell, W. (1983). The Iron Cage Revisited: Institutional Isomorphism and Collective Rationality in Organizational Fields. *American Sociological Review* 48/2, 147–160.

Do or Die, eds. (2000): *Do or Die volume 8: voices from the ecological resistance*. Brighton: Do or Die.

Domine, V. (2011) Think Global, Act Local: Expanding the Agenda for Media Literacy Education in the United States. *Library Trends* 60/2, p. 440–453.

Dorner, D. G. and Gorman, G. E. (2011). Contextual factors affecting learning in Laos and the implications for information literacy education. *Information Research* 16/2.

Douglas, Mary (1986): *How Institutions Think*, Syracuse UP: Syracuse.

Downing, J. D. (1988). Trouble in the backyard: Soviet media reporting on the Afghanistan conflict. *Journal of Communication* 38/2, 5–32.

Dudziak, E. A. (2010). Competência Informacional: análise evolucionária das tendências da pesquisa e produtividade científica em âmbito mundial. *Informação & Informação* 15/2.

Easterby-Smith, M., Snell, R. and Gherardi, S. (1998) Organizational Learning: Diverging Communities of Practice? *Management Learning* 29/3, 259–272.

Edwards, S. L. (2006). *Panning for gold: Information literacy and the net lenses model*. Adelaide: Auslib Press.

Eisenberg, M. B., & Berkowitz, R. E. (1990). *Information Problem Solving: The Big Six Skills Approach to Library & Information Skills Instruction*. Norwood, NJ: Ablex.

Eisenberg, M. B., Lowe, C. A., & Spitzer, K. L. (2004). *Information literacy: Essential skills for the information age*. Westport, CT: Greenwood.

Elmborg, J. (2002). Teaching at the desk: toward a reference pedagogy. *Portal* 2/3, 455–464.

Elmborg, J. (2006). Critical information literacy: Implications for instructional practice. *Journal of Academic Librarianship* 32/2, 192–199.

Elmborg, J. (2011). Libraries as the Spaces Between us. *Reference and User Services Quarterly*, 50/4, 338–350.

Engeström, Y., Miettinen, R. and Punamäki, R.-L. (eds) (1999) *Perspectives on Activity Theory*. Cambridge, UK: Cambridge University Press.

Evans, J. (1989) *Bias in Human Reasoning: Causes and Consequences.* Mahwah, NJ: Lawrence Erlbaum.

Eubanks, V. (2011). *Digital dead end: Fighting for social justice in the information age.* Cambridge, MA: MIT Press.

Eubanks, V. (2013). Keynote speech at *How to Avoid Digital Dead Ends: A Teaching and Learning Conference,* Blackburn College, UK.

Fay, B. (1975). *Social Theory and Political Practice.* London: Allen & Unwin.

Feenberg, A. (2002) *Transforming Technology: A Critical Theory Revisited.* Oxford, UK: Oxford University Press.

Ferguson, S. (2012). Are Public Libraries Developers of Social Capital? A Review of Their Contribution and Attempts to Demonstrate It. *The Australian library journal,* 61/1, 22.

Fleck, L. (1935). *The Genesis and Development of a Scientific Fact.* Chicago, IL: University of Chicago Press.

Forester, J., ed. (1985). *Critical Theory and Public Life.* Cambridge, MA: MIT Press.

Foster, S. (1993) Information Literacy: Some Misgivings. *American Libraries* 24, 344.

Foucault, M. (1980) *Power/Knowledge.* New York, NY: Random House.

Foucault, M., & Miskowiec, J. (1986). Of other spaces. *diacritics,* 16(1), 22–27.

Fourie, I. (2009). Learning from research on the information behaviour of healthcare professionals: a review of the literature 2004–2008 with a focus on emotion. *Health information and libraries journal,* 26/3, 171–186.

Fourie, I. (2011). Personal information management (PIM), reference management and mind maps: the way to creative librarians? *Library Hi Tech* 29/4, 764–771.

Fransella, F. and Dalton, P. (2000) *Personal Construct Counselling in Action.* London: Sage.

Franz, J. (1994) Managing intricacy in phenomenographic inquiry. In *Phenomenography: philosophy and practice.* Brisbane, Centre for Applied Environmental and Social Education (pp. 175–182).

Fraser, N. (1992). Rethinking the Public Sphere: A Contribution to the Critique of Actually Existing Democracy. In C. Calhoun, ed.: *Habermas and the Public Sphere.* Cambridge, MA: MIT Press. (pp. 109–142).

Freeman, J. (1984). The Tyranny of Structurelessness. In *Untying the Knot: Feminism, Anarchism and Organization.* London: Dark Star Press.

Freire, P. (1970). *Pedagogy of the Oppressed*. Harmondsworth: Penguin.

Friedland, R. and Alford, R. (1991). Bringing Society Back In: Symbols, Practices and Institutional Contradictions. In W. Powell and P. DiMaggio, eds.: *The New Institutionalism in Organizational Analysis*. Chicago: University of Chicago Press.

Frisch, A., Camerini, L., Diviani, N. and Schulz, J. (2011). Defining and measuring health literacy: how can we profit from other literacy domains? *Health Promotion International*, 27/1, 117–126.

Fry, H., Ketteridge, S., & Marshall, S. (Eds.). (2008). *A handbook for teaching and learning in higher education: enhancing academic practice*. London: Routledge.

Gardiner, M. E. (2004). Wild publics and grotesque symposiums: Habermas and Bakhtin on dialogue, everyday life and the public sphere. *The Sociological Review*, 52/1, 28–48.

Gardner, D. P. (1983). *A nation at risk*. Washington, D. C.: The National Commission on Excellence in Education, US Department of Education.

Garnett, F., & Ecclesfield, N. (2012). Towards a framework for co-creating open scholarship. *Research in Learning Technology*, 19.

Garvey, T. G. (2000). The value of opacity: A Bakhtinian analysis of Habermas's discourse ethics. *Philosophy and Rhetoric* 33/4, 370–390.

Gastil, J. (1993). *Democracy in Small Groups: Participation, Decision Making and Communication*. Philadelphia: New Society.

Geijer, L. and Olstedt, E. (2009) Vocational Education and Academia: Focus group discussions over time. In Junefelt, K. and Nordin, P., eds: *Proceedings from the Second International Interdisciplinary Conference on Perspectives and Limits of Dialogism in Mikhail Bakhtin*, Stockholm, June 3–5. 2009. (pp. 157–170).

Gherardi, S., Nicolini, D. and Odella, F. (1998). Toward a Social Understanding of How People Learn in Organizations: The Notion of Situated Curriculum. *Management Learning* 29/3, 273–297.

Gibson, J. J. (1979) *The Ecological Approach to Visual Perception*. Boston, MA: Houghton Mifflin.

Goldacre, B. (2008). *Bad Science*. London: HarperCollins.

Graeber, D. (2012). *Debt: The first 5,000 years*. New York: Melville House.

Gramsci, A. (1971). *Prison Notebooks*. London: Lawrence & Wishart.

Grafstein, Ann (2007). Information Literacy and Technology: An Examination of Some Issues. *Portal* 7/1, 51.

Grix, J. (2002). Introducing students to the generic terminology of social research. *Politics* 22/3, 175–186.

Gunton, L. (2011). Religious information literacy: Using information to learn in church community. *Australian Library Journal*, 60(2), 155–164.

Gustavsen, B. (2001) Theory and Practice: The Mediating Discourse, in Reason, P. and Bradbury, H. (eds) *Handbook of Action Research*. London: Sage (pp. 17–26).

Gwyer, R., Stubbings, R. and Walton, G. (eds.) *The Road to Information Literacy: Librarians as Facilitators of Learning*. Berlin, de Gruyter.

Habermas, J. (1984). *The Theory of Communicative Action vol 1: Reason and the Rationalization of Society*. London: Heinemann.

Habermas, J. (1987). *The Theory of Communicative Action vol 2: Lifeworld and System – A Critique of Functionalist Reason*. Cambridge, UK: Polity Press.

Habermas, J. (1989). *The Structural Transformation of the Public Sphere: An Inquiry into a Category of Bourgeois Society*. Cambridge, MA: MIT Press.

Habermas, J. (1993) *Justification and Application: Remarks on Discourse Ethics*. Cambridge, UK: Polity Press.

Habermas, J. (1996). *Between Facts and Norms: Contributions to a Discourse Theory of Law and Democracy*. Cambridge: Polity Press.

Hall, E. T., et al (1968). Proxemics. *Current anthropology* 1968, 83–108.

Hamelink, C. (1976). An alternative to news. *Journal of Communication* 20, 120–123.

Harding, S. (1995). "Strong objectivity": A response to the new objectivity question. *Synthese*, 104/3, 331–349.

Harris, B. R. (2008). Communities as Necessity in Information Literacy Development: Challenging the Standards. *Journal of Academic Librarianship*, 34/3, 248–255.

Hasselgren, B. and Beach, D. (1997) Phenomenography — a "good-for-nothing brother" of phenomenology? Outline of an analysis. *Higher Education Research and Development* 16/2, 191–202.

Hepworth, M. and Walton, G. (2009). *Teaching information literacy for inquiry-based learning*. Oxford: Chandos.

Herman, E. (1998). The propaganda model revisited. In McChesney, R., Meiksins Wood, E. and Foster, J. B. (Eds.). *Capitalism and the information age: the political economy of the global communication revolution*. (pp. 191–205). New York, NY: Monthly Review Press.

Hess, C. and Ostrom, E. (eds) (2007) *Understanding Knowledge as a Commons: From Theory to Practice*. Cambridge, MA: MIT Press.

Hirschkop, K. (2004). Justice and drama: on Bakhtin as a complement to Habermas. *The Sociological Review, 52/1*, 49–66.

Hoffmann, D. A., and LaBonte, K. (2012). Meeting information literacy outcomes: Partnering with faculty to create effective information literacy assessment. *Journal of Information Literacy*, 6(2), 70–85.

Holub, R. (1992). *Antonio Gramsci: Beyond Marxism and Postmodernism*. London: Routledge.

Holquist, M. (2002). *Dialogism: Bakhtin and his world*. London: Routledge.

Holquist, M. (2009) The role of chronotope in dialogue. In Junefelt, K. and Nordin, P., eds: *Proceedings from the Second International Interdisciplinary Conference on Perspectives and Limits of Dialogism in Mikhail Bakhtin*, Stockholm, June 3–5 2009. (pp. 9–17).

Horkheimer, M. and Adorno, T. (1972). *The Dialectic of Enlightenment*. New York: Seabury.

Horton Jr, F. W. (2011). Information Literacy Advocacy—Woody's Ten Commandments. *Library Trends* 60/2, 262–276.

Hughes, H., Bruce, C. and Edwards, S. (2007) Models for reflection and learning: A culturally inclusive response to the information literacy imbalance. In S. Andretta, ed. *Change and Challenge: Information literacy for the 21st century*. Adelaide: Auslib (pp. 59–84).

Hultgren, F. (2009) *Approaching the Future: A study of Swedish school leavers' information-related activities*. Borås: Valfrid.

Huvila, Isto (11/2010). Information sources and perceived success in corporate finance. *Journal of the American Society for Information Science and Technology*, 61/11, 2219.

Inhaber, H. (1976) *Environmental Indices*. New York: Wiley.

Ipri, T. (2010). Introducing transliteracy: What does it mean to academic libraries? *College & Research Libraries News* 71/10, 532–567.

Julien, H., and Pecoskie, J. J. (2009). Librarians' experiences of the teaching role: Grounded in campus relationships. *Library & Information Science Research*, 31/3, 149–154.

Julien, H. and Williamson, K. (2011). Discourse and practice in information literacy and information seeking: Gaps and opportunities. *Information Research* 16(1).

Kakkonen, A. and A. Virrankoski (2010). Implementation of the Finnish University Libraries National Information Literacy Recommendation into academic studies at the Kumpula Science Library, University of Helsinki. *New Library World* 111/11–12, 493–502.

Kammer, J. and Thompson, T. (2011) Information Literate Avatars: Resource-Based Learning in Second Life. In Mackey, T. and Jacobson, T. (eds): *Teaching Information Literacy Online*, New York NY, Neal-Schulman. (pp. 109–132).

Kanyengo, C. (2010). Information and communication: a library's local response to HIV/AIDS in Zambia. *Health information and libraries journal*, 27/1, 57.

Kapitzke, C. (2003) Information literacy: a positivist epistemology and a politics of outformation. *Educational Theory* 53/1, 37–53.

Keen, A. (2007) *The Cult of the Amateur: How Today's Internet Is Killing Our Culture and Assaulting Our Economy*. London: Nicholas Brearley.

Kelly, G. (1963). *A theory of personality: The psychology of personality constructs*. New York: Norton.

Kemmis, S. (2001) Exploring the relevance of critical theory for action research: Emancipatory action research in the footsteps of Jürgen Habermas. In Reason, P. and Bradbury, H. (eds) *Handbook of Action Research*. London: Sage (pp. 91–102).

Kemmis, S. and Grootenboer, P. (2008) Situation praxis in practice. In Kemmis, S. and Smith, T.J. (Eds), *Enabling Praxis*, Sense Publishers, Rotterdam (pp. 37–62).

Kempcke, K. (2002): The Art of War for Librarians: Academic Culture, Curriculum Reform, and Wisdom from Sun Tzu: *Portal* 2/4.

Kenny, P. (2009). *News agencies as content providers and purveyors of news: A mediahistoriographical study on the development and diversity of wire services*. Doctoral dissertation: University of Stellenbosch.

Klein, H. and Truex, D. (1996). Discourse Analysis: An Approach to the Investigation of Organizational Emergence. In B. Holmqvist, P. Andersen, H. Klein and R. Posner, eds: *Signs of Work: Semiotics and Information Processing in Organizations*. Berlin: de Gruyter.

Knight, P. (2000) *Conspiracy Culture: From the Kennedy Assassination to the X-Files*. London, UK: Routledge.

Korten, D. (1990). *Getting to the 21st Century: Voluntary Action and the Global Agenda*. Westview, CT: Kumarian.

Kuhlthau, C.C. (1993). *Seeking meaning: A process approach to library and information services*. Westport, CT: Greenwood.

Kuhn, T. (1970) *The Structure of Scientific Revolutions*, 2nd edn. Chicago, IL: University of Chicago Press.

Kurbanoğlu, S. (2012). An Analysis of Concept of Information Literacy. Paper delivered at the IFLA/UNESCO conference on Media and Information Literacy, June 2012, Moscow.

Lancaster, F.W. (1970) User Education: The Next Major Thrust in Information Science. *Journal of Education for Librarianship* 11, 55–63.

Landry, C., Morley, D., Southwood, R. and Wright, P. (1985) *What a Way to Run a Railroad: An analysis of radical failure*. London: Comedia.

Laurillard, D. (2002) *Rethinking University Teaching*, 2nd edn. London, UK: Routledge Falmer.

Lavoie, D., Rosman, A. and Sharma, S. (2011) Information Literacy by Design: Recalibrating Graduate Professional Asynchronous Online Programs. In Mackey, T. and Jacobson, T. (eds): *Teaching Information Literacy Online*, New York NY, Neal-Schulman. (pp. 133–158).

Leckie, G. J. (1996). Desperately seeking citations: Uncovering faculty assumptions about the undergraduate research process. *The Journal of Academic Librarianship* 22/3, 201–208.

Leckie, G. and Fullerton, A. (1999) The Roles of Academic Librarians in Fostering a Pedagogy for Information Literacy. *Proceedings of the ACRL Ninth National Conference* (pp. 8–11).

Levine, P. (2007). Collective Action, Civic Engagement and the Knowledge Commons. In C. Hess and E. Ostrom (eds.): *Understanding Knowledge as a Commons: From Theory to Practice*. Cambridge, MA: MIT Press (pp. 247–276).

Limberg, L., Sundin, O., and Talja, S. (2012). Three theoretical perspectives on information literacy. *Human IT* 11/2, 93–130.

Lin, P., Cheng, H., Liao, W. and Yen, Y. (2012) A Study of the Mobile Technology Literacy Indicators in Taiwan. *Proceedings of the International Conference on Emerging Computation and Information teChnologies for Education (ECICE 2012)*.

Linell, P. (2009). *Rethinking language, mind, and world dialogically: Interactional and contextual theories of human sense-making*. IAP, Charlotte, NC.

Lloyd, A. (2006): Information literacy landscapes: an emerging picture. *Journal of Documentation* 62/5, 570–583.

Lloyd, A. (2007): Learning to Put Out the Red Stuff: Becoming Information Literate through Discursive Practice. *Library Quarterly* 77/2, 181–198.

Lloyd, A. (2010). *Information literacy landscapes: Information literacy in education, workplace and everyday contexts*. Oxford: Chandos.

Lloyd, A. (2010b). Framing information literacy as information practice: site ontology and practice theory. *Journal of documentation*, 66/2, 245.

Lloyd, A. (2012). Information literacy as a socially enacted practice: Sensitising themes for an emerging perspective of people-in-practice. *Journal of Documentation* 68/6, 772–783.

Lloyd, A. (2013) Lost in Translation? Interactions, impact and practice of information literacy. What does this mean for the workplace? Keynote speech, *i3: Information: interactions and impact*, Robert Gordon University, Aberdeen, June 25–28, 2013.

Lloyd, A., & Williamson, K. (2008). Towards an understanding of information literacy in context: Implications for research. *Journal of Librarianship and Information Science* 40/1, 3–12.

Lonka, K. (2012) Engaging Learning Environments for the Future. In R. Gwyer, R. Stubbings and G. Walton (eds.) *The Road to Information Literacy: Librarians as Facilitators of Learning*. Berlin, de Gruyter (pp. 15–29).

Loughran, J. J. (2002). *Developing reflective practice: Learning about teaching and learning through modelling*. London: Routledge.

Luckin, R. (2010): *Redesigning Learning Contexts: Technology-rich, learner-centred ecologies*, London, Routledge.

Luckin, R., Clark, W., Garnett, F., Whitworth, A., Akass, J., Cook, J., Day, P., Ecclesfield, N., Hamilton, T. and Robertson, J. (2010). Learner-generated contexts: A framework to support the effective use of technology to support learning. In Lee, M. W. and McLoughlin, C. (eds): *Web 2.0- Based E-Learning: Applying Social Informatics for Tertiary Teaching*. Hershey PA: IGI Global.

Luna-Reyes, L. F., Zhang, J., Gil-García, J. R., & Cresswell, A. M. (2005). Information systems development as emergent socio-technical change: a practice approach. *European Journal of Information Systems*, 14/1, 93–105.

Lundh, A., Limberg, L. and Lloyd, A. (2013) Swapping settings: researching information literacy in workplace and in educational contexts. *Information Research* 18/3.

Lupton, M. (2004): The *Learning Connection: Information Literacy and the Student Experience*. Adelaide: Auslib.

Luyt, B. and Azura, I. (2010). The sigh of the information literate: an examination of the potential for oppression in information literacy. *Information Research* 15/3.

Lyotard, F. (1984). *The Postmodern Condition: A report on knowledge*. Minneapolis: University of Minnesota Press.

Macevičiūtė, E. (2006). Information needs research in Russia and Lithuania, 1965–2003. *Information Research* 11/3.

Mackey, T. and Jacobson, T. (eds): *Teaching Information Literacy Online*, New York NY, Neal- Schulman.

March, J., Olsen, J. and Christensen, S. (1976) *Ambiguity and Choice in Organizations*. Bergen, Norway: Universitetsforlaget.

Marcum. J. (2002) Rethinking information literacy. *Library and Information Quarterly* 72/1.

Marcuse, H. (1964). *One-Dimensional Man: Studies in the Ideology of Advanced Industrial Society*. London: Routledge and Kegan Paul.

Mark, A. E. (2011a). Privileging Peer Review: Implications for Undergraduates. *Communications in Information Literacy* 5/1, 4–8.

Mark, A. E. (2011b). Format as a false judge of credibility. *Communications in Information Literacy*, 5/1, 21–37.

Markless, S. (2009). A New Conception of Information Literacy for the Digital Environment in Higher Education. *Nordic Journal of Information Literacy in Higher Education*, 1/1.

Markless, S. and Streatfield, D. (2007) Three decades of information literacy: redefining the parameters. In Andretta, S. (ed.), *Change and Challenge: Information Literacy for the 21st Century*. Adelaide, Australia: Auslib; pp. 15–36.

Marton, F. (1981). Phenomenography—describing conceptions of the world around us. *Instructional science*, 10/2, 177–200.

Marton, F. (1995). Cognosco ergo sum. Reflections on reflections. *Nordisk Pedagogik*, 15/3, 165–180.

Marton, F. and Booth, S. (1997) *Learning and awareness*. Mahwah, NJ: Lawrence Erlbaum.

Marton, F., Dall'Alba, G. and Beaty, E. (1993). Conceptions of learning. *Journal of Educational Research* 19, 277–299.

Matusov, E. (2011). Irreconcilable differences in Vygotsky's and Bakhtin's approaches to the social and the individual: An educational perspective. *Culture & Psychology* 17/1, 99–119.

McCarthy, T. (1984). *The Critical Theory of Jürgen Habermas*. Cambridge: Polity Press.

McCrank, L. J. (1991). Information literacy: A bogus bandwagon? *Library Journal* 116/8, 38–42.

McFarlane, A. (ed.) (1997) *Information Technology and Authentic Learning*. London, UK: Routledge.

McGuinness, C. (2007). Exploring Strategies for Integrated Information Literacy: From "Academic Champions" to Institution-Wide Change. *Communications in information literacy* 1/1, 26–38.

Medvedev, P. N. (1985). *The Formal Method in Literary Scholarship: A Critical Introduction to Sociological Poetics*, tr. A. J. Wehrle. Cambridge MA: Harvard University Press.

Melucci, A. (1989) *Nomads of the Present: Social Movements and Individual Needs in Contemporary Society*. London: Century Hutchinson.

Melucci, A. (1996). *Challenging Codes: Collective action in the information age.* Cambridge: Cambridge University Press.

Meyer, J. and Rowan, B. (1991) Institutionalised Organizations: Formal Structure as Myth and Ceremony. In Powell, W. and DiMaggio, P., eds: *The New Institutionalism in Organizational Analysis,* Chicago: University of Chicago Press.

Mezirow, J. (Ed.). (1990): *Fostering critical reflection in adulthood: A guide to transformative and emancipatory learning.* San Francisco, CA: Jossey-Bass.

Miller, C. R. (1984). Genre as social action. *Quarterly Journal of Speech,* 70, 151–167.

Mintzberg, H. (1989) *Mintzberg on Management.* London, UK: Collier Macmillan.

Misztal, B. A. (2003). Durkheim on Collective Memory. *Journal of Classical Sociology* 3/2, 123–143.

Morgan, G. (1999) *Images of Organization,* 2nd edn. London, UK: Sage.

Morson, G. S. and Emerson, C. (1990). *Mikhail Bakhtin: Creation of a Prosaics.* Stanford, CA: Stanford University Press.

Mutch, Alistair (1997): Information Literacy: An exploration. *International Journal of Information Management* 17/5, 377–386.

Nara, Yumiko (2007). Information Literacy and Everyday Life Risks in *Knowledge-Based Intelligent Information and Engineering Systems: KES 2007-WIRN 2007: 11th International Conference,* Vietri sul Mare, Italy, September 12–14, 2007.

Nevison, J. (1976). Computing in the liberal arts college. *Science* 194: 396–402.

Ngoh, L. N. (2009). Health literacy: A barrier to pharmacist–patient communication and medication adherence. *Journal of the American Pharmacists Association* 49/5, 132–149.

Nielsen, G. M. (2002). *The Norms of Answerability: Social Theory Between Bakhtin and Habermas.* Albany, NY: SUNY Press.

Norton, F. (2008) Using library and museum materials in the pursuit of scientific literacy and public engagement, keynote speech, *LILAC '08 conference,* Liverpool, UK.

O'Connor, L. (2009). Information literacy as professional legitimation: a critical analysis. *Journal of Education for Library and Information Science* (50/2), 79–89.

O'Farrill, R. T. (2008). Information Literacy and Knowledge Management: Preparations for an Arranged Marriage. *Libri* 58, 155–171.

O'Farrill, R. (2008b). *Conceptions of effective information use and learning in a tele-health organization: a phenomenographic study of information literacy and knowledge management at work.* PhD thesis, Robert Gordon University, Aberdeen, Scotland.

Oladokun, O. and Aina, L. (2011) ODL and the Impact of Digital Divide on Information Access in Botswana. *International Review of Research in Open and Distance Learning* 12/6.

Orlikowski, W. J., and Yates, J. (1994). Genre repertoire: The structuring of communicative practices in organizations. *Administrative Science Quarterly* 39/4, 541–574.

Orwell, G. (1950). Politics and the English Language. In *Shooting an Elephant: Collected Essays*, London, Secker & Warburg.

Outhwaite, W., ed. (1996) *The Habermas Reader.* Cambridge: Polity Press.

Owens M. (1976). State, government and libraries. *Library Journal* 101/1, 19–28.

Partridge, H., Bruce, C. and Tilley, C. (2008). Community information literacy: developing an Australian research agenda. *Libri* 58/2, 110.

Patterson, D. (2009). Information Literacy and Community College Students: Using New Approaches to Literacy Theory to Produce Equity. *The Library Quarterly*, 79/3, 343.

Pawley, C. (2003). Information Literacy: A Contradictory Coupling. *The Library Quarterly* 73/4, 422–452.

Pilerot, O., and Lindberg, J. (2011). The concept of information literacy in policy-making texts: an imperialistic project? *Library Trends* 60/2, 338–360.

Pinto, M., Cordon, J. and Diaz, R. (2010): Thirty years of information literacy (1977–2007): A terminological, conceptual and statistical analysis. *Journal of librarianship and information science*, 42/1, 3.

Pinto, M., Escalona-Fernández, M. and Pulgarín, A. (2013). Information literacy in social sciences and health sciences: a bibliometric study (1974–2011). *Scientometrics* 1–24.

Polanyi, M. (1962). Tacit knowing: Its bearing on some problems of philosophy. *Reviews of Modern Physics*, 34/4, 601–615.

Ponjuan, G. (2010). Guiding principles for the preparation of a national information literacy program. *The International Information and Library Review* 42, 91–97.

Pope, A. and Walton, G. (2011). Introduction. In A. Pope and G. Walton, eds: *Information Literacy: Infiltrating the Curriculum, Challenging Minds.* Oxford: Chandos (pp. 1–15).

Prague Declaration (2003). *Towards an information literate society.* Prague, Czech Republic: UNESCO.

Purdue, J. (2003) Stories, Not Information: Transforming Information Literacy. *Portal* 3/4.

Rader, H. (2002) Information literacy 1973–2002: a selected literature review. *Library Trends* 51/2.

Ragains, P. (2001). Infusing information literacy into the core curriculum: a pilot project at the University of Nevada, Reno. *Portal* 1/4, 391–407.

Ray, L. J. (1993). *Rethinking Critical Theory: Emancipation in the Age of Global Social Movements*. London: Sage.

Reason, P. and Bradbury, H. (eds) (2001). *Handbook of Action Research*. London, UK: Sage.

Reffell, P. and A. Whitworth (2002). Information fluency: critically examining IT education. *New Library World* 102/11–12, 427–35.

Riddle, J. S. (2003). Where's the library in service learning? Models for engaged library instruction. *Journal of Academic Librarianship* 29/2, 71–81.

Robins, K. and F. Webster (1987). *The Technical Fix: Education, Computers and Industry*. Basingstoke, UK: Macmillan.

Rockman, I. (ed.) (2004) *Integrating Information Literacy into the Higher Education Curriculum*. San Francisco, CA: Jossey-Bass.

Rockquemore, K. A. and Schaffer, R. H. (2000): Toward a Theory of Engagement: A Cognitive Mapping of Service-Learning Experiences, *Michigan Journal of Service Learning* 7, 14–24.

Rose, N. (1996). The death of the social? Reconfiguring the territory of government. *Economy and Society* 25/3, 327–356.

Roszak, T. (1994) *The Cult of Information*, 2nd edn. Berkeley, CA: University of California Press.

Russell, C. L. (2003). Minding the gap between methodological desires and practices. *OISE papers in STSE education*, 4, 125–134.

Russell. P., & O'Brien, T. (2009). The Irish Working Group on Information Literacy (WGIL), Part II: Report of cross-sector activity 2006–2008 and recommendations for action. *SCONUL Focus* 46, 101–104.

Sadler, E. and Given, L. M. (2007). Affordance theory: a framework for graduate students' information behavior. *Journal of documentation*, 63/1, 115.

Säljö, R. (1994). Minding action: Conceiving of the world versus participating in cultural practices. *Nordisk Pedagogik* 14/2, 71–80.

Säljö, R. (1997). Talk as data and practice—a critical look at phenomenographic inquiry and the appeal to experience. *Higher Education Research & Development* 16/2, 173–190.

Samson, P. and Pitt, D. (eds) (1999) *The Biosphere and Noösphere Reader: Global Environment, Society and Change.* London, UK: Routledge.

Saracevic, T. (1975). Relevance: A review of and a framework for the thinking on the notion of information science. *Journal of American Society for Information Science,* 26/6, 321–343.

Saracevic, T. (2007a). Relevance: A Review of the Literature and a Framework for Thinking on the Notion in Information Science: Part II: Nature and Manifestations of Relevance. *Journal of the American Society for Information Science and Technology* 58/3, 1915–1933.

Saracevic, T. (2007b). Relevance: A Review of the Literature and a Framework for Thinking on the Notion in Information Science. Part III: Behavior and effects of relevance. *Journal of the American Society for Information Science and Technology,* 58/3, 2126–2144.

Sayyad Abdi, E., Partridge, H., & Bruce, C. (2013). Website designers: how do they experience information literacy? *The Australian Library Journal,* 62/1, 40–52.

Schatzki, T. (2006), On organizations as they happen, *Organization Studies* 27/12, 1863–73.

Schön, D. (1991): *The Reflective Practitioner: How Professionals Think in Action.* Aldershot: Ashgate.

Schotter, A. (1981) *The Economic Theory of Social Institutions,* Cambridge: Cambridge University Press.

Schutz. A. (1964) *Alfred Schutz: collected papers.* Den Haag: Martinus Nijhoff.

Scoble, B. (2011). Contemporary technologies' influence on learning as a social practice. In A, Pope and G. Walton, (eds). *Information literacy: infiltrating the agenda, challenging minds.* Oxford: Chandos (pp. 219–252).

Scott, J. C. (1990). *Domination and the Arts of Resistance.* New Haven, CT: Yale University Press.

Seale, J. (2010). Digital Inclusion. A research briefing by the Technology Enhanced Learning Phase of the Teaching and Learning Research Programme. London Knowledge Lab, London, [online] Available at: *http://www.tlrp.org/docs/DigitalInclusion.pdf.*

Secker, J. and Coonan. E., eds. (2013) *Rethinking Information Literacy: a practical framework for supporting learning.* London: Facet.

Shapiro, J. J. and Hughes, S. K. (2004). Information Literacy as a Liberal Art: Enlightenment Proposals for a New Curriculum. *Educom Review* 31/2, 31–35.

Shenk, D. (1997). *Data Smog: Surviving the Information Glut*. New York, NY: Harper Collins.

Shenton, A. K. and Hay-Gibson, N. (2011). Information behaviour and information literacy: The ultimate in transdisciplinary phenomena? *Journal of librarianship and information science* 43/3, 166.

Shor, I. (1996): *When Students Have Power: Negotiating Authority in a Critical Pedagogy*, Chicago, IL: Chicago University Press.

Simmons, M. H. (2005) Librarians as Disciplinary Discourse Mediators: Using Genre Theory to Move Toward Critical Information Literacy. *Portal* 5/3.

Simon, N. (2010). *The participatory museum*. Museum 2.0.

Simon, R. (1991) *Gramsci's Political Thought: An Introduction*. London: Lawrence and Wishart.

Skagen, T., Torras, M. C., Kavli, S. M., Mikki, S., Hafstad, S., & Hunskår, I. (2009). Pedagogical Considerations in Developing an Online Tutorial in Information Literacy. *Communications in Information Literacy* 2/2, 84–98.

Smith, M. and Hepworth, M. (2012) Young people: A phenomenographic investigation into the ways they experience information. *Libri*, 62/2, 157–173.

Snavely, L. and Cooper, N. (1997). The information literacy debate. *The Journal of Academic Librarianship* 23/1, 9–14.

Špiranec, S., & Zorica, M. B. (2010). Information Literacy 2.0: hype or discourse refinement? *Journal of Documentation*, 66(1), 140–153.

Spurlock, M. (2005). *Don't Eat This Book*. London, UK: Penguin.

Standing Conference of National and University Libraries. (1999). *Information skills in higher education*. London: SCONUL. (A SCONUL Position Paper.)

Star, S. L. (1989). The structure of ill-structured solutions: heterogeneous problem-solving, boundary objects and distributed artificial intelligence. *Distributed artificial intelligence*, 2, 37–54.

Sturges, P. and Gastinger, A. (2010) Information literacy as a human right. *Libri* 60/3, 195–202.

Sundin, O. (2008). Negotiations on information-seeking expertise: A study of web-based tutorials for information literacy. *Journal of documentation* 64/1, 24–44.

Steinerová, J. (2010) Ecological dimensions of information literacy. *Information Research* 15/1.

Stevens, C. R. (2007) Beyond Preaching to the Choir: Information Literacy, Faculty Outreach, and Disciplinary Journals. *The Journal of academic librarianship* 33/2, 254.

Streatfield, D. and Markless, S. (2008). Evaluating the Impact of Information Literacy in Higher Education: Progress and Prospects. *Libri* 58, 102–109.

Tagliaventi, M., & Mattarelli, E. (2006). The role of networks of practice, value sharing, and operational proximity in knowledge flows between professional groups. *Human Relations* 59/3, 291– 319.

Tavares, R., Hepworth, M. and de Souza Costa, S. N. (2011). Investigating citizens' information needs through participative research: a pilot study in Candangolandia, Brazil. *Information development*, 27/2, 125.

Taylor, R. S. (1979): Reminiscing about the Future. *Library Journal* 104, 1875.

Teilhard de Chardin, P. (1959) *The Phenomenon of Man*. London: Collins.

Thompson, D. (2008). *Counterknowledge*. London: Atlantic.

Thompson, K. M. (2007). Furthering understanding of information literacy through the social study of information poverty. *Canadian journal of information and library science*, 31/1, 87.

Thornton, S. (2010). From 'Scuba Diving' to 'Jet Skiing'? Information Behavior, Political Science, and the Google Generation. *Journal of Political Science Education* 6, 353–368.

Tiemensma, L. (2012). Information Literacy Education in Higher Education Institutions in South Africa. In R. Gwyer, R. Stubbings and G. Walton (eds.) *The Road to Information Literacy: Librarians as Facilitators of Learning*. Berlin, de Gruyter (pp. 155–168).

Tippett, J., Handley, J. F. and Ravetz, J. (2007). Meeting the challenges of sustainable development—A conceptual appraisal of a new methodology for participatory ecological planning. *Progress in Planning*, 67(1).

Tolonen, E. and Toivonen, L. (2010). *Information Literacy State-of-the Art Report – Nordic Countries*. Online at *http://www.ifla.org/publications/information-literacy-state-of-the-art-reports* [*last accessed 6th Dec 2013*].

Tomic, T. (2010). The philosophy of information as an underlying and unifying theory of information science. *Information Research*, 15/4.

Torras i Calvo, M. (2012) Access to Knowledge as a Social Practice: Information Literacy Education for MA Students. In Lau, J., Tammaro, A. M., & Bothma, T. J. (Eds.). *Libraries driving access to knowledge*. Berlin: de Gruyter.

Tuominen, K., Savolainen, R. and Talja, S. (2005). Information Literacy as a Sociotechnical Practice. *Library Quarterly* 75/3, 329–345.

Turner, B. A. (1971). *Exploring the Industrial Subculture*. Basingstoke: Macmillan.

Urbinati, N. (1998) From the Periphery of Modernity: Antonio Gramsci's Theory of Subordination and Hegemony. *Political Theory* 26/3, 370–391.

Urquhart, C. (2010). Systematic reviewing, meta-analysis and meta-synthesis for evidence-based library and information science. *Information Research* 15/3.

Urquhart, C. and Rowley, J. (2007) Understanding student information behavior in relation to electronic information services: Lessons from longitudinal monitoring and evaluation, Part 2. *Journal of the American Society for Information Science and Technology*, 58/8, 1188.

van Dijck, J. (2010). Search engines and the production of academic knowledge. *International Journal of Cultural Studies* 13/6, 574.

Virkus, S. (2003). Information literacy in Europe: a literature review. *Information Research* 8/4.

Voloshinov, V. (1973) *Marxism and the Philosophy of Language*, tr. L. Matejka and I. Titunik, New York: Seminar.

Vygotsky, L. (1978): *Mind in society: The development of higher psychological processes*. Cambridge, MA: Harvard University Press.

Wall, D. (1999). *Earth First! and the Anti-Roads Movement: Radical environmentalism and comparative social movements*. London: Routledge.

Wandersee, J. H. (1990). Concept mapping and the cartography of cognition. *Journal of research in science teaching* 27/10, 923–936.

Ward, D. (2006) Revisioning Information Literacy for Lifelong Meaning. *Journal of Academic Librarianship* 32/4, 399.

Warschauer, M. (1999) *Electronic Literacies: Langauge, Culture and Power in Online Education*. Mahwah, NJ: Lawrence Erlbaum.

Watkins, J. and Russo, A. (2005) *Developing communities and collections with new media and information literacy*. In Proceedings 8th International Conference on Asian Digital Libraries (pp. 390–394).

Webber, S. (2010) Information literacy for the 21st century. *INFORUM* 16.

Weber, M. (1947). *The Theory of Social and Economic Organization*. Oxford: Oxford University Press.

Webster, F. (2002) *Theories of the Information Society*, 2nd edn. London, UK: Routledge.

Weiner, J. (2011) Is There a Difference Between Critical Thinking and Information Literacy? A Systematic Review 2000–2009. *Journal of Information Literacy* 5/2, 81–92.

Weiner, S. A. (2012) Institutionalising Information Literacy. *The Journal of Academic Librarianship*, 38(5), p. 287.

Wellmer, A. (1985) Reason, Utopia and *The Dialectic of Enlightenment*. In Bernstein, R., ed: *Habermas and Modernity*. Cambridge: Polity Press.

Wellmer, A. (1991). *The Persistence of Modernity. Aesthetics, Ethics and Postmodernism*. Cambridge: Polity Press.

Wenger, E. (1999). *Communities of practice: Learning, meaning and identity*. Cambridge: Cambridge University Press.

Wenger, E., White, N. and Smith, J. D. (2009) *Digital Habitats: Stewarding Technology for Communities*. Portland OR: CPSquare.

Wertsch, J. V. (1998). *Mind as Action*. Oxford: Oxford University Press.

Wertsch, J. (2009) Text and Dialogism in the Study of Collective Memory. In Junefelt, K. and Nordin, P., eds: *Proceedings from the Second International Interdisciplinary Conference on Perspectives and Limits of Dialogism in Mikhail Bakhtin*, Stockholm, June 3–5 2009. (pp. 33–38).

White, E. J. (2009) Polyphonic Portrayals: A Dostoevskian dream or a researcher's reality? In Junefelt, K. and Nordin, P., eds: *Proceedings from the Second International Interdisciplinary Conference on Perspectives and Limits of Dialogism in Mikhail Bakhtin*, Stockholm, June 3–5 2009. (pp. 87–96).

Whitworth, A. (2007). Communicative competence in the information age: towards a critical pedagogy. In S. Andretta, ed. *Change and Challenge: Information literacy for the 21st century*. Adelaide: Auslib (pp. 85–114).

Whitworth, A. (2009): *Information Obesity*. Oxford: Chandos.

Whitworth, A. (2009b). Teaching in the relational frame: the Media and Information Literacy course at Manchester. *Journal of Information Literacy* 3/2, 25–38.

Whitworth, A. (2010) Empowerment or Instrumental Progressivism? Analyzing Information Literacy policies. *Library Trends* 60/2, 312–337.

Whitworth, A. (2012). The reflective information literacy educator. *Nordic Journal of Information Literacy in Higher Education*, 4/1.

Whitworth, A., Fishwick, I. and McIndoe, S. (2011). Framing Multiliteracies: A Blended and Holistic Approach to Digital Technology Education. In Mackey, T. and Jacobson, T. (eds): *Teaching Information Literacy Online*, New York NY, Neal-Schulman. (pp. 47–64).

Whitworth, A., Garnett, F. and Pearson, D. (2012). Aggregate-then-Curate: How digital learning champions help communities nurture online content. *Research in Learning Technology*, 20, 399–415.

Whitworth, A., Torras i Calvo, M., Moss, B., Amlesom Kifle, N. and Blåsternes, T. (2014): Facilitating self-reflection and action research in the face of organizational change – the Bibliotek i Endring (Changing Libraries) project. Forthcoming in *New Review of Academic Librarianship*.

Williams, R. and Edge, D. (1996). The Social Shaping of Technology. *Research Policy* 25/6, 865–99.

Williamson, K. and Asla. T. (2009). Information behavior of people in the fourth age: Implications for the conceptualization of information literacy. *Library & Information Science Research*, 31/2, 76.

Wilson, P. (1983). *Secondhand Knowledge: An inquiry into cognitive authority*, Greenwood Press, London.

Winner, L. (1986) Do Artefacts Have Politics? In *The Whale and the Reactor: A Search for Limits in an Age of High Technology*. Chicago, IL: University of Chicago Press (pp. 19–39).

Wyer, P. C. and Silva, S. (2009) Where is the wisdom? A conceptual history of evidence-based medicine. *Journal of Evaluation in Clinical Practice*, 15/6, 891.

Wynne, B. (1989). Sheepfarming after Chernobyl: A case study in communicating scientific information. *Environment: Science and Policy for Sustainable Development*, 31/2, 10–39.

Yates, C., Partridge, H. L., & Bruce, C. S. (2009). Learning wellness: how ageing Australians experience health information literacy. *The Australian Library Journal* 58/3, 269–285.

Zhang, X., Majid, S. and Foo, S. (2010) Environmental Scanning: An application of information literacy skills at the workplace. *Information Research* 17/2.

Zurkowski, P. G. (1974): *The Information Service Environment: Relationships and Priorities*, Report presented to the National Commission on Libraries and Information Science, Washington DC.

Index

As well as concepts, this index lists references to the authors whose previously published ideas have featured most prominently in this book. Non-appearance on this list is not meant to indicate insignificance in the fields of information literacy, LIS or any other academic discipline.

Lightning Source UK Ltd.
Milton Keynes UK
UKOW05f1545250215

246872UK00003B/43/P